T0407592

PRAISE FROM BUTEYKO METHOD, OXYGEN ADVANTAGE®, AND MYOTAPE USERS

In researching this book, we reached out to our global network of Buteyko Clinic, Oxygen Advantage®, and MyoTape customers, clients, and social media followers, inviting them to complete an online survey or share their stories in an interview.

We were overwhelmed by the responses we received. You will see accounts from those who responded peppered throughout the book to illustrate just how simple, effective, and life-changing these approaches can be. Some respondents were happy to include their name, age, and the country where they live, while others preferred to remain anonymous. Here is just a small selection of the responses we received:

"After years of struggling with snoring and poor sleep quality, I discovered the transformative effects of breathing techniques and mouth taping. These practices didn't just help me stop snoring; they significantly improved the quality of my sleep and overall well-being. By supporting natural nasal breathing, mouth taping has helped me feel more rested and energized each morning, and my stress levels have also balanced out. Today, I enjoy a more consistent, restful sleep that makes a real difference in my daily life, giving me greater focus, calm, and vitality."

Kamila, 46, Poland

"Mouth taping changed my life! I went from waking up tired (which left me fatigued for the whole day) with a dry mouth, waking up to use the loo in the night, and breathing heavily as I slept, to sleeping through the night without disruption and feeling well rested and refreshed each morning. If I ever forget to tape my mouth I notice it."

Jessica, 33, Australia

"I suffered from insomnia and apnea. Today, my sleep is restful, and my focus and energy are improved. I practice LSD [light, slow, and deep breathing] and breath holds before sleep. Slipping into sleep is much easier."

Anonymous

"Since childhood, I struggled with snoring. I had my adenoids removed, but it didn't help because I was still sleeping with my mouth open. After completing the Buteyko course and taping my mouth at night, my sleep improved 100%.

Occasionally, I still snore through my nose, but only when I sleep on my back, and it's much quieter now.

I used to wake up feeling unrested almost every day, and I often had nightmares. Today, I only experience nightmares when it's too warm in the bedroom, and my breathing noticeably speeds up. The same thing happens if I have a very stuffy nose and wake up without a mouth tape; I can clearly feel a huge difference in how unrefreshed I feel. . . .

Every day before bed, I habitually do breathing reduction [*Breathe Light*] exercises while reading, followed by a five-second breath-hold exercise right before falling asleep. Thanks to these exercises, I fall asleep very quickly and wake up feeling refreshed in the morning without needing an alarm to get up."

Anonymous

"I have struggled with waking up frequently and waking up earlier and earlier. Since this [Buteyko] training, my sleep has improved a ton! I can catch myself over-breathing, practice the soft breathing techniques, and calm down. It has been very effective and a big blessing."

Anonymous

THE
BREATHING
CURE FOR
BETTER SLEEP

Also by Patrick McKeown

*The Breathing Cure: Develop New Habits
for a Healthier, Happier, and Longer Life*

*The Breathing Cure for Yoga: Apply Science
Behind Ancient Wisdom for Health and Well-Being*

*Mouth Breather—Shut Your Mouth:
The Self-Help Book for Breathers*

Atomic Focus

The Oxygen Advantage

Anxiety Free: Stop Worrying and Quieten Your Mind

Buteyko Meets Dr. Mew: Buteyko Method for Children and Teenagers

Always Breathe Correctly (children's book)

Asthma-Free Naturally

Close Your Mouth

Support App

Download the ButeykoClinic app to support practice
of the Buteyko Method exercises.

Buteyko Training Courses and Online Clinics

The Buteyko Clinic offers an online course on
Buteyko Breathing for Better Sleep and Snoring,
one-to-one clinics, a *Live Online Clinic for Snoring, Sleep Apnea,
and Insomnia,* and training courses for anyone interested in
becoming a certified Buteyko Breathing Instructor.
Check out ***https://buteykoclinic.com/*** for more details.

THE
BREATHING
CURE FOR
BETTER SLEEP

7 DAYS TO QUALITY SLEEP
USING THE BUTEYKO METHOD

PATRICK McKEOWN

AND

CATHERINE BANE, PH.D.

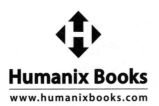

Humanix Books
www.humanixbooks.com

Humanix Books, P.O. Box 20989, West Palm Beach, FL 33416, USA
www.humanixbooks.com | info@humanixbooks.com

Humanix Books titles may be purchased for educational, business, or sales promotional use. For information about special discounts for bulk purchases, please contact the Special Markets Department at info@humanixbooks.com.

Cover Illustration by iStockPhoto/artsholic
Illustrations by Bex Burgess
Editing by Dr. Catherine Bane

Disclaimer: The information presented in this book is not specific medical advice for any individual and should not substitute medical advice from a health professional. If you have (or think you may have) a medical problem, speak to your doctor or a health professional immediately about your risk and possible treatments. Do not engage in any care or treatment without consulting a medical professional.

ISBN: 978-1-63006-306-1 (Hardcover)
ISBN: 978-1-63006-307-8 (E-book)

Printed in the United States of America
10 9 8 7 6 5 4 3 2 1

CONTENTS

SECTION 2
ADULT SLEEP

INTRODUCTION

Imagine falling asleep effortlessly tonight, breathing quietly and steadily, and waking up feeling truly refreshed. Picture yourself enjoying deep, uninterrupted sleep—no more frequent awakenings, no more tossing and turning. Imagine your breathing becoming light, smooth, and silent, so natural that snoring is significantly reduced or even eliminated.

Over the past 23 years, I've witnessed something truly remarkable: when people learn to change their breathing, most notice a dramatic improvement in their sleep, often within just a few days. If you've been waking frequently, snoring, or breathing heavily at night, there's a good chance this approach could help you too.

For anyone who breathes heavily, wakes frequently, or snores, the physician-developed Buteyko Method offers a practical, evidence-based solution. This book will help you to understand how your everyday breathing habits affect your sleep and guide you step-by-step in retraining your breath for better rest. When breathing becomes slower, lighter, lower, more regular—and through the nose—sleep improves significantly.

Children and adults alike experience better focus, improved mood, and renewed energy. Partners who were once kept awake by noisy breathing, or forced to sleep in a separate room, can finally experience peaceful shared nights, undisturbed by snoring or gasping.

In the field of sleep medicine, we often hear about sleep quality—how it affects health, cognition, and performance. Countless books, articles, and experts stress the importance of good sleep; yet they frequently overlook a critical factor: *breathing patterns*.

What could be more straightforward than getting a good night's sleep? And yet, why do so few of us truly experience it?

If you've been struggling with insomnia, snoring, or sleep apnea, you've probably been offered the usual solutions: maybe medication, maybe a device that's uncomfortable or hard to stick with. And if those haven't worked for you, you're not alone.

What often gets overlooked is something surprisingly simple: your breathing. Unlike so many aspects of sleep, breathing is something you can directly influence. With a few gentle practices, you can calm the body and quiet the mind addressing some of the root causes of sleepless nights.

But the benefits go beyond easing insomnia. The same breathing techniques can help reduce airway turbulence and the negative pressure in your throat that contributes to snoring, upper airway resistance syndrome (UARS), and even obstructive sleep apnea.

What's more, when I talk about breathing, it's important to remember that not all breathing exercises are the same. Different techniques can produce completely opposite effects. And let's be realistic—it's not feasible to rely on practicing breathing exercises for the rest of your life. The real question is: what can we incorporate into our normal, everyday routines to naturally improve our sleep? After all, sleep isn't just about rest; it's about restoring the very functions that help us think, focus, and thrive in daily life.

Cognitive performance is arguably the most vital function of being human. It encompasses our ability to make decisions, analyze situations, plan a course of action, and direct attention. It enables us to achieve our goals and cultivate a sense of purpose. Yet this critical function diminishes when sleep is less than optimal. Even something as seemingly minor as a stuffy nose has been shown to impact sleep and impair cognitive function—a clear example of the intricate connection between airways, breathing, and sleep.

Breathing lies at the very core of sleep-disordered breathing—it's even in the name—yet it is frequently neglected, even by health professionals working in the field. For many, myself included, breathing is the missing link. My own journey involved years of struggle and a touch of serendipity before I fully understood just how deeply connected breathing and sleep really are.

MY STORY

Before I share my story, let me say this: parts of it may sound familiar. Maybe you've lived with low energy too. Maybe your mind races at night or your focus seems to vanish just when you need it most. I'm 51 now, and sleep has been a journey—one that took me from a childhood marked by low energy levels to discovering the transformative power of proper breathing.

As a child, I was dealing with asthma, a perpetually stuffy nose, and a mind that felt like it was always racing. Every morning, I'd wake up feeling tired, and it would take me a few hours to get going. My concentration was terrible.

By the time I reached high school, I just wasn't paying much attention to what the teacher was saying. And when I did manage to focus, it felt forced and I couldn't sustain it for very long. I spent most of my time living in my head, drifting into thoughts that had nothing to do with the school curriculum. My mind would often wander in class, but no one ever asked why—and honestly, I didn't ask myself either. It was just the way things were, and I learned to push through it.

Teachers saw a distracted kid, and over time, I began to believe it too—maybe I just wasn't as smart as everyone else. That quiet sense of self-doubt crept in early, even though I was driven to do well. Looking back, I don't think I was hyperactive. It wasn't that I couldn't sit still—I just had poor concentration. I probably had some degree of attention deficit, though I was never given a label. That was nearly forty years ago. I often wonder whether I would have received a diagnosis if I were a student today. Possibly. But would it have helped me? I'm not so sure. Maybe it would've just left me stuck, quietly accepting that this was simply how my brain worked and that there was little I could do to change it.

In my early teens, I left school. I felt that the traditional education path just wasn't for me. I began working as a trainee shop manager, learning the ropes of retail, something I'd already been doing part-time since the age of eleven. I genuinely enjoyed the work: chatting with customers, organizing stock, stacking shelves, and working at the checkout.

This was 1980s Ireland, and while it probably broke every labor law on the books, it was a great experience and taught me a lot. But about a year into my new career, the shop was sold. The new owners took over, but I was still too young to be officially employed, so I had no choice but to return to school.

Looking back, working full-time matured me and taught me that nothing was going to be handed to me. If I wanted a relatively comfortable life, I'd have to work for it. I threw myself into studying, determined to succeed. And while I was still spending plenty of time living in my head, I made up for it by putting in the work. In the end, I got the results I needed to make it to university—Trinity College Dublin. It's funny how life can take unexpected turns. From leaving school at fourteen to walking through the gates of Trinity—it wasn't the usual path, but it was mine.

One memory stands out from my time at university. While I was an exchange student at Uppsala University in Sweden, I shared a room with a friend from back home after a late night out. The next morning, he was half complaining and half teasing me, saying my snoring had kept him awake all night, and that in between, I'd stop breathing altogether for stretches of time. At one point, he even said he thought I was dead! Well, twenty-year-olds can have a decent sense of humor. He didn't really understand what was going on and neither did I. I kind of laughed it off as the aftereffects of a night out, but his comment stuck with me. Could there be something more to it? Was my chronic tiredness somehow connected to my breathing?

At the time, I didn't have a clue what that could mean, but the thought lingered, sparking questions I didn't yet know how to answer.

After university, I started my first job, but by then, tiredness had become such a normal part of my life that I barely thought about it. I chalked it up to being bad at handling stress, struggling with concentration, and losing my calm under work pressures. It never occurred to me that there could be an underlying issue.

How is it that we can go through life feeling exhausted, anxious, or on edge, yet never stop to question why? We assume this is just how things are—part of the deal, the way life is meant to be. We push forward, caught up in the momentum of daily demands, rarely stepping back to ask: "Could it be different? Could it be better?"

The truth is, we often don't realize something is affecting us until we experience life without it. It's only when we step outside our usual patterns, when we compare the "before" with the "after" that we gain real clarity.

Looking back now, I see how much better things could have been. There were two things shaping my reality, influencing my health, energy, and focus—two things I had never truly paid attention to: *my breathing and my sleep.*

DISCOVERING NASAL BREATHING AND DR. BUTEYKO

A turning point came years later when I stumbled upon an article about Dr. Konstantin Buteyko, a Ukrainian physician who developed a unique breathing technique to normalize breathing patterns. In reading about Buteyko's method, something clicked. I was drawn to try his techniques—not out of any firm belief they'd work, but out of a sense that I had nothing to lose.

The first exercise I tried was simple enough: clearing my nose using a breath-hold technique. It worked almost immediately. That initial success was exactly what I needed to motivate me to continue practicing. Had the exercise not worked, I likely would have dismissed breathing techniques altogether as a load of nonsense. But the *Nose Unblocking Exercise* changed my perspective entirely.

I'd like you to try it yourself now. The version below is gentle and suitable for everyone:

1. Take a normal, silent breath in and out through your nose. (Although your nose may feel congested, it's unlikely that both sides of your nose are completely blocked.)
2. Pinch your nose with your fingers to hold your breath.
3. Slowly nod your head up and down five to ten times while holding your breath.
4. Repeat six times with 30-second to 1-minute rests between each.

Give it a try and see how it works for you!

This exercise was a small victory for me, and it made me curious. Next, I tried practicing *Breathe Light*, where I intentionally took in less air and held back a little from the instinct to take a big breath. It was strange at first—feeling air hunger is uncomfortable—but something else happened too: I felt a calmness of mind and quiet warmth spread through my body. By practicing the exercises, I noticed my hands got warmer. They had never been warm before, and this small change was a clear signal to me that breathing exercises can be truly powerful.

I'm going to include a very simple explanation of *Breathe Light* here, as I'd like you to give this a try too. This exercise is one of the most important for improving sleep quality.

1. Bring your attention to your breathing.
2. Take a short, silent breath through your nose—only about 70% of your normal breath.
3. Allow a slow, relaxed breath out.
4. You're doing it correctly if you feel a tolerable sensation of not getting enough air.

Practice this for two to three minutes and see if your hands start to warm up. The goal is to keep the exercise stress-free. If you begin to feel a little stressed, take a short break, just 30 seconds or so, and then return to the exercise.

Give it a go and see how it feels!

That night, I decided to try taping my mouth shut with a small strip of paper tape and used a nasal dilator to keep my nose open. I wasn't sure what to expect, and on the first morning, I didn't notice much of a difference. However, I kept breathing through my nose throughout the day and continued practicing the exercises.

On the second night, I applied the paper tape and nasal dilator again. This time, I woke up feeling more refreshed than I had in years. After a lifetime of grogginess, it felt as if I had stumbled upon a key to unlocking truly restful sleep!

Breathing through the nose was a game-changer for me. However, in hindsight, the tape I should have used would have allowed me to breathe out through the mouth if necessary. Ideally, mouth tape should surround or partially cover the mouth without sealing it completely.

Fully covering the mouth prevents exhalation through the mouth during sleep. For some people, especially those with moderate to severe sleep apnea, it's crucial to have the option to exhale through the mouth if needed—an escape hatch. Using a tape that completely seals the mouth could actually worsen their breathing during sleep and potentially increase the severity of their sleep apnea.

BREATHING AND SLEEP: THE OVERLOOKED CONNECTION

That initial experience transformed my understanding of sleep. Here was something simple, natural, and completely free that had been missing all my life. I realized that breathing wasn't just a detail in the mechanics of sleep; it was *foundational*. This revelation set me on a path to explore how breathing affects not only sleep but also concentration, stress, and overall health.

For so many people, the story is the same. They suffer from sleep disorders, low energy, and a racing mind; yet they go undiagnosed or struggle with solutions that feel more like Band-Aids than cures. We've come to accept a cycle of poor sleep and fatigue, not knowing there might be an underlying issue in how we breathe. Most resources about sleep do focus on the importance of quality and quantity, but they overlook this essential component.

What if the way you breathe could transform the way you sleep? That's what this book explores; not just breathing exercises, but simple daily shifts that could change how you feel when you wake up, how clearly you think, and how deeply you rest.

This book is the culmination of over twenty years of research, experience with thousands of clients, and insights from a global network of more than 13,000 instructors trained in the Buteyko Method and Oxygen Advantage®. Our instructors come from all walks of life—many are health professionals like sleep doctors, dentists, psychiatrists, psychologists, and physiotherapists, all bringing a wealth of expertise to the field of breathing and sleep.

To ensure this book reflects real-life experiences, we reached out to our global community of Buteyko Clinic, Oxygen Advantage®, and MyoTape clients and followers, inviting them to share their stories through an online survey or an interview with our research team. Throughout these pages, you'll find brief quotes from those who responded, as well as in-depth accounts from individuals who kindly shared their journeys.

My hope is that these personal experiences will bring these practices to life—showing just how quick, simple, effective, and truly transformative they can be—in as little as seven days!

As I share these breathing techniques, I hope that you'll find a way to make them part of your own journey to better sleep and health. In a world where so much is complex, expensive, or temporary, breathing is something we can change ourselves, every day, to achieve better health. Let's explore how these simple adjustments can make a profound difference in your life, just as they did for me.

SECTION 1

AN OVERVIEW OF SLEEP AND BREATHING

CHAPTER 1

BREATHING AND SLEEP— HOW DAYTIME HABITS AFFECT NIGHTTIME REST

Breathing is, at its core, a simple rhythm—a breath in, a breath out. But within that simplicity lies a set of foundational principles that shape how we feel, how we cope, and how well we sleep. In essence, breathing comes down to a few key principles: *how fast, how deeply, how regularly,* and *where* we breathe. Understanding these basics reveals how breathing, though natural and instinctive, can dramatically impact our quality of life.

As we get started, you might wonder, "What's the connection between the way I breathe during the day and how I breathe at night?" Simply put, our breathing patterns during wakefulness set the *foundation* for our breathing during sleep. The mechanics behind every breath are the same, whether it's midday or midnight. But when breathing patterns during the day become dysfunctional—such as breathing quickly, heavily, or through the mouth—these habits carry over into sleep and can have a huge impact on rest quality and subsequently on health and well-being.

For many of us, the way we breathe day-to-day has quietly shifted without us even noticing. The breath might be a little too fast, a little too effortful, and sitting high in the chest. We might even be breathing through an open mouth, not just during exercise or stress, but as a regular habit. It's common, yes, but it's far from ideal.

This kind of breathing isn't just something that shows up when we're anxious; it's become the norm for a lot of people. And when it becomes the norm, it doesn't stay confined to daytime. It follows us into sleep.

You might not be aware of it, but if your breath is fast, shallow, or high up in the chest, your brain could be receiving a subtle but persistent message: something's not right. Even if your life is calm, your body might still be breathing like it's under threat.

In the chapters ahead, we'll explore how this happens and more importantly, how to change it. Because once you shift the way you breathe, the way you sleep can shift too.

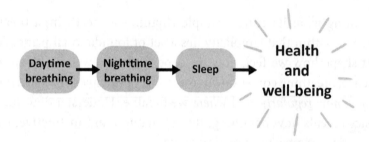

As you read this, take a moment to check in with your breathing. Is it a little faster than it needs to be? Do you feel your breath rising high into your chest? Is your mouth open, even when you're just sitting quietly? No need to change anything yet. Just observe. That awareness alone is a powerful first step.

These may seem like small details, but they can have a big impact. Just by noticing how you breathe during the day, you might start to see connections between your breathing and how well you sleep, how tired you feel, or how tense your body tends to be.

Maybe someone's even pointed it out before, mentioning that your breathing sounded quite heavy, or that you seemed to sigh a lot. Often, we brush those comments off, but they can be gentle clues that something's a little out of balance.

The goal is simple: *soften the inhale, slow down the speed of the exhale,* and *lower each breath* to the diaphragm. With this trifecta—*light, slow, and deep*—you can activate the body's "rest, digest, and repair" mode, the state needed to unwind after a busy day, relax the nervous system, and ease into sleep. In addition, breathing through the nose, instead of the mouth, encourages a steady, efficient airflow that reduces airway turbulence and the potential for airway obstruction. When these principles are consistently practiced, snoring and sleep apnea can lessen, and quality, uninterrupted sleep becomes more achievable.

How do we achieve this goal? Changing breathing patterns isn't as complicated as it may sound. This book is about small, simple steps you can take each day to gradually shift your breathing patterns so that the way you breathe naturally supports calm, energy, and better sleep.

You might wonder, if changing breathing can have such an impact, why isn't it more widely discussed? I don't have a perfect answer to that, especially given how the sleep industry continues to search for lasting solutions. Medications for insomnia can lead to next-day drowsiness, and surgeries for snoring or sleep apnea don't always address the root cause of the issue. Even continuous positive airway pressure (CPAP) machines, the standard treatment for sleep apnea (and highly effective when used consistently), are often abandoned; not because they don't work, but because they can feel uncomfortable, noisy, or restrictive. Breathing re-education, however, is simple, entirely natural, free of charge, and completely accessible. Perhaps it's this very simplicity that holds it back?

UNDERSTANDING THE ROLE OF CO_2 AND YOUR SENSITIVITY TO IT

We're about to dip a little into the science; but don't worry, the goal isn't to complicate things. It's just to give you a basic understanding of what actually determines how you breathe.

Most people assume that we breathe because our bodies are craving oxygen. But surprisingly, it's not oxygen that drives our urge to breathe; it's carbon dioxide, or CO_2.

CO_2 is a natural byproduct of metabolism; the process your body uses to turn food and oxygen into energy. Every time you move, think, or even rest, your cells are producing CO_2. From there, it travels into your blood, makes its way to the lungs, and some of it is released when you exhale.

But here's something you might not expect: CO_2 isn't just a waste gas. In fact, we only exhale about 15% of what we produce. The rest stays in the body, playing important roles; helping to regulate your breathing, your blood's pH level, and how efficiently oxygen is delivered to your cells.

The rate and depth of each breath are determined by how sensitive your body is to CO_2. As CO_2 levels rise in the blood, it causes a slight drop in pH. That's when your brainstem, the part of your brain responsible for essential life functions, steps in. It sends a signal to your diaphragm, the main breathing muscle, prompting you to take a breath.

The brainstem acts like the body's quiet autopilot. It's always there in the background, managing your breathing, heartbeat, and blood pressure day and night; constantly working to keep everything in balance.

Some of us have a heightened sensitivity to CO_2. This can lead to breathing that is faster and harder than necessary, even when resting. While we may not be experiencing a panic or hyperventilation attack, it does mean we're taking in more air than we need. And remember, how you breathe during the day determines how you breathe at night. If your breathing tends to be fast, heavy, or through the mouth, this pattern usually doesn't stop when you go to bed.

The Impact of Fast, Heavy, and Mouth Breathing on Sleep

Let's look at what happens when you carry over these daytime breathing habits into sleep:

1. **Fast and heavy breathing.** Even a slightly faster and harder breathing pattern can increase turbulence in the airways, particularly in the nose and throat. This subtle shift—breathing just a bit more quickly or harder than normal—can be enough to create extra resistance in the airway. Maybe someone has told you that you snore or you've woken up with a dry mouth or a sore throat. Snoring might seem harmless or just something your partner complains about, but it's often a sign of increased airway pressure. And in more serious cases, it can progress into obstructive sleep apnea.

   The airway isn't made of bone; it's soft and flexible. Under enough pressure, it can partially or even fully collapse. When that happens during sleep, breathing temporarily stops. This is what happens in obstructive sleep apnea; a condition where airflow is repeatedly interrupted, often without the person even knowing it.

2. **Mouth breathing.** When we breathe through the mouth, our breathing tends to become faster and heavier and moves to the upper chest. Try it yourself—if you're currently breathing through your nose, switch to breathing in and out through an open mouth. Notice how your breaths naturally become quicker and more pronounced, engaging the upper chest.

   Mouth breathing during sleep brings its own set of challenges. When the mouth falls open, the jaw relaxes and drops, and the tongue can fall back toward the throat, partially blocking the airway. Unlike the nose, which filters, humidifies, and warms the air, the mouth doesn't offer these benefits. As a result, mouth breathing leads to cooler, unfiltered air flowing into the throat, often drying out both the mouth and throat, which can cause inflammation and irritation.

Maybe you've had mornings where you wake up with a dry mouth or a sore throat, feeling groggy despite a full night's sleep. I've been there too. For me, it often happened after breathing through my mouth all night. I'd wake feeling anything but rested.

Understanding Airway Resistance— It's Not Just About Size

To understand how breathing affects sleep, it helps to think a little like an engineer. Imagine air flowing through a tube. An engineer wouldn't just focus on how wide the tube is; they'd also consider how quickly the air is moving, how much pressure is building, and how much volume is passing through.

Sleep medicine needs this same kind of perspective. Yes, the diameter of your airway matters, but just as important is how air moves through it.

Airway resistance refers to the effort it takes to pull air in and push it out of the lungs. When resistance is high, your body has to work harder to breathe, even when you're asleep. As that effort increases, the brain senses something isn't quite right and may react by nudging you out of deep sleep into a lighter stage. You may not remember waking, but these brief disruptions, known as micro-awakenings, can happen over and over again, breaking up your sleep without you realizing it.

A narrow airway makes this more likely. There is simply less space for the air to flow. And when you're asleep, the muscles around the airway naturally relax, making the space even smaller. The tighter the airway, the more resistance your body has to push against just to breathe.

Now add in poor breathing habits like breathing through the mouth, using the upper chest, or breathing too quickly. For many people, these patterns have been there for years, quietly becoming their default way of breathing.

This is where things really start to compound. A narrowed airway is already more prone to collapsing, which alone increases resistance. The body responds by trying to pull in more air to compensate, and this leads to faster, more forceful breathing. But the harder we try to breathe, the more turbulence we create in the airway, which increases negative pressure and pulls the airway walls inward.

So now we have two issues working together: the physical structure of the airway and the way a person breathes. When both are out of balance, breathing during sleep becomes strained and unstable.

It turns into a loop. The airway is narrow. Breathing is inefficient. The body instinctively tries to breathe harder and faster to compensate, which only makes the airway more likely to collapse. This leads to disturbed sleep, lighter stages of rest, and frequent awakenings. For many people, this shows up as loud snoring, gasping at night, or even full-blown obstructive sleep apnea.

The key takeaway is this: it is not just about the size or shape of your airway, and it is not just about how you breathe. But when both are working against you, your sleep is almost certainly going to suffer.

The good news is that while you may not be able to completely change your anatomy, you can absolutely influence both the openness of your airway and how it functions, especially during sleep, by improving your breathing patterns. With small and consistent changes, you can calm your breath, reduce resistance, and create a more stable and restful night's sleep. And it all starts with how you breathe right now.

Stress, Breathing, and Sleep

In today's fast-paced world, stress has become part of the background noise. We're constantly juggling packed schedules, endless notifications, and a stream of responsibilities that never quite seems to pause. It's no wonder so many of us feel wired, tired, and overstimulated, all at the same time. This constant state of alertness affects far more than just our mood; it deeply impacts how we breathe and how well we sleep.

Stress is the body's natural response to pressure or challenge. In small doses, it can help us stay sharp and focused. But when stress becomes chronic, as it so often does these days, it keeps the nervous system stuck in a high-alert setting. This is often called the "fight, flight, or freeze" state. Over time, being stuck in this mode takes a toll on both the body and the mind, and one of the first things to suffer is sleep.

Have you ever found yourself lying in bed, unable to switch off? The day is done, but your mind keeps going, running through to-do lists, replaying conversations, or worrying about tomorrow. Your heart might feel like it's beating a little too fast, and your body refuses to settle, even though you're completely exhausted. That is the stress response at work. It floods your system with cortisol, your main stress hormone, and throws your natural sleep rhythm off course.

When this happens night after night, it becomes harder to fall asleep and stay asleep. Racing thoughts, restlessness, and elevated cortisol levels can disrupt the body's internal clock, your circadian rhythm, and lead to broken sleep, headaches, poor concentration, and a low mood that lingers throughout the day. Over time, this can feed into anxiety, depression, and a sense of being constantly out of sync.

Then there is the role of technology. Let's be honest, most of us check our phones one last time before bed. A quick scroll through emails, messages, or the news often feels harmless, but it adds to the mental stimulation when we most need to wind down. The glow of the screen tricks the brain into thinking it's still daytime, and the never-ending stream of information keeps the mind alert when it should be settling.

If better sleep is your goal, here's a small but meaningful shift: when you go to bed, put your phone to bed too. And in the morning, let your phone have a lie-in. It's a quiet act of kindness, not just for your sleep, but for your nervous system and your peace of mind. Please see Chapters 7 and 8 for a deep dive into this subject.

THE BUTEYKO METHOD: HOW CHANGING YOUR BREATHING CAN CHANGE YOUR SLEEP

Sleep medicine has made strides with tools like CPAP and mandibular advancement devices (MADs). If you've been diagnosed with sleep apnea, chances are you've heard of these or maybe even tried one yourself. Here's how they work:

- **CPAP machines.** These devices use continuous positive airway pressure to keep the airway open. Think of it like blowing air through a paper tube, keeping just enough pressure so it doesn't cave in. That steady airflow helps keep the airway open during sleep, preventing the collapses that happen with sleep apnea.
- **MADs.** These move the lower jaw forward, increasing the airway's diameter. This device aims to reduce resistance by widening the passage to breathe.

But here's the missing piece: CPAPs and MADs focus on the airway's physical structure alone. They don't address how you're breathing. Even with these devices, your sleep may still feel disrupted if you're breathing through your mouth, taking fast or shallow breaths, or relying on your upper chest instead of your diaphragm. These habits can reduce how effective the treatment is, and in some cases, make it harder to stick with it. If the underlying breathing pattern isn't addressed, even the best equipment can only go so far.

The Core Principles of the Buteyko Method

The physician-developed Buteyko Method focuses on re-educating your breathing patterns during the day so that, over time, these healthier habits carry over automatically into sleep. By practicing gentle adjustments to your everyday breathing, you create a foundation for deeper, quieter, and more restorative sleep each night. At the heart of this method is nasal breathing.

Let's explore the core principles:

- **Nose.** Nasal breathing is one of the most powerful supports for healthy sleep. It naturally encourages light, slow and deep breathing. Breathing through the nose also protects the airways by keeping them moist and reducing irritation that can happen when dry air flows in through the mouth. When you breathe through your nose, your tongue rests in its ideal position, lightly against the roof of the mouth. This helps open up space at the back of the throat, making it easier for air to move in and out. At least half of the clients I have worked with over the past 23 years have reported waking up with a dry mouth, a clear sign of mouth breathing during sleep.

- **Light.** Breathing light is about retraining your everyday breathing pattern so that your body's natural drive to breathe is calmer and more efficient. When your breathing is gentle and quiet throughout the day, it naturally becomes light and slow at night. This reduces turbulence in the airways, helping to minimize snoring, lessen sleep disruptions, and improve oxygen delivery. Over time, breathing less rather than more helps your body maintain balance, keeping you calmer, more focused, and more resilient both during the day and while you sleep.

- **Slow.** When each breath is slower, there's less suction pulling on the airway walls. The result? Fewer disruptions and a better chance of sleeping through the night undisturbed.

- **Deep.** Deep breathing with optimal use of the diaphragm, instead of the upper chest, not only improves oxygen transfer; it also gives physical support to the throat muscles that help keep your airway open. This natural connection between the diaphragm and the throat muscles is often overlooked, yet it plays a key role in reducing snoring and sleep apnea.

With regular practice, these principles nose, light, slow, and deep start to feel effortless. You're not just doing breathing exercises now and then; you're changing your default pattern. And when healthy breathing becomes second nature during the day, it carries over into the night, helping you breathe more quietly, sleep more deeply, and wake feeling genuinely refreshed.

Here is a selection of quotes from our online community that have successfully implemented these breathing principles.

"Since starting to use MyoTape and doing Buteyko breathing exercises my sleep health has completely turned my health and energy around. I now awake rested not like I've run a marathon or fought for my life overnight.

I don't struggle to stay awake when I'm seated anymore, i.e., driving, telephone conversations, hairdresser or other appts, dining out, I'm not sick as much, my immune system seems stronger. More strength and endurance with my fitness in all of my sports and activities.

I'm even a happier person all of the time. So every part of my life changed."

"I was a chronic mouth breather. Two years ago [I] started mouth taping—first night, weird adjustment. Second night—best sleep of my life.

Since then, I have a lot more energy, wake up alert, and my dental health has improved (no more lower teeth plaque buildup).

My husband [was] very congested, [but] mouth tape has given [him] his nose back, reduced his snoring significantly . . . , and he also reports increased energy."

BUTEYKO EXERCISES FOR ADULTS

The Buteyko Method is a powerful and effective physician-developed approach to improving sleep. However, these exercises are not suitable to practice *during pregnancy*.

Its main exercise, *Breathe Light*, involves consciously breathing less air into your body for short periods throughout the day. The key is to practice in a way that feels comfortable and stress-free. The exercises are designed to be manageable, much like walking at a pace where you feel tolerably breathless.

If you have a serious medical condition, it's important to keep your breathing under good control at all times. For instance, when practicing the *Nose Unblocking Exercise,* only hold your breath until you experience a comfortable level of air hunger.

If you are unsure whether these exercises are appropriate for you, please consult with your family doctor before beginning the practice.

Breathing Test Using the Control Pause

The primary measure of progress in the Buteyko Method is the *Control Pause* (CP). It's a simple, easy-to-do test that gives insight into how well your breathing is functioning and improving with practice.

What Is the Control Pause?

In simple terms, it's the number of seconds you can comfortably hold your breath after a normal exhale without strain and without gasping when you resume breathing. A low CP indicates faster, harder, and upper chest breathing, while a CP above 20 seconds reflects light, slow, and deep breathing patterns.

Each 5-second improvement in your CP score corresponds to an improvement in your breathing.

It's normal for the CP to increase by about 3 seconds per week until it reaches around 20 seconds. Beyond this, progress continues but at a slower rate.

The goal here isn't to get obsessed with your CP or turn it into a competition. Instead, think of it as a gentle way to track your progress over time. It's just one tool, not the whole picture.

Alongside checking your CP once a week, start tuning in to how your breathing feels in daily life. Are your breaths becoming a little lighter? A little slower? Are they starting to settle lower in your body? These simple observations matter just as much, if not more. They're signs that your breathing is beginning to shift in the right direction.

Measuring the CP will not directly change your breathing patterns, but it serves as a useful tool to gauge your progress. You can find a short, easy-to-follow video demonstration of the CP by simply scanning the QR code. It walks you through each step and shows you exactly how to do it correctly.

Here's how to measure your CP:

1. Take a normal, silent breath in and let it out through your nose.
2. After exhaling, gently pinch your nose to hold your breath.
3. Time, in seconds, how long it takes until you feel the first definite urge to breathe or the first involuntary movement of your breathing muscles.
4. Release your nose and breathe in through your nose, ensuring your breathing remains calm and controlled after the breath hold.
5. Use this measurement as a benchmark to monitor improvements in your breathing over time.

Here's what to expect (breathing patterns relative to CP score):

CP Score of 11 Seconds (or Lower)	CP Score of 20 Seconds (or Higher)
Faster respiratory rate	Normal respiratory rate
Irregular breathing, including frequent sighing and yawning	Regular breathing with less breathlessness
Harder breathing	Normal, light breathing
Upper chest breathing	Breathing is driven by the diaphragm
A feeling of air hunger/suffocation	Effortless breathing
A mixture of mouth and nose breathing	Full-time nasal breathing
No natural pause following exhalation	Natural pause following exhalation

Nose Unblocking Exercise

Nasal congestion often leads to mouth breathing, which disrupts the sleep cycle and reduces sleep quality. I always explain to my clients that having a stuffy nose is never just about the nose. It often goes hand in hand with poor sleep and increased tiredness. The good news is, there's a simple exercise that can help clear your nasal passages. It's easy to do and can make it much easier to switch to nasal breathing not just during the day, but while you sleep too.

Steps

1. Take a normal breath in and let it out through your nose.
2. Pinch your nose with your fingers to hold your breath.
3. While holding your breath, gently nod your head up and down 5–15 times depending on how comfortable you are with air hunger.
4. Repeat 6 times, resting for 30–60 seconds between each repetition.

Use this exercise as needed to relieve nasal congestion.

The most important thing about the nose is that the more you use it, the better it works. With regular practice, this exercise helps keep nasal passages clear, reduces reliance on mouth breathing, and supports deeper, more restful sleep.

Adapting to Nasal Breathing

It's important that the *Nose Unblocking Exercise* gives you some relief because that can be a good motivator. It also gives you a sense of control. You realize you can do something to help clear your nose. Chances are, you've already tried all sorts of remedies: eucalyptus oil, menthol rubs, nasal sprays from the pharmacy, maybe even prescriptions from your doctor. And while some of those might have brought temporary relief, they often don't get to the root of the issue. This exercise is different; it's simple, natural, entirely free of charge and puts the control back in your hands.

If you're used to mouth breathing, switching to nasal breathing might feel strange at first. You might notice a mild sensation of air hunger, like you're not getting quite enough air. That's completely normal.

This feeling can come from a partially blocked nose, but it can also happen if your breathing pattern has become a bit off over time—too fast, too shallow, or stuck in the chest.

The key here isn't to force anything. The goal is to gently guide your body back toward nasal breathing, one step at a time. With a little practice, nasal breathing starts to feel more natural and you'll notice the difference not just in your sleep, but in your energy levels.

If the feeling of air hunger remains strong, even after doing the *Nose Unblocking Exercise*, it can help to use a nasal dilator, a simple strip or plastic device that gently flares the nostrils to make breathing easier. This can be particularly useful during sleep or physical activity, when nasal airflow needs to be at its best.

But if that sensation continues to feel intense, even after regular practice, it could be a sign of a mechanical issue inside the nose.

In children, this might be due to enlarged adenoids. In adults, it could be something like a severely deviated septum or other structural obstruction. In these cases, breathing exercises alone may not be enough to restore full nasal airflow.

The Buteyko Method can do a lot to support healthy breathing function, but it can't correct structural blockages. If you suspect that something might be physically limiting your ability to breathe through your nose, the best next step is to consult with an ear, nose, and throat (ENT) doctor for a proper assessment.

The ultimate goal is to restore nasal breathing because that's the foundation for better sleep, more energy, and long-term health. It's worth taking the steps to get there.

From personal experience, when I first made the shift to nasal breathing, I needed a nasal dilator during sleep to help keep my nasal passages open. My airway was too compromised at the time, and the feeling of air hunger would have made it too uncomfortable without that support. Over time, as my breathing improved, my need for the nasal dilator during sleep gradually reduced. That said, I still find it helpful during my morning exercise routine, especially due to my deviated septum and naturally limited nasal airway.

A higher CP—above twenty seconds—signals a decongested nose and a naturally lighter, slower breathing pattern. This makes it much easier to maintain continuous nasal breathing, both at rest and during movement

Breathe Light Exercise

This exercise is *foundational* for improving breathing patterns by reducing air intake volume, activating the body's "rest, digest, and repair" response, making it easier to fall asleep, and enhancing tolerance to carbon dioxide. Earlier, we discussed how carbon dioxide is the primary driver of breathing. With consistent practice, your tolerance to carbon dioxide will improve, resulting in lighter everyday breathing, even during sleep.

Light breathing lowers resistance in the airways, which can help reduce snoring and sleep apnea. Regular practice of this exercise promotes relaxation and enhances oxygen delivery throughout the body, offering support for insomnia, snoring, upper airway resistance syndrome, and sleep apnea.

Steps

1. **Sit comfortably.** Place one hand on your chest and the other on your abdomen to monitor your breathing.
2. **Shorter inhale.** Breathe in softly through your nose, taking only about 70–80% of your usual breath (a shorter inhale).
3. **Relaxed exhale.** Breathe out slowly and calmly, letting the breath flow out naturally.
4. **Reduce air intake.** Aim to breathe so lightly that approximately 20–30% less air enters your lungs than usual.
5. **Feel air hunger.** Allow yourself to experience a tolerable feeling that you'd like to take a deeper breath.
6. **Rest if needed.** If the sensation of air hunger becomes too strong, or you experience jerking in your breathing, take a short 15–20 second rest; then resume the exercise.

Practice goal. Practice for five minutes, 4–6 times daily, and aim for a full 10 minutes before bed.

While the exercises that follow such as *Breathe Slow* and *Breathe Deep* are both excellent for calming the body and mind, my personal preference, especially when it comes to sleep, is the *Breathe Light Exercise* outlined earlier.

Why? Because breathing light gently slows your breathing, increases your tolerance to carbon dioxide, and directly supports deeper, more stable sleep. It also improves blood flow and oxygen delivery to the brain, which has a calming effect.

That is not to say the other exercises are not valuable. They absolutely are. But if you are short on time and want the most impact, *Breathe Light* gives you the most return. It helps you feel like you are heading in the right direction.

If you only choose to practice one exercise, let it be *Breathe Light*. And if you combine it with nasal breathing throughout the day, you will naturally slow your breath, reduce effort, and start engaging the diaphragm more effectively. These are all essential steps toward better sleep and better health.

Breathe Slow Exercise

Slow, steady breathing is a powerful way to balance the body and mind, reducing stress and calming the autonomic nervous system. Research shows that slowing your breathing rate to around 4.5–6.5 breaths per minute brings a sense of calm and promotes restful sleep. By practicing this breathing rhythm regularly, you can support your body's natural relaxation response and prepare for better-quality sleep.

Steps

1. Inhale gently and silently through your nose to a count of four.
2. Exhale slowly and quietly through your nose for a count of six.
3. Repeat this pattern, aiming to reach a calm and steady rhythm that brings your breathing rate to about six breaths per minute.

   Practice. Use *Breathe Slow* throughout the day, especially during moments of stress or as part of your pre-sleep routine.

Breathe Nose, Slow, and Deep Exercise

This exercise is designed to engage the diaphragm, supporting a light, slow, and nasal-driven breathing pattern. Practicing daily helps reinforce stable, calming breathing, setting the foundation for better breathing both day and night. You could try this exercise as part of your bedtime routine. Once you're in bed, lie on your back and bring your attention to the lower ribs. It can help to place one hand on the area just above your navel or on either side of your lower ribs. As you breathe in, feel the tummy gently rise beneath your hand.

As you breathe out, notice it gently fall. It is not about pushing or pulling the tummy; it is about allowing the breath to guide it up during inhalation and down during exhalation.

This simple awareness helps shift your breathing away from the chest and back toward the diaphragm. Practicing even for a few minutes can bring a sense of calm to both the body and mind, creating the right conditions for sleep to come more easily.

Steps

1. **Lie on your back.** Bend your knees to allow for better engagement of the diaphragm.
2. **Place hands on lower ribs.** Rest your hands on either side of your lower ribs, tuning in to the movement as you breathe.
3. **Inhale gently through your nose.** Feel your lower ribs gently expand outward as you breathe in.
4. **Exhale softly through your nose.** Feel your lower ribs move back inward with each exhale.
5. **Engage the diaphragm.** Aim to let 80% of the movement come from the diaphragm, with minimal movement in the upper chest.
6. **Maintain a calm, steady flow.** Keep your breathing light, slow, nasal, and deep, focusing on a gentle rhythm.

Practice. Aim to practice this exercise for five minutes, once or twice a day.

Note: This exercise isn't about filling your lungs to capacity; instead, the goal is soft, gentle, and deep breathing into the lower lungs, keeping it calm and natural.

Breathing to Activate Relaxation

This is one of my favorite go-to exercises. I use it myself all the time. Anytime I'm about to step into something that feels a little challenging, like giving a public talk or heading into a meeting, I bring my attention to the breath and focus on slowing down the exhalation. It's simple, but it works.

One of the reasons I like this exercise so much is that you can use it at any time, without anyone noticing. That can be especially helpful in situations where showing stress might not work in your favor. For example, in a job interview, the people across the table may not be consciously watching your breathing, but they'll pick up on it. If you're sighing often or taking large, deep breaths, it not only increases your own stress response, but it can give the impression that you're uncomfortable or not confident. That might lead them to question whether you're ready for the job or able to manage pressure. Don't let your breathing give you away.

That's why it's helpful to have something you can use discreetly. Slowing your breath sends a message to your body that you're okay, and it does so without making it obvious to anyone else. Just a quiet breath in and a longer, softer breath out. And there's reassurance in knowing that you have something practical to fall back on when things feel tense. Sometimes, just knowing you have that option is enough to help you stay steady.

There's no need to count or follow a set pattern. What matters is keeping the breath soft on the way in, and slowing down the speed of the exhalation. Let the breath out gently and gradually, as if you are trying not to disturb the quiet around you.

The more you practice this during everyday moments, times when the stakes are low, the easier it becomes to use when things are more intense. You're teaching your body what to do, so when the pressure rises, you can settle yourself more quickly. A gentle breath in, followed by a slower breath out, tells the brain that the body is safe. And when the brain gets that message, it responds by sending signals of calm back through the body, relaxing the nervous system and easing the stress response.

Applying Buteyko Breathing for Insomnia

Insomnia is a common sleep issue, often caused by an overactive nervous system (hyperarousal) and/or disruptions in breathing during sleep. Problems like heavy snoring, upper airway resistance, sleep apnea, or needing to use the bathroom during the night can repeatedly wake you up, preventing deep rest. Even breathing too fast or too hard during sleep can keep your body in a state of alertness, making it harder to stay asleep.

For some, insomnia is temporary, perhaps triggered by stress or a major life event. But for others, it becomes a long-term struggle, lasting months or even years. The result? Endless tossing and turning, waking up feeling drained, brain fog, and difficulty functioning throughout the day. Over time, poor sleep can take a serious toll on both mental and physical health.

By improving your breathing habits and practicing good sleep hygiene, you can create the right conditions for deeper, more restorative sleep.

Sleep hygiene is the term often used to describe the everyday habits and environment that support healthy sleep. It includes things like when you go to bed, how you wind down in the evening, your use of screens, your bedroom setup, and even how consistent your sleep and wake times are. In simple terms, it's the routine and setting that either helps you sleep well or makes it harder.

The good news is that small changes in sleep hygiene, combined with Buteyko breathing, can make a big difference. When your body feels safe and your breathing is calm, your nervous system starts to let go. You're no longer trying to sleep; you're allowing it to happen.

Insomnia usually takes two main forms: one is trouble falling asleep, and the other is waking up in the middle of the night.

1. **Difficulty falling asleep.** Struggling to fall asleep often stems from an overstimulated mind, whether it's caused by a stressful day,

anxiety, work overload, or perhaps endless scrolling on social media before bed. Additionally, a breathing pattern that is too fast or too hard signals to the brain that the body might be under threat.

The brain's primary job is to protect. It won't allow the body to drift off into sleep if it senses that something isn't right. From an evolutionary point of view, this makes complete sense. Falling asleep when there's danger nearby would have left us vulnerable.

One of the main ways the brain picks up on whether we're safe or not is through our breathing. It's constantly monitoring how fast we're breathing, how hard we're working to breathe, and where in the body that breath is coming from. If the breathing is fast, effortful, or stuck high in the chest, the brain may interpret that as a sign of stress or threat, even if there's nothing around us to worry about.

To help quiet the mind and ease into sleep, it's important to breathe light and slow. This sends a powerful signal to the brain that the body is safe and that it's okay to let go. Activating this rest response is one of the key steps to falling into a peaceful, natural sleep.

Here are a few ways to achieve this:

- **Commit to nasal breathing.** Practice breathing through your nose consistently throughout the day, during rest, exercise, and sleep. Nasal breathing naturally encourages a calm, steady breath that carries into the night.
- **Work toward a Control Pause score of 20+ seconds.** A Control Pause score over 20 seconds is a reliable indicator of breathing stability, which plays an important role in sleep.
- **Practice *Breathe Light* for 10 minutes before bed.** This exercise helps to calm both the mind and body by slowing down your breathing rate and activating the body's "rest, digest, repair" response, preparing you for sleep.

- For ease, you might try listening to my free guided audio for insomnia, which incorporates the *Breathe Light Exercise*. You can access it using the QR code.

2. **Waking in the middle of the night.** Waking up after a few hours of sleep can be even more challenging than struggling to fall asleep initially. It's incredibly frustrating, especially when you know you have a busy day ahead. This realization adds pressure to fall back asleep quickly, as you're aware that a lack of rest will impact your concentration and energy levels throughout the day. Unfortunately, this pressure often makes it even harder to relax and drift back to sleep.

   Traditionally, when working with my clients, I recommended focusing on softening and slowing their breath while lying awake. This approach is effective for calming the mind and activating the body's relaxation response. However, I've found that listening to the guided audio for insomnia can enhance these effects even further.

   - **Listen to a guided audio for insomnia.** This audio guides you into the *Breathe Light Exercise*, which activates the body's natural relaxation response. It removes the pressure of "trying" to fall back asleep. The effort to "try" implies tension, whereas listening allows you to ease back into rest without forcing it. By simply following the instructions, you'll find yourself growing sleepier until you nod off. Simply scan the QR code to download it to your phone.
   - **Listen to the Yoga Nidra guided audio.** Tiger Bye, breath educator, yoga instructor, and co-founder of Better Yoga, guides you through a relaxing Yoga Nidra. Through slow, gentle breathing, visualization, and focused attention, Yoga Nidra calms the nervous system and shifts you from a state of stress or hyperarousal to a state of deep rest. Scan the QR code to download it to your phone.

Additional Tips for Restful Sleep

- **Breathe only through the nose during sleep.** Nasal breathing at night helps to ensure a lighter, slower breath driven by the diaphragm. If you often wake with a dry mouth, consider using MyoTape or a similar nasal breathing support that does not cover the mouth to help ensure nose breathing.
- **Improve your everyday breathing.** As your Control Pause score gradually improves, so does your breathing stability. Each 5-second increase in your Control Pause score reflects progress in your breathing patterns, and a score of 20 seconds or more can significantly reduce turbulence in the nasal passages and throat, supporting deeper, uninterrupted sleep and fewer awakenings.

By incorporating these practices into your routine, you'll build a strong foundation for deep, restorative sleep. As your breathing stabilizes and your Control Pause score improves, you'll experience fewer nighttime disruptions, better sleep quality, and more energy to greet each morning. For a deeper dive into the topic of insomnia, check out Chapter 10A.

Understanding Snoring and How Breathing Plays a Role

Snoring—it's something we may blame on our partners, or get nudged awake for in the middle of the night. But have you ever stopped to wonder *why* we snore? That loud, rumbling noise isn't just an annoyance; it's a sign that airflow is *restricted* somewhere in your airway. And when air has to fight to get through, it creates turbulence, making tissues in the throat, nose, or mouth vibrate. That vibration? That's the unmistakable sound of snoring.

Snoring isn't a one-size-fits-all issue. In fact, there are different types of snoring. Some occur without any restriction to airflow, while others involve a reduction in airflow, where breathing becomes more effortful and disruptive. For the purpose of this book, we'll keep things simple and focus on two main types of snoring based on where the turbulence begins—through the mouth or the nose:

- **Mouth snoring.** This happens when air flows through an open mouth during sleep, causing the soft palate and tissues in the throat to vibrate. The simple fix? Keep your mouth closed! It's almost impossible to snore through the mouth if it stays shut, which is why nasal breathing is so important for quiet, restful sleep.
- **Nose snoring.** This type occurs when airflow struggles to pass smoothly through the nasal passages, often due to congestion, a deviated septum, or naturally narrow airways. When air moves too fast or forcefully through a restricted nasal passage, it creates turbulence, leading to snoring, especially where the nose meets the throat (the nasopharynx).

It's worth noting that snoring isn't only about the size of the airway. The speed and depth of your breathing play a big role too. If you think back to the engineer analogy from earlier in the chapter, this makes perfect sense. Just like airflow through a narrow tube, when you breathe too fast or too forcefully, the increased pressure can cause soft tissues in the airway, such as the soft palate to vibrate more easily. The result is more turbulence, more vibration, and more snoring. To understand how this works, try a simple exercise. Make a snoring sound through your nose by slightly tightening the back of your throat and speeding up your breathing. You will notice the distinct sound of snoring through the nose which is quite different from that of mouth snoring. (A tip for partners who are lying awake having to listen to a rattle every night—try and identify where the snoring is coming from—nose or mouth.)

Next, practice breathing light and slow. Gradually slow down each breath until it becomes almost imperceptible, with barely any air moving through your nose. While doing this, try to snore through your nose as you continue to breathe light and slow. You'll notice it's much harder to create a snoring sound when breathing gently at a slower pace.

This illustrates an important point: snoring isn't solely caused by anatomical challenges. Breathing patterns, such as a faster breathing rate and greater air volume, can create turbulence in the upper airway, contributing to snoring. While most snoring remedies focus exclusively on airway structure, they often neglect the role of airflow. Any engineer assessing resistance would consider both the diameter of the airway and the speed and volume of airflow—and the same principle applies to snoring.

Practical Tips for Reducing Snoring

To Stop Mouth Snoring

- **Use a gentle nasal breathing support tape.** MyoTape can help keep the mouth closed during sleep, encouraging nasal breathing. Since snoring through the mouth isn't possible when the mouth is closed and breathing is exclusively through the nose, I can confidently say that mouth snoring stops 100% under these conditions.

To Reduce Nasal Snoring

If you're dealing with nasal snoring, the tips below can make a real difference. And while it might seem like a lot at first glance, these steps are actually very accessible. Later in the chapter, I'll show you how to bring them into your daily life so they become part of your routine, not just another list of things to do.

Here are the key steps you can start with:

- **Clear the nose with the *Nose Unblocking Exercise*.** Practicing this exercise reduces nasal congestion, making nasal breathing easier and reducing nose snoring.
- **Establish consistent nasal breathing.** Practice nasal breathing throughout the day, whether at rest or during physical exercise, to reinforce the habit and make it easier to maintain at night.

- **Consider using a nasal dilator at night.** Not everyone will need one, but if your nasal breathing feels a bit restricted at night, a nasal dilator might help. It gently opens the nostrils to reduce resistance and make breathing through the nose easier. That said, a nasal dilator only works if you're actually breathing through your nose.
- **Adapt the correct tongue resting posture.** Place three-quarters of your tongue against the roof of your mouth, avoiding contact with the top front teeth. Resting the tongue in this position helps ensure a more open airway, particularly where the back of the mouth meets the throat.
- **Normalize breathing volume with the *Breathe Light Exercise.*** Practicing *Breathe Light* for 10 minutes, four times daily, helps make nasal snoring less intense.
- **Improve your Control Pause score.** Aim for a score above 20 seconds, which can significantly reduce the speed and volume of airflow, lowering the intensity of snoring.

While some people may eliminate nasal snoring entirely, those with narrower airways might still experience it, albeit with significantly reduced volume and intensity, making it far less disruptive. By focusing on both breathing techniques and airflow, you can create a more restful, quieter sleep environment. Please see Chapter 10B for more on snoring.

Upper Airway Resistance Syndrome and Buteyko Breathing

Upper airway resistance syndrome (UARS) is a sleep disorder that often goes unnoticed, yet it can have a significant impact on daily life. It occurs when the throat (upper airway) narrows just enough to create resistance to airflow, making it harder to breathe during sleep. Although this resistance doesn't cause full airway collapse, as it does in obstructive sleep apnea, the increased effort required to breathe is enough to trigger frequent micro-arousals—brief interruptions in sleep that prevent the body from reaching deep, restorative sleep stages. The result? Waking up feeling unrefreshed and experiencing persistent fatigue throughout the day.

Because UARS doesn't always involve snoring or obvious breathing pauses, it is often misdiagnosed or completely overlooked. It can be especially frustrating if you're feeling the symptoms, but your test results come back "normal." One of the biggest challenges with UARS is that it can affect people who don't fit the typical profile of a sleep disorder patient. While obstructive sleep apnea is commonly associated with older, overweight men, UARS frequently affects women; often younger, thinner, and otherwise healthy-looking who find themselves exhausted but dismissed. Many people with UARS also have certain anatomical features, such as a high and narrow palate or a small airway, which make breathing more effortful during sleep. Some even have a history of orthodontic treatments, like wisdom tooth extractions, that may have contributed to airway narrowing. For many, there's no obvious explanation for their fatigue, only a sense that sleep never quite does what it's supposed to. This makes diagnosis tricky, as traditional sleep studies often focus on detecting apneas rather than the subtler breathing struggles seen in UARS.

The effects of UARS go beyond just feeling tired. Many individuals with UARS also experience anxiety, difficulty concentrating, and even symptoms resembling chronic fatigue syndrome or fibromyalgia. This is because the body remains in a state of heightened alertness due to repeated sleep disruptions. Over time, the cycle of poor sleep and increased stress can make it even harder to rest properly, creating a feedback loop that worsens symptoms. Addressing UARS is not only about sleeping better; it's about feeling like yourself again. The Buteyko Method can make a meaningful difference, whether used on its own or alongside traditional treatments. It supports nasal breathing, reduces over-breathing, and helps calm the nervous system—key factors that promote more stable breathing patterns and better quality sleep.

1. Supporting Nasal Breathing and Airway Function
    *   **Decongest your nose and practice nasal breathing.** Nasal congestion can worsen airway resistance, but the *Nose Unblocking Exercise* can help clear nasal passages and promote consistent nasal breathing. Pairing this with proper tongue posture—resting the tongue on the roof of your mouth during sleep—helps keep the airway open and reduces resistance.
    *   **Engage the diaphragm.** Diaphragmatic breathing stabilizes the throat muscles, minimizing collapses and making it easier for air to flow smoothly. Practicing the *Breathe Deep Exercise* during the day reinforces proper breathing mechanics for sleep.
    *   **Consider nasal dilators or snore strips.** For individuals with significant nasal resistance, these tools physically open the nasal passages, easing airflow and reducing breathing effort during sleep.
    *   **Weight loss (if appropriate).** Reducing excess weight, particularly around the throat, can improve breathing mechanics and reduce airway collapses.
2. Normalizing Breathing Volume and Patterns
    *   **Increase your Control Pause score.** The CP score is a simple way to assess your breathing patterns and how well they are regulated. A CP of 20 seconds or more indicates stabilized breathing, reducing airway resistance and lowering the risk of waking up unnecessarily.
    *   **Practice light, slow, and deep breathing.** Nasal breathing is key to fostering light, slow, and deep breathing, each of which plays an important role in stabilizing the airways and promoting better sleep. Breathing through the nose helps regulate airflow, encouraging light breathing, which means less forceful and

intense airflow through the airways. By reducing negative pressure, airway resistance is lowered, making it less likely to cause sleep disruptions. Light and slow breathing means the body doesn't have to work as hard to draw air in, which helps keep the airway more open. At the same time, this gentle breathing rhythm calms the nervous system, making it easier to relax and drift into restful sleep.

Finally, deep breathing supports better movement of the diaphragm, which is directly connected to the throat muscles. When the diaphragm is working well, it helps keep the upper airways more open and stable, reducing the risk of them collapsing during sleep.

Remember, every five-second improvement in your CP score reflects progress in achieving lighter, slower, and deeper breathing.

3. Balancing the Autonomic Nervous System

The heightened sympathetic drive seen in UARS and insomnia often leaves the body in a constant state of hyperarousal. This makes it difficult to relax, unwind, and stay asleep. Many people describe it as feeling tired but wired; your body is exhausted, but your nervous system hasn't quite gotten the message.

The Buteyko Method exercises are especially helpful here, as they encourage a shift toward the parasympathetic, or "rest, digest, repair," state by gently slowing the breath, lowering the heart rate, and letting the brain know the body is safe.

This balance improves sleep quality and reduces sensitivity to minor breathing disturbances. The *Breathe Light* and *Breathe Slow* exercises are practical tools that help bring the nervous system back into balance, making it easier to fall asleep and stay asleep.

For a detailed overview of UARS, check out Chapter 10C.

Obstructive Sleep Apnea and Buteyko Breathing

Obstructive sleep apnea (OSA) is a sleep disorder in which breathing repeatedly stops and starts during sleep because your airway becomes blocked. This happens when the muscles in your throat relax too much, causing your airway to collapse and cut off airflow. Your brain senses the lack of oxygen and jolts you awake sometimes with a gasp, snore, or choking sound so you can start breathing again. This cycle can happen dozens or even hundreds of times a night, preventing you from reaching deep, restful sleep.

The problem is that most people don't remember waking up because these episodes are brief. But the effects show up during the day—feeling exhausted no matter how many hours you spend in bed, struggling with brain fog, or feeling irritable. OSA is thought to affect approximately *1 billion adults worldwide*,[1] and many don't even realize they have it. Left untreated, OSA can increase the risk of high blood pressure, heart disease, stroke, diabetes, and mental health conditions.

Let's talk about something that's often overlooked in both CPAP and mandibular advancement device (MAD) therapy: mouth breathing.

Research shows that nasal obstruction is one of the biggest reasons people stop using their CPAP machines early.[2] When the nose is blocked, users often revert to mouth breathing. That alone can reduce the effectiveness of therapy, especially for those using nasal or nasal pillow masks.

It's estimated that 30–50% of CPAP users breathe through an open mouth while they sleep. That's why many are prescribed full-face masks. But here's the problem: this approach can introduce its own set of challenges.

A large study found that people using full-face CPAP masks are twice as likely to be non-adherent as those using nasal masks.[3] That's a big difference.

And when you think about it, it makes perfect sense. Mouth breathers are typically prescribed oronasal (full-face) masks with

CPAP, but this often introduces new challenges. Mouth breathing increases the likelihood of air leaks, raises pressure requirements, causes dry mouth, and can lead to fragmented sleep. In short, the therapy becomes harder to tolerate and less effective. In sleep medicine, it's becoming increasingly clear that supporting nasal breathing is essential for CPAP to work as intended. When the mouth stays open, air escapes and the airway may no longer be properly supported. Even if you're currently using a full-face mask, learning to breathe through your nose and retraining your breathing habits can make CPAP therapy feel easier and more comfortable.

That's where Buteyko and MyoTape can help. MyoTape is a soft, skin-friendly tape worn around the lips, not over them. It gently brings the lips together to encourage nasal breathing, while still allowing you to exhale through the mouth if needed. This makes it a safer and more comfortable option for CPAP users.

A MAD is a custom-fitted oral appliance worn in the mouth during sleep. It works by holding the lower jaw forward, helping to keep the airway open and reducing the risk of airway collapse. MADs are typically fitted by dentists trained in airway health and sleep-disordered breathing. They are commonly used for people with mild to moderate OSA and can be an effective option for improving airway stability during sleep. A recent study on mouth taping for MAD wearers revealed that 76% of participants reduced their apnea events to fewer than 10 per hour with mouth tape, compared with 43% without it.[4]

Improving OSA severity with the Buteyko Method focuses on two essential areas:

1. **Open Your Airway to Prevent Collapse**
    *   **Nose breathe during sleep.** Breathing through the nose during sleep creates less resistance compared with mouth breathing. In contrast, mouth breathing pushes the soft palate backward and moves the jaw downward, narrowing the airway in the throat and weakening the muscles that keep it open. This can worsen the severity of OSA.[5]

- **Maintain proper tongue posture.** Keep three-quarters of your tongue resting on the roof of your mouth during sleep to help maintain an open airway.
- **Engage the diaphragm.** Breathing low and engaging the diaphragm helps to stabilize the throat muscles, reducing the risk of airway collapse.[6]
- **Consider weight loss.** For individuals carrying excess weight, losing fat can help improve airway function. Reducing fat deposits around the throat can open the airway, while losing fat from the torso can relieve pressure on the diaphragm, allowing for increased lung volume and more stable airways. In a study of 72 predominantly male patients with mild apnea and an average weight of 97 kg, an 11-kilogram (about 24 pounds) weight loss reduced the risk of OSA by 76% compared with the control group, which lost only 2 kilograms (about 4 pounds).[7]

2. Normalize Your Breathing Volume
   - **Raise your Control Pause score.** Incremental improvements in your CP score indicate normalized breathing volume. Aim to gradually reach a CP of 20 seconds or more.

Sleep apnea can only be diagnosed through clinical sleep studies. These studies are carried out in hospitals and sleep centers all over the world. You might have already completed one and been prescribed a CPAP machine if your apnea-hypopnea index (AHI), a measure of sleep apnea severity, was over 20 events per hour as an adult. Or perhaps you're preparing for your very first sleep study.

Either way, it's worth remembering that how you breathe during the study can influence the results. If you spend the night breathing hard and fast through your mouth, it's likely your results will reflect a higher level of disordered breathing than if you go into the study with nasal breathing, good tongue posture, and a CP above 20 seconds. These simple changes can help reduce airway resistance and improve breathing stability during sleep—and that can make a real difference to how your sleep is measured.

If you've already completed a sleep study and have since applied the Buteyko Method, it's fascinating to reflect on the difference those breathing changes may have made. You may even be surprised by how much your sleep has improved, simply by changing how you breathe. And if this is your first time doing a study, why not bring everything you've learned in this book with you? Think of it as giving yourself the best possible foundation for a clearer picture of what's really going on.

Practicing consistently, ideally reaching a CP of 20 seconds or more before your study is a practical way to see how much impact better breathing can have on sleep quality.

Expected Results: Many individuals find that these breathing adjustments can reduce their AHI score by 50% or more.

If you're using mouth tape to support nasal breathing at night, I recommend MyoTape, as it's designed to allow for mouth puffing when needed. You might not recognize the term "mouth puffing," but you've likely experienced it. It refers to those moments during sleep when air escapes through the mouth, even if you're mostly breathing through your nose. Sometimes it's a full breath out through the mouth, other times it's just a short puff; your body's way of relieving pressure when it needs to.

If the body needs to mouth puff during sleep, it will find a way. Blocking that reflex entirely can actually make things worse, especially for someone with sleep apnea. That's why it's important not to seal the mouth shut. MyoTape helps encourage nasal breathing while still allowing a release of air if needed. It keeps the mouth gently supported without sealing it shut. This makes it a safe and comfortable option to keep your mouth closed during sleep.

By consistently following the Buteyko Method, you can expect gradual improvements in sleep quality, breathing stability, and overall well-being. For more information on OSA, please see Chapter 10D.

DAILY PRACTICE PROGRAM: A SIMPLE PATH TO BETTER BREATHING AND SLEEP

Integrating the following breathing practices into your daily routine is easier than it may seem. Just like brushing your teeth, breathing exercises can become a natural part of your day.

This program is designed to gradually shift your breathing patterns to support improved sleep quality and address common sleep-related issues. By following these simple steps, you'll foster lighter, slower, nasal-driven breathing that promotes restful, uninterrupted sleep.

Key Daily Practices

1. **Commit to nasal breathing throughout the day.** Aim to breathe only through your nose during rest, physical activity, and ideally, throughout the night. Nasal breathing is essential to reduce airway resistance, as it naturally humidifies, filters, and warms the air. Make a conscious effort to keep your mouth closed during the day, especially during exercise, to reinforce nasal breathing and help regulate your breathing volume.

2. **Maintain correct tongue posture.** Proper tongue posture supports an open airway and encourages nasal breathing. Rest about three-quarters of your tongue on the roof of your mouth, with the tip positioned gently behind the upper front teeth without touching them. This position supports the upper palate, helping to reduce snoring and mitigate sleep apnea.

3. **Monitor your Control Pause regularly.** Your CP score is a key measure of breathing stability. Aiming for a CP score of at least 20 seconds indicates improved CO_2 tolerance and a more regulated breathing volume.

4. **Practice the *Breathe Light Exercise* (5 minutes, 4–6 times daily).** The *Breathe Light Exercise* is at the core of the Buteyko Method, helping to recalibrate your breathing volume and foster a sense of calm. Practicing this exercise multiple times throughout the

day, with a focused 10-minute session before bed, prepares your body for the night ahead.

5. **Engage in physical activity with your mouth closed.** Daily physical activity with nasal breathing builds CO_2 tolerance and reinforces breathing patterns that support restful sleep. Aim for 30–60 minutes of light exercise daily, breathing only through your nose. Maintain a pace that makes you feel comfortably breathless without needing to open your mouth. If you feel the need to breathe through your mouth, slow down your pace to re-establish nasal breathing.

6. **Use MyoTape at night (if needed).** If you wake up with a dry mouth, it may indicate mouth breathing during sleep. MyoTape can gently encourage nasal breathing by bringing your lips together without fully sealing the mouth. If mouth taping feels uncomfortable, try wearing MyoTape for 20 minutes before bed to become accustomed to the sensation

A note on MyoTape: This product is my own creation, originally developed to help children transition from mouth to nasal breathing. It quickly became popular with adults, and to date, over 11 million strips have been sold. It's incredible to think that something I started practicing over 23 years ago—once considered unconventional—is now becoming mainstream.

Your progress depends on several key factors:

1. **Your Control Pause score.** Each 5-second improvement reflects lighter, slower, and more efficient breathing.

2. **Your ability to breathe through your nose.** Nasal breathing, supported by correct tongue posture, helps maintain an open and stable airway during sleep.

3. **The lightness of your breathing.** Gentle, quiet breathing indicates a balanced breathing pattern and reduced respiratory effort.

4. **How refreshed you feel upon waking.** Restorative sleep is one of the best signs that your breathing is improving.

Having worked with thousands of people over the years, I'm confident that you, too, will experience a positive shift in sleep quality.

Ultimately, this book is designed to help you sleep better, which is why I've front-loaded it with practical information you can apply right away. Enjoy the journey, and here's to a restful night's sleep.

BUTEYKO EXERCISES FOR CHILDREN AND ADOLESCENTS

The natural and healthiest way for us humans to breathe, no matter our age, is through the nose. Our noses are designed to filter, warm, and humidify the air we breathe, which helps protect the lungs and supports overall health. However, sometimes issues like blockages in the airways can force someone to switch from nose breathing to mouth breathing. These blockages can happen for different reasons, such as structural problems in the nose or inflammation caused by allergies or infections.

When it comes to children, there are some common signs of mouth breathing that parents or caregivers can look out for. These include:[8]

- Sleeping with their mouth open (seen in about 86% of children who mouth breathe)
- Snoring during sleep (79%)
- Rubbing or scratching an itchy nose frequently (77%)
- Drooling on their pillow while sleeping (62%)
- Tossing and turning or appearing restless during sleep (62%)
- Complaints about having a blocked or stuffy nose (49%)
- Being irritable or cranky during the day (43%)

Another clear sign is when a child regularly breathes through an open mouth during the day, especially when relaxed or focused on something, like watching TV or reading. Ideally, a child's mouth should not hang open for more than three minutes at a time, and this should not happen often. If it does, it may indicate an issue that needs attention.

Interestingly, there isn't an official definition of what exactly makes someone a "mouth breather," especially in children. But careful observation by parents, teachers, or caregivers can often provide enough clues to recognize the problem.

Studies looking at how common mouth breathing is in children have produced very different results, with estimates ranging anywhere from 7 to 60%.[9-11] This wide range may be because of differences in how the studies were done or the populations they looked at.

The main reasons children breathe through their mouths are:[12]

- **Allergies (81%).** These can cause nasal congestion, making it hard to breathe through the nose. The child may have an allergy to common triggers like dust mites in the home or pollen from plants, which can lead to a stuffy nose and difficulty breathing through the nose.
- **Enlarged adenoids (79%).** The adenoids are tissue in the back of the nasal airway, and when they swell, they can block airflow.
- **Enlarged tonsils (13%).** Large tonsils can block airflow at the back of the throat, forcing a child to breathe through their mouth.
- **A crooked nasal septum (1%).** The septum is the wall that divides the two sides of the nose, and if it's not straight, it can obstruct airflow.

The most common reason children breathe through their mouths is *nasal congestion*, often caused by allergies such as allergic rhinitis or hay fever. These allergies lead to swelling and inflammation of the nasal passages, resulting in a stuffy nose that makes nasal breathing difficult. Another common cause is enlarged adenoids, located at the back of the nasal cavity where the nose meets the throat. When enlarged, they can block this area, reducing the space for air to pass from the nose to the lungs and making nasal breathing challenging or even impossible.

When a child experiences discomfort breathing through their nose, such as a sensation of air hunger or feeling they aren't getting enough air, it is natural for them to switch to mouth breathing as a coping mechanism. The more a child breathes through their mouth, the less their nose is used and functions effectively, reinforcing the habit of mouth breathing. Over time, this behavior can become deeply ingrained, making it more challenging for the child to return to nasal breathing, even after the initial cause of the nasal obstruction has been resolved.

The transition from mouth to nasal breathing is often more complex for children than adults, particularly if structural issues like enlarged adenoids or tonsils are involved. For children with nasal congestion caused by rhinitis, the Buteyko Method can be an effective tool for relieving nasal obstruction.

If the Buteyko exercises quickly decongest the nose within 10–15 minutes of practice, allowing the child to breathe comfortably through their nose, it suggests that allergic rhinitis or another inflammatory condition is the likely cause. However, if the child continues to feel discomfort or has difficulty breathing through their nose despite practicing the exercises, this may point to an underlying structural issue, such as enlarged adenoids.

This approach has been the primary way I've identified which children can successfully transition to nasal breathing by practicing the Buteyko exercises alone, and which may require professional intervention. For those who respond quickly to the exercises and achieve nasal breathing comfort, the exercises are often enough to support lasting improvements.

From my experience working with thousands of children, approximately 75% are able to transition to comfortable nasal breathing after practicing the Buteyko Method. Many of these children came to my clinics with stuffy or runny noses, and in most cases, they were able to achieve nasal breathing through the exercises alone.

However, for the remaining 25%, persistent difficulty in nasal breathing may require further investigation. If your child shows signs of sleep-disordered breathing—such as snoring, pauses in breathing during sleep (sleep apnea), or ongoing nasal obstruction—it's important to consult an ENT specialist. An ENT evaluation can help identify and address structural issues, such as enlarged adenoids, that may be preventing the child from successfully transitioning to nasal breathing. Early intervention is critical, as untreated sleep-disordered breathing can negatively impact a child's brain development, intelligence, and overall well-being. Ensuring your child can breathe comfortably through their nose and sleep well is essential in supporting their growth and long-term health.

Teaching Children Nasal Breathing: A Step-by-Step Approach

The Buteyko Method focuses on establishing permanent nasal breathing during both wakefulness and sleep. This involves keeping the lips gently closed, the jaws relaxed, and the tongue resting in its correct position on the roof of the mouth. These foundational habits support healthy breathing patterns and promote better sleep quality.

Restoring healthy breathing patterns in children, even very young ones, starts with simple exercises that help decongest the nose and encourage nasal breathing. These exercises are particularly beneficial for children with rhinitis or nasal congestion due to allergies. Teaching and motivating children to adopt nasal breathing is a crucial part of this process.

The exercises that follow are designed to make the process simple and encouraging. They start with gentle techniques to help clear the nose, so your child can experience what it feels like to breathe comfortably through it. From there, the exercises gradually build in movement and play, helping your child learn to breathe through their nose even when they're active.

The goal is to give your child the tools and the confidence to breathe well, not just during quiet moments, but throughout the day and night.

Preparing for Success

Before starting the exercises, gently guide your child to place a strip of one-inch 3M Micropore tape (or a similar gentle paper tape) across their lips. This helps encourage nasal breathing by preventing air from being drawn in through the mouth.

To keep things comfortable and safe, fold a small tab at one end of the tape so your child can remove it easily if they feel any discomfort. It's a simple step that gives them a clear sense of what nose breathing feels like and helps build awareness in a calm, non-invasive way.

The first goal is to help clear your child's nose using the Buteyko exercises and then simply see how well they can breathe through it afterward. In other words, you're just checking if they can breathe comfortably through their nose once the exercises are done.

This early step gives you a sense of how effective the exercises are on their own or whether your child might need a little more support to maintain nasal breathing, especially during sleep.

If your child has nasal issues, they may initially feel uncomfortable breathing through their nose. This is a normal response, and the best approach is to begin the exercises promptly to minimize the time they spend in discomfort. These gentle exercises help clear the nose, making it easier to breathe, reducing the sensation of air hunger.

That said, if your child feels quite uncomfortable breathing through their nose from the outset, and the air hunger is particularly strong, it may be better to practice the exercises without the tape initially. This allows your child to get used to the breathing techniques without feeling overwhelmed. Once your child feels more comfortable, you can reintroduce the tape to encourage exclusive nasal breathing.

Below is a brief summary of the exercises. A detailed description is provided later in this chapter. You might also find it helpful to watch the exercises online, especially if you're guiding your child through them for the first time. A few years ago, I recorded these exercises while teaching my daughter, Lauren, who was nine years old at the time. You can follow along with the same videos for free by simply scanning the QR code. They are easy to follow and perfect for kids and teenagers alike.

Logical Progression of Exercises

1. **Breath Recovery Exercise (Many Small Breath Holds).** This exercise introduces your child to the technique of gently holding their breath. It helps them become familiar with the sensation of holding their nose while staying relaxed and calm. Encourage your child to practice this exercise for three minutes, ensuring they remain at ease throughout the process. This foundational step is key to building comfort and confidence with the breathing exercises that follow.

2. **Magic Nose Unblocking Exercise.** Move on to the *Magic Nose Unblocking Exercise,* which is specifically designed to clear nasal congestion. Perform six repetitions to help your child breathe more freely through their nose.

3. **Dolphin Breathing Exercise (Steps Exercise).** Introduce the *Steps Exercise,* which combines physical movement with breath- holding to create a moderate-to-strong sensation of air hunger. Begin with walking short distances while holding the breath. As your child gains confidence, you can turn it into a fun challenge; counting steps together or turning it into a game. Progress to jogging while holding the breath. Record the number of paces completed during each attempt to track their progress. Repeat six times.

4. **Sitting with mouth closed.** Next, have your child sit quietly for three minutes with their mouth taped. Observe whether they can breathe comfortably through their nose during this time. Listen to their breathing—is it silent or audible? Does your child want to remove the tape due to air hunger? Are they breathing fast? Ideally, your child should be able to breathe in and out through their nose silently and comfortably.

5. **Physical activity with mouth closed (Racehorse Breathing).** If your child is comfortable breathing through their nose while at rest for

three minutes, progress to physical activity while keeping their mouth closed. Start with walking for one minute while your child wears a strip of paper tape across their lips to encourage nasal breathing. If your child remains comfortable breathing through their nose while walking, gradually increase the intensity by having them jog for one minute. Repeat this cycle several times, aiming for a total of five to ten minutes of activity.

Observe whether your child's breathlessness is proportional to the intensity of the activity. It is normal for the child to feel some breathlessness when transitioning to nasal breathing during exercise, particularly if they are new to this practice. However, if your child struggles significantly, slows their pace, or removes the tape due to air hunger—despite completing the *Nose Unblocking* and *Steps Exercises*—it may indicate they are unable to functionally breathe through their nose. In such cases, an ENT evaluation is recommended to assess potential structural issues, that may be obstructing nasal breathing. Keep in mind, every child moves at their own pace. What matters most is consistency, patience, and encouragement. Even small improvements can make a big difference over time.

While this observation isn't clinical or diagnostic, I've seen it time and again in practice. Based on my experience working with many children, if your child can breathe through their nose with good breath control while jogging, it's a very good sign that their nose is working well for everyday nasal breathing.

It's a simple but practical way to check how efficient their breathing really is and gives you confidence that all the small steps you're taking are paying off.

Transitioning to Nasal Breathing Full-Time

It's important to note that the *Nose Unblocking* and *Steps Exercises* will only temporarily decongest the nose. If your child has a history of a stuffy or runny nose, their nasal passages may become congested again after a few hours. Stay with me here—this is just the starting point. As your child breathes more and more through their nose and continues practicing the exercises, their nasal passages will start to function more effectively over time.

With regular daily practice, most parents notice that their child's nasal symptoms, such as a stuffy or runny nose, ease by about 50% within two weeks. This improvement lays the foundation for long-term nasal breathing and a significant reduction in nasal discomfort.

One of the most effective exercises I use is *Dolphin Breathing*, also called the *Steps Exercise*. This exercise serves two purposes: it helps decongest the nose and acts as a measurement tool. I always explain to children and teenagers with stuffy noses that they will continue to have nasal congestion if their *Steps* score is below 40 paces. For younger children, the target score may be slightly lower, but in general, reaching 40 paces is a solid benchmark and the minimum goal to aim for.

Want to see how it's done? You can watch a free video demonstration of how to perform and measure your child's Steps Score by scanning the QR code. It's simple to follow and perfect for kids or teens who want to start retraining their breathing in a gentle and structured way.

In the first week of switching to nasal breathing, the focus should be on helping the child consistently breathe through their nose during the day. Keep in mind that a child or teenager with a history of nasal congestion is also likely to have developed a mouth-breathing habit. This habit forms over months or even years of breathing through an open mouth. While decongesting the nose is crucial, it's equally important to address and change the mouth-breathing behavior.

Motivating Children and Teens

In helping children and young people to change their breathing habits, they need to understand the importance of breathing through the nose. When I work with young people, I ask them which reasons they consider the most important when it comes to breathing nasally. The most popular replies tend to focus on athletic performance and developing a good-looking face. I've found it more effective to avoid focusing on the negatives of mouth breathing when talking to children. Instead, I find they respond well to hearing about the many benefits of nasal breathing. The following ideas may be helpful:

- **Nasal breathing makes you more intelligent.** You can explain to your child that people who breathe through their noses tend to have better focus, energy, and brain power. Nasal breathing improves cognition, concentration, alertness, and energy levels because it promotes better sleep and delivers more oxygen to the brain. This helps your child focus better in class so learning will be easier and more enjoyable.
- **Nasal breathing improves sports performance.** Children who breathe through their mouths often become breathless quickly during physical activity, which can make them shy away from sports they might otherwise enjoy. Nasal breathing helps build stamina and better recovery. Professional athletes, Olympians, and some world-famous musicians all use Buteyko breathing techniques to improve their performance during training.
- **Mouth breathing causes crooked teeth and bad breath.** Let's be honest; no teenager wants to have bad breath. Nasal breathing helps to maintain a healthy mouth and prevents smelly breath. It can also avert problems in facial development, such as narrow jaws, crooked, overcrowded teeth, and small upper airways.
- **Breathing through the nose helps you sleep better and gives you more energy.** Mouth breathing interferes with a good night's sleep, and you will have less energy to enjoy life. Children who

sleep poorly are also up to ten times more likely to develop learning difficulties.[13]

- **Mouth breathing is bad for posture.** Persistent mouth breathing during early childhood can lead to changes in posture. The head often shifts forward in an attempt to open the airway, which can throw off the body's natural alignment. Over time, this can affect the stability of the spine, especially if combined with upper chest breathing. These things may not be particularly motivating for children, but parents will understand their importance.

- **Nasal breathing leads to good table manners.** When your child has a blocked nose, even eating can become difficult. Nasal congestion makes it tricky to coordinate breathing and swallowing, so the child may need to stop chewing or chew faster to breathe through the mouth. This breathlessness may look like bad table manners as the child sniffs and gulps their way through each meal.[14]

In all cases, the best place to start is by encouraging nasal breathing both day and night. Children under five years of age may find it difficult to practice breathing exercises, so it's important for parents to take the lead by avoiding habits that encourage over-breathing. Children mirror the adults around them, even when it comes to breathing. If you're walking around with your mouth open, sighing or panting without noticing it, chances are your child will copy you. The same goes for everyone else in the house. I've often seen situations where a child's progress stalls simply because those around them haven't changed their own habits.

That's why leading by example is key. When the whole household gets on board, the benefits are shared and everyone starts to feel the difference.

Help your child understand what "breathing too much" means, and explain that over-breathing is often behind tiredness, wheezing, coughing, and a stuffy nose. The best way to do this is by giving a physical demonstration. Ask your child to hold out a finger and blow a big puff of air onto it. Let them feel the strength and quantity of air on their finger. Explain that this is "big breathing." Then, ask your child to blow a tiny, gentle stream of air onto their finger. It should be so light they can barely feel it. Explain that this is what healthy, quiet breathing should feel like.

You can also ask your child to explain these ideas to others in the household. This gives your child a chance to reflect on what they've learned and to express it in their own words. By listening to how your child describes it, you'll get a good sense of how well they've understood the key ideas.

The Role of the Buteyko Method

The Buteyko Method helps decongest the nose and improve breathing patterns so your child can comfortably breathe through their nose. To change the mouth-breathing habit, I have found that using a nasal breathing support tool, such as MyoTape, is highly effective. This gentle support, worn for just 30 minutes daily, can guide your child from mouth breathing to more consistent nasal breathing. As mentioned earlier in the chapter, I want to be transparent in saying that I am the creator and owner of MyoTape. I developed this product because there was no tool on the market designed to be worn surrounding the mouth, gently bringing the lips together to encourage nasal breathing. MyoTape helps children safely transition to nasal breathing during wakefulness and, once established, maintain it during sleep.

The design of MyoTape ensures that the mouth is never covered, allowing mouth breathing if needed. Another important consideration? Children love to talk. That's why it was essential to create a nasal breathing support they can wear while chatting, eating, or drinking, without needing to take it off. At the same time, if your child's mouth tends to hang open and they start breathing through it, the tape gives a gentle elastic reminder to switch back to nasal breathing. This reduces the need for parents to constantly remind or nag their child to "breathe through your nose." Let MyoTape do the reminding for you. Once your child has been consistently breathing through their nose during the day for a week or more and has practiced the exercises, they can begin using MyoTape during sleep to promote nasal breathing throughout the night. MyoTape is only suitable for children over the age of five, and only when nasal breathing already feels comfortable and natural.

It's important to remember that we never want to force nasal breathing, especially in children. If your child is still very congested or struggling to breathe through the nose, we don't push through it. Nasal breathing should feel easy and comfortable.

Before introducing nasal breathing during sleep, it's essential to make sure your child can breathe comfortably through their nose while at rest. If they're still having difficulty nasal breathing, even after working with the Buteyko Method, or if they appear to be putting in a lot of effort just to breathe, then it's best to hold off on using any kind of mouth tape during sleep. Ensuring the child is ready for this step helps create a safe and effective transition to consistent nasal breathing.

If you're a parent reading this, my suggestion is to start by practicing the exercises yourself first. Work on switching to nasal breathing during rest, during exercise, and—when comfortable—during sleep. If you find yourself waking up with a dry mouth in the morning, it's a clear sign that you've been mouth breathing during sleep. And here's something I've learned over the years: children make much better progress when a parent leads by example. For a child to successfully switch to nasal breathing, it's just as important for the parent to put these practices into action.

That said, the *Steps Exercise* may not always be suitable for parents. For instance, it's not recommended for individuals with high blood pressure, serious medical conditions, panic disorder, or anxiety. Additionally, if the mother is pregnant, she should not perform any of the exercises designed for children.

Remember, before starting the exercises, encourage your child to wear paper tape across their lips to help ensure nasal breathing throughout the entire sequence. Begin with the *Breathing Recovery Exercise*, and then go on to *Nose Unblocking*, then *Steps*, then nasal breathing during rest for three minutes, then nasal breathing during walking, followed by nasal breathing during jogging or running.

Breath Recovery Exercise (Many Small Breath Holds)

Here's a step-by-step way to explain the exercise to your child:

1. Take a gentle breath in through your nose; then gently breathe out through your nose.
2. Pinch your nose with your fingers to hold your breath for 3–5 seconds. The parent can count down out loud: 5, 4, 3, 2, 1.
3. After letting go of your nose, breathe normally through your nose for about 10–15 seconds. Keep your breathing nice and calm.
4. Repeat this for about 2–3 minutes. The parent can let the child know when the exercise is complete.

Once your child is confident and comfortable with this exercise, move on to the *Magic Nose Unblocking Exercise* as the next step in their practice. Remind your child that these exercises are designed to make breathing through their nose easier and to take their time while learning.

Magic Nose Unblocking Exercise

Here's a simple step-by-step guide to help your child with this exercise:

1. Ask your child to take a normal breath in and out through their nose.
2. Have them gently pinch their nose with their fingers to hold their breath.
3. While holding their breath, encourage them to gently nod their head up and down five times.

4. After five head nods, have them release their nose and breathe calmly through it. Remind them to breathe softly and avoid gasping or breathing heavily.
5. Let them rest for 30–60 seconds to allow their breathing to return to normal.

Progression

This exercise involves holding the breath until your child feels a moderate-to-strong sensation of air hunger, but they should still be able to recover their breathing through the nose within a couple of breaths. Once your child is comfortable with this exercise, gradually increase the breath hold to 10 head nods. Over time, they can progress to 15 head nods or more, depending on their comfort level. As your child holds their breath for longer periods, it's normal for their breathing to feel slightly harder when they resume.

The key is ensuring that your child remains relaxed and can recover their breathing within two breaths. With regular practice, your child will likely be able to hold their breath for 20 head nods or more. This progression not only builds their confidence but also helps improve their ability to breathe comfortably through their nose.

How Often

Guide your child to repeat this exercise six to eight times in one session, with a 30–60 second rest between repetitions.

This consistent practice can make a big difference in clearing nasal congestion and promoting healthy nasal breathing habits. The next exercise, the *Dolphin Breathing Exercise*, also known as *Steps* is another excellent way to help decongest the nose. In fact, it tends to be a little stronger than this exercise and often works more quickly. That said, it's still valuable for your child to learn and use both techniques, as each can be helpful in different settings.

Dolphin Breathing Exercise (Steps Exercise)

Steps Exercise: A Guide for Parents to Teach Their Child
This exercise is a valuable tool for children and teenagers to improve their breathing and measure progress. It involves holding the breath while walking, jogging, or running and can be easily adapted for beginners and advanced practice.

Precautions
- **Serious medical conditions.** If your child has pulmonary hypertension, epilepsy, or any other serious medical condition, they must not practice the *Steps Exercise*. Holding the breath to create a moderate-to-strong air hunger can temporarily activate a stress response, which should be avoided in these cases.
- **Diabetes.** For children with diabetes, breath-hold exercises can lower blood sugar levels. Make sure your child has a snack before practicing, and monitor their blood sugar levels frequently during the exercise.
- **Asthma or wheezing.** If your child is wheezy or coughing, limit the *Steps Exercise* to 10–20 paces. While this exercise can significantly improve asthma symptoms within just a few weeks, it's important not to overdo it. The key is to make sure that your child's breathing returns to normal shortly after each breath hold. If your child starts breathing heavily after a breath hold, it may trigger wheezing, chest tightness, or a cough. It's not the breath hold itself that triggers these symptoms; it's the heavier breathing that can follow if it isn't kept under control.

Beginners' Steps Exercise

Introduce small children (ages four to six) to the *Steps Exercise* by having them walk a short distance (about five paces) while holding their breath. Use the help of another adult or an older sibling to make this more engaging. Position yourselves as helpers at either end of the walking distance to guide the child.

Example setup:

Adult one ← Distance of five paces → *Adult two*

Here's how to teach the *Steps Exercise*:

1. Ask your child to breathe in and out gently through their nose.
2. After they exhale, have them pinch their nostrils closed with their fingers to hold their breath.
3. While holding their breath, they should walk the five-pace distance between the two helpers.
4. Once they've walked the distance, have them release their nose and resume gentle nasal breathing.
5. Wait 30–60 seconds to allow their breathing to normalize; then repeat the exercise.

Advanced Steps Exercise

Once your child is comfortable holding their breath over a short distance, gradually increase the number of paces. You can do this in two ways:

- Increase the distance between the two helpers.
- Keep the five-paces distance but have the child walk back and forth multiple times before releasing their breath, similar to swimming laps underwater.

As the child becomes more advanced, they can incorporate jogging or even running while holding their breath. Encourage them to gradually increase the number of steps they take with their breath held, building up to a point where they feel a strong air hunger.

After the breath hold, your child should:

- Take their first breath in through the nose.

- Calm their breathing immediately. While the first and second breaths may be larger than usual, the third breath should be under good control.

Practice Schedule

- Perform six repetitions of the *Steps Exercise* in one session, with 30–60 seconds of rest between each repetition.
- Practice two to three sets per day.
- Count the number of steps your child takes during each breath hold and record their scores.

Using the ButeykoClinic app can make tracking progress even easier. The app allows you to record your child's best *Steps* score, compare results over time, and set goals for improvement.

Motivation Tips

- Compare weekly scores to monitor improvement.
- Use a star chart to reward your child for reaching new milestones.
- Incorporate the *Steps Exercise* into other activities like skipping, jogging, or running to make it more fun and engaging.

The *Steps Exercise* is highly effective at decongesting the nose—arguably even more powerful than the *Magic Nose Unblocking Exercise* practiced earlier. Beyond clearing nasal passages, it helps your child improve their breathing patterns and provides a sense of accomplishment as they track their progress over time.

Young children tend to have a strong response to the buildup of carbon dioxide in the blood, although this sensitivity decreases as they grow older. A child's ability to hold their breath is largely determined by how sensitive they are to carbon dioxide, not by willpower or lung size. Because of this, the *Steps Exercise* should be adapted based on the child's age to ensure it remains safe and effective.

Here are the general targets for the *Steps Exercise:*

- **Children aged 5 to 7 years.** Aim to achieve 50 to 60 paces.

- **Children aged 8 to 9 years.** Aim to achieve 60 to 70 paces.
- **Children aged 10 and over.** The goal is to reach 80 paces.

Don't worry if your 10-year-old isn't hitting 80 paces straight away. Most children start off reaching around 20 to 30 paces, and that's perfectly normal. What matters most is that they're doing the exercise correctly. That alone means they're making progress. How quickly they improve depends on things like genetics and their breathing history. The key is regular practice and a willingness to breathe through the nose.

If you're a parent teaching your own child, you'll know it's not always easy. Children are often much more open to learning from someone other than their parent. That said, it's well worth sitting down with your child to watch the free demonstration videos; just scan the QR code or find them in the ButeykoClinic app. These simple resources can make a big difference.

Every bit of practice helps, and with a little patience and encouragement, your efforts will absolutely pay off. A lifetime of mouth breathing is not a good option. Helping your child transition to healthy nasal breathing now will benefit them for years to come.

Incorporating Nasal Breathing into Everyday Life

Let's face it—no child or teenager is going to practice these exercises indefinitely. The key is to integrate nasal breathing into their daily routine, making it a natural part of their life while helping them understand why it's important. Here are some key tips:

- **Be mindful of your child's breathing.** Pay attention to your child's breathing throughout the day. If you hear your child breathing audibly or notice their mouth is open, gently remind them to breathe through their nose with their tongue resting on the roof of their mouth. Encourage them to keep their lips sealed and ensure no air is "sneaking" in through the mouth.

You might even turn it into a playful moment by saying, "Let's catch the sneaky air together." Framing it as a game helps avoid it feeling like a correction and keeps your child engaged in learning to breathe through their nose.

- **Make practice fun.** Children love games, so keeping things fun and varied is essential. If your child becomes bored with practicing the exercises, you can bring breath-holding into games instead such as playing hopscotch, doing jumping jacks, or bouncing on a trampoline. Incorporating these activities keeps practice enjoyable while encouraging healthy breathing habits.

- **Recognize the importance of nasal breathing during sleep.** Switching to nasal breathing during sleep is just as important as doing so during the day. It supports better oxygenation, reduces snoring, and promotes deep, restorative rest. It also helps to maintain good dental health, as mouth breathing can dry out the mouth and increase the risk of cavities and gum disease.

  Once your child has established nasal breathing during the day, gradually introduce tools like MyoTape at night to gently keep their lips together and encourage nasal breathing throughout sleep.

- **Motivate children and teenagers.** Help your child understand the many benefits of nasal breathing, such as improving sports performance by enhancing endurance, focus, and recovery; supporting proper jaw development and healthier teeth; and reducing the risk of orthodontic problems. Nasal breathing isn't just healthier; it also looks and feels better. It's a sign of strength, calm, and confidence.

  Explaining these benefits in terms that resonate with your child, especially teenagers who may be more focused on sports or appearance, can motivate them to adopt these habits.

- **Get professional guidance.** If you feel that you need additional guidance or assistance in teaching your child, reach out to a certified Buteyko Clinic Instructor. Many instructors offer online training sessions and are also certified myofunctional therapists. This means they can combine breathing exercises with good oral habits, including correct tongue posture, proper swallowing techniques, and more. You can visit ***https://buteykoclinic.com*** for a list of certified instructors who work specifically with children and teenagers.

By supporting your child to breathe through their nose during wakefulness and sleep, you'll be setting them up with healthy habits that can last a lifetime.

CHAPTER 2

UNDERSTANDING AND ASSESSING YOUR SLEEP

There's nothing quite like the feeling of waking up truly refreshed—the mind clear, your energy high, and your body ready to take on the day. But the reality is that many of us experience the exact opposite. Instead of bouncing out of bed, we drag ourselves up and spend the day feeling groggy, grumpy, and foggy, with a sense of fatigue that lingers throughout the day. Sound familiar?

The truth is, good sleep isn't just about how many hours you spend in bed—it's about the *quality* of that sleep. You might be getting enough hours, but if your sleep is disrupted by snoring, upper airway resistance, insomnia, or sleep apnea, your body won't get the deep rest it craves. As a result, you can still wake up feeling terrible.

Sleep deprivation, also known as "sleep insufficiency" or "sleeplessness," happens when the duration or quality of sleep is not enough to maintain proper alertness, performance, and overall health. In today's fast-paced world, lack of sleep has become the norm, especially among working adults. According to the Centers for Disease Control and Prevention (CDC), over a third of adults in the United States don't get enough sleep. This figure rises to a staggering 46% among African American adults.[1]

The numbers are also high among business owners and managers, who often run on fumes. Total sleep time has declined significantly over the last decade. Among American employees, 30% report sleeping less than six hours per night, and this percentage rises to 41% among managers and entrepreneurs.[2] And this isn't just an American problem—countries like the UK, Finland, China, and South Korea all see similar sleep struggles. For instance, the *Sleep Index Report* of China in 2015 revealed that 31% of Chinese residents experienced low sleep quality, with 38% of working individuals reporting sleep problems that impacted their daytime work efficiency.[3]

We all know that sleep affects our mood, focus, and energy levels, but did you know it can also influence our *morals*? When employees don't get enough rest, the effects go far beyond feeling tired. Poor sleep can lead to decreased job performance, tense workplace relationships, and even lapses in ethical judgment.[4,5]

Professor Christopher M. Barnes from the University of Washington's Foster School of Business has explored this surprising link between sleep and moral awareness. His research reveals that when people face demanding circumstances—like long work hours or personal conflicts that disrupt sleep—they're less likely to recognize ethical dilemmas.[6] In other words, exhaustion doesn't just cloud thinking; it can blur the line between right and wrong.

Ethical behavior means acting in a way that aligns with legal standards and society's moral values. Unethical behavior, on the other hand, includes actions that are illegal or widely considered wrong—things like theft, sexual harassment, or even falsified performance reporting.[7-9] Studies show that sleep-deprived employees are more likely to engage in these behaviors because fatigue weakens their self-control and decision-making abilities.

Sleep deprivation also significantly impairs cognitive functions, making it harder to make sound decisions, especially when the most immediately gratifying or "prepotent" choice—the one that feels instinctive or rewarding—is also the less ethical option.[10] For example, taking credit for someone else's work might offer immediate recognition but is clearly unethical. When sleep-deprived, individuals struggle to recognize such dilemmas, identify better alternatives, and act appropriately, meaning integrity takes a major hit.

Brain imaging studies of sleep-deprived individuals reveal that the prefrontal cortex, located just behind the forehead, experiences the most significant decline in cerebral metabolic rate.[11,12] Often referred to as the brain's "control center," the prefrontal cortex is responsible for "executive functions" such as decision-making, problem-solving, self-control, and regulating social behavior. These complex thought processes require significant energy, and when sleep is insufficient, the prefrontal cortex doesn't receive enough glucose, its primary energy source. This energy deficit impairs its ability to weigh consequences, suppress impulsive actions, and manage ethical reasoning.

The takeaway? Prioritizing sleep isn't just about personal health—although that's undoubtedly important—it's also about maintaining integrity, fostering a positive work environment, and making better decisions every day.

Research further highlights the severity of these sleep-related impairments, demonstrating that sleep deprivation can affect cognitive and motor performance to levels comparable to alcohol intoxication. A study by Williamson and Feyer conducted in 2000 found that after 17–19 hours without sleep, performance on certain tests was equivalent to or worse than having a blood alcohol concentration of 0.05%. After 24 hours of wakefulness, performance dropped to levels comparable to a blood alcohol concentration of 0.10%, which is legally classified as drunk in many regions.[13]

Now, imagine the consequences of this level of impairment: how comfortable would you be with a sleep-deprived doctor performing surgery, a lawyer representing your case, or an investment banker managing your finances? Sleep deprivation doesn't just compromise individual performance; it severely affects the brain's ability to function ethically and effectively.

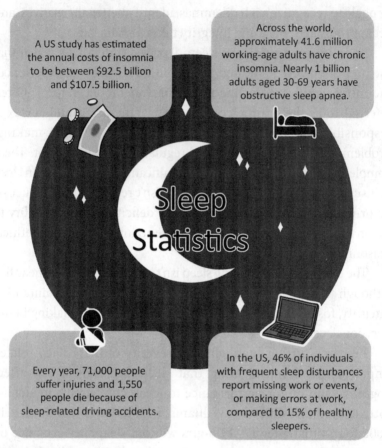

A US study has estimated the annual costs of insomnia to be between $92.5 billion and $107.5 billion.

Across the world, approximately 41.6 million working-age adults have chronic insomnia. Nearly 1 billion adults aged 30-69 years have obstructive sleep apnea.

Sleep Statistics

Every year, 71,000 people suffer injuries and 1,550 people die because of sleep-related driving accidents.

In the US, 46% of individuals with frequent sleep disturbances report missing work or events, or making errors at work, compared to 15% of healthy sleepers.

Sleep statistics sources[14,15]

Sleep quality is deeply connected to overall well-being, serving as a partial mediator in the relationship between stress and mental health. Research by Hamilton et al. found that individuals with insomnia symptoms experienced significantly lower psychological and subjective well-being.[16] Addressing sleep insufficiency is critical not just for individual health but also for the productivity and functionality of workplaces and society at large.

If your goal is to live a longer, healthier life and make the most of your energy and focus each day, one of the most important steps you can take is to get consistent, restorative sleep.

But let's be honest; how often does sleep quietly slip to the bottom of the list?

Maybe you're staying up late to finish work, or just needing a little quiet time after a long day. Or maybe it's catching up with friends, watching that extra episode, or scrolling a little longer than planned.

Now, I'm not here to be a killjoy; life's meant to be lived, and we all need a bit of fun. But it's worth knowing that even just two or three late nights a week can leave a lasting imprint on how you feel for the rest of the week.

This isn't just about feeling groggy or irritable the next day. Sleep is foundational to health and well-being, and the consequences of insufficient sleep can be profound. As noted earlier, poor sleep has been linked to reduced productivity, increased risk of accidents, and a cascade of physical and mental health issues. Chronic sleep deprivation doesn't just diminish quality of life—it shortens lifespan. Research shows that men and women with high-quality sleep live significantly longer: 4.7 years more for men and 2.4 years more for women compared with those with poor sleep.[17] Now, you might think 2.4 or 4.7 years doesn't sound like a lot, so why bother? But I can promise you, when your time is running short, those extra years start looking pretty good. That's more time with your family, more laughs, more stories told (and retold), and maybe even a few extra birthdays. When we've got just a little time left, we tend to appreciate it a whole lot more.

Recognizing the impact of insufficient sleep, the CDC has classified it as a "public health epidemic." Sleep issues such as insomnia and snoring aren't just nuisances to push through; they are warning signs that action is needed. Ignoring these signs can lead to long-term health consequences, affecting not only your immediate well-being but also your longevity.

I'm not here to be a harbinger of doom, but rather to emphasize how vital sleep is to every aspect of your health. By understanding the importance of sleep, we can make intentional choices to prioritize it—choices that improve our health, extend our lifespan, and enhance our quality of life. It's time to take sleep seriously, for ourselves and for the people who rely on us.

Sleep is a vast subject. Over the 23 years of seeing clients and running sleep clinics, I have heard some common questions:

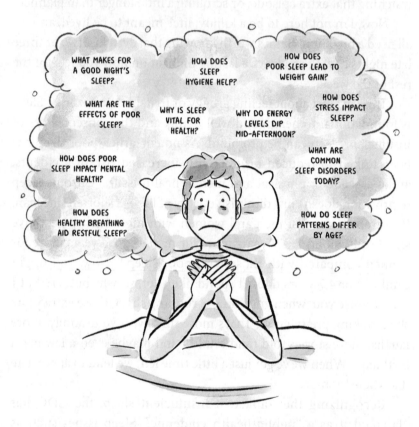

To gain a deeper understanding of sleep, we will explore all these questions (and more) in an approachable, easy-to-digest manner in the upcoming chapters. As we progress, I'll take you deeper into the vital role of the breath in sleep health and share effective strategies to enhance your sleep. But first, let's begin by exploring the different *stages of sleep* and some of the foundations of healthy sleep: *quality, quantity,* and *consistency.*

SLEEP STAGES

Think of sleep as a journey. Your brain and body go through a series of stages, each with a different purpose. Some help you lock in memories, others repair muscles, and some even balance your mood so you wake up feeling refreshed instead of groggy or irritable.

Your night isn't just one long stretch of sleep; instead, you cycle through different sleep stages about four to six times a night, with each cycle lasting 90 to 110 minutes.[18,19] You start in light sleep, move into deep, restorative sleep, and finally enter REM sleep, where most dreaming happens.

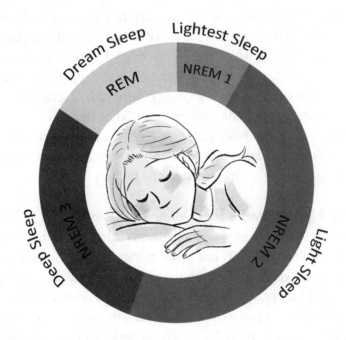

There are two main types of sleep:

- **NREM** (non-rapid eye movement) sleep
- **REM** (rapid eye movement) sleep, also known as "dream sleep"

Each sleep stage has a unique role, and getting enough of all of them is what makes you feel truly rested. If you want better sleep, it's not just about spending more hours in bed—it's about making sure you're getting the right balance of these stages for deep, restorative rest.

What Happens During Non-Rapid Eye Movement Sleep?

Non-rapid eye movement (NREM) sleep might not get as much attention as its better-known cousin, REM sleep, but it's just as important, possibly even more so when it comes to deep restoration. Let's be honest, REM kind of stole the spotlight. Maybe it was the band, with Michael Stipe at the mic, that helped put it on the map. But while REM sleep gets the fame, NREM is the quiet workhorse in the background. It's where the real recovery happens: tissue repair, immune support, memory consolidation, and deep physical rest. If you've ever woken up feeling groggy, unrefreshed, cranky, or just "off," chances are you didn't get enough NREM sleep.

Sleep is like the body's nightly housekeeping service. It goes through different stages, each with its own specific role in repairing, refreshing, and resetting your body and brain.

Stage 1: Lightest Sleep—The "Dozing Off" Phase (5%)

This is that "in-between" stage when you're drifting off but can still be easily woken up. It only lasts a few minutes, and it's basically your body shifting gears, slowing down your heart rate, relaxing your muscles, and preparing for deeper sleep. If you've ever felt like you were falling just as you were nodding off—that sudden "jerk"—this is when it happens. It's called a "hypnic jerk," and while it can feel dramatic, it's completely normal. Think of it as your brain double-checking that it's okay to fully let go.

If you're spending more time in Stage 1 sleep, it could be that you have a "low arousal threshold," meaning you're more easily woken up by noises, movements, or even just a shift in your own breathing.[20]

Low arousal threshold can fragment your sleep and is linked with insomnia as well as being a subtype of OSA.

Stage 2: Light Sleep—The Processing Stage (45%)

Now, your body is fully committed to sleep, but you're not in deep sleep just yet. This stage of sleep is moderately easy to wake from, meaning you can still be disturbed by external noises or movements.

Your body temperature drops, your heart rate and breathing slow down, and the body eases into a more stable rhythm, reducing levels of the stress hormone cortisol and setting the stage for deep, restorative sleep. Your brain starts producing bursts of activity called "sleep spindles," which help with learning and protect your sleep from disturbances.[21]

This stage is about mental fine-tuning. It helps the brain clear out unnecessary details and strengthen and integrate the important ones, making it easier to recall what truly matters the next day.[22,23] Think of it as your brain's "auto-save" function—converting short-term experiences from the day into long-term memories, ensuring that important experiences and knowledge don't just fade away.

Stage 3: Deep Sleep—The Body's Repair Mode (25%)

This is the powerhouse of sleep when it comes to feeling refreshed and rejuvenated. As you progress through the stages of NREM sleep, your body enters a deeper state of relaxation. Your body is in its most restorative state, and your brain activity has slowed significantly. In fact, it's also known as "slow-wave sleep" because of the very slow, synchronized brain waves that take over. Your heart rate and breathing also slow, and your body temperature drops.

This stage is the hardest stage to wake up from, meaning it has the highest arousal threshold.[24] If you do wake up during deep sleep, you'll likely feel disoriented, sluggish, and groggy, as your brain was still in full recovery mode. The downside? As you get older, your body naturally spends less time in this deep, restorative sleep and more time in lighter NREM Stage 2 sleep, which isn't as refreshing.[25] That's why prioritizing good sleep habits becomes even more important as you age! More on this in Chapter 9.

During this phase:

- Your body goes into full repair mode—muscle growth, tissue healing, and immune system strengthening all happen here.
- Growth hormone is released, which is why kids and teenagers need so much deep sleep.[26] But growth hormone isn't just important to children—adults need it for nighttime muscle repair, fat metabolism, bone strength, tissue regeneration, immune function, and brain health. Also, growth hormone stimulates collagen production, which keeps skin firm, elastic, and youthful-looking.
- Thanks to the glymphatic system—the brain's built-in waste removal system—your brain flushes out toxins (including the ones linked to Alzheimer's), making this stage crucial for long-term brain health. Please see the section "Brain Health" in Chapter 4 for more on the glymphatic system.

What Happens During REM Sleep?

Unlike NREM sleep, during REM sleep your brain gets very active—almost like it's awake! Your eyes dart around (hence the name "rapid eye movement"), your breathing may become more erratic and irregular, and your brain processes lots of information. It's the stage where most of your vivid dreams happen. You also experience atonia, which is a temporary paralysis of your muscles, with two exceptions: the eyes and the muscles that control breathing. This is helpful, as it prevents you from acting out your dreams.[27] Overall, you spend *about 25% of your sleep time in REM sleep.*

A Nightly Therapy Session

Throughout the day, we go through ups and downs—stress at work, happy moments with friends, and minor frustrations like getting stuck in traffic. All these emotions get stored in the brain. But if they just piled up with no sorting system, we'd feel overwhelmed all the time.

That's where REM sleep comes in! Think of it as your *brain's emotional detox*—it sorts through the day's feelings and helps you make sense of them. It decides what's worth keeping (like an important life lesson) and what's okay to let go of (like the irritation of spilling coffee). This process helps us wake up feeling more balanced and less emotionally drained.

If you skimp on REM sleep (due to stress, poor sleep habits, or disruptions), your brain struggles to regulate emotions properly. You might wake up feeling cranky, anxious, or just "off" without knowing why. Over time, a lack of REM sleep is linked to mood disorders like anxiety and depression.

REM sleep is a bit like your brain's nightly therapy session—it helps you process emotions, so you wake up refreshed and ready to tackle the next day.

A Librarian to Sort and Store Information

REM sleep doesn't just help with emotional regulation; it also plays important roles in learning and memory consolidation. It helps you learn new things, store important information, and even connect the dots between ideas.

Throughout the day, your brain takes in tons of information— what you read, conversations you had, and skills you practiced. But if this info just sat in your brain like a messy pile of papers, it would be useless.

During REM sleep, your brain:

- Sorts and organizes memories
- Strengthens important connections
- Discards unnecessary information

It's like cleaning up your mental workspace so you don't wake up with a cluttered brain.

REM sleep also helps you think creatively and solve problems. It takes all the random pieces of knowledge in your brain and connects them in new ways. You can thank REM sleep for those "aha" moments—when you wake up with newfound clarity on a problem that seemed impossible to solve the day before!

The first period of REM sleep is short, but as the night goes on, you spend progressively more time in REM sleep and less in deep sleep.[28] This varies among persons due to diverse factors, which include age, recent sleep patterns, physical activity, and even alcohol and drug consumption.

Nocturia: Are Nighttime Bathroom Trips Stealing Your Deep Sleep?

Waking up to use the bathroom—also known as "nocturia"—is one of the biggest sleep disruptors. It pulls you out of whatever sleep stage you're in, and if it happens during deep sleep (Stage 3), you're losing out on some of the most restorative rest your body needs. This is why frequent nighttime trips to the bathroom can leave you feeling less refreshed, even if you think you got enough hours in bed.

> "I've been using the Oxygen Advantage® app for over a year. It's reduced my breathing rate and volume and has helped with my meditation practice.
>
> I also taped my mouth during sleep for about 6 months, improving my sleep and my daytime energy levels.
>
> Before, I'd wake up 2–3 times throughout the night to use the restroom, and it would take me some time to fall back asleep.
>
> Now, I wake up once at most to use the restroom and generally fall back asleep immediately. . . ."
>
> *Hadi, 39, Spain*

Nocturia becomes more common with age—about 50% of adults between 50 and 79 experience it.[29] It starts with occasional wake-ups in your fifties and can increase to twice a night or more for men in their 70s. The real problem? Falling back asleep. If you wake up fully, your brain resets back to Stage 1 sleep, making it take longer to return to deep sleep and REM sleep, which can seriously impact overall sleep quality.

Want an easy way to spend more time in deep sleep? Focus on nasal breathing. Breathing through your nose during sleep helps your body stay in a deeper sleep state. If you struggle with this, using a nasal breathing aid like MyoTape can bring significant benefits. I always remind my clients: if you wake up with a dry mouth, it means you've been mouth breathing—and that's a sign your sleep quality is suffering.

Check out Lisa's story in Chapter 10C to find out how using MyoTape freed her from a lifetime of nighttime bathroom visits and lying awake for hours.

OPTIMIZING YOUR SLEEP: THE IMPORTANCE OF QUALITY, QUANTITY, AND A REGULAR SLEEP SCHEDULE

Most sleep advice focuses on how many hours you should be getting—but optimal sleep isn't just about *quantity*; it's about *quality* and *consistency* too. You could be clocking in a full night's sleep and still wake up feeling drained. I know this firsthand—I used to sleep 10 hours a night and still feel exhausted every morning. It wasn't until I discovered the critical role of breathing in achieving truly restorative, quality sleep that everything changed.

Sleep Quantity: How Much Sleep Do You Need?

You've probably heard that adults should aim for *seven to nine hours of sleep per night*—and that's solid advice from health organizations.[30] Babies, kids, and teenagers need even more since their bodies and brains are still developing. But here's the thing: sleep needs aren't one-size-fits-all.

Take Margaret Thatcher, for example—the former UK Prime Minister reportedly functioned on just four hours of sleep a night. But before you try to copy her schedule, there's a catch: she was known to sneak in a midday nap, sometimes even in her official limousine.[31]

Thatcher was what's known as a "short sleeper"—a rare group of people who can thrive on much less sleep than the rest of us. But let's be honest—this isn't the norm, and forcing yourself to survive on minimal sleep will likely lead to burnout, brain fog, and long-term health issues. Bottom line? Listen to your body—it'll tell you how much rest you actually need.

Sleep Quality: It's Not Just About How Long You Sleep

Getting enough sleep is important, but if you're tossing, turning, and waking up throughout the night, those hours might not be doing enough for you. And deep down, most of us already know this. You can feel the difference between a morning when you wake up clear-headed and ready to go, and a morning where you need two coffees and a couple of hours just to get going.

Truly restorative sleep is deep, uninterrupted, and refreshing—and sleep experts break it down into four key dimensions:[32]

- **Sleep latency.** How long it takes you to actually fall asleep.
- **Awakenings.** How often you wake up during the night.
- **Wake after sleep onset.** The total time you spend awake *after* initially falling asleep.

- **Sleep efficiency.** The ratio of time you spend *actually sleeping* versus just lying in bed.

Take Emily, for example. She spends over an hour trying to fall asleep (poor sleep latency), wakes up multiple times throughout the night (too many awakenings), and once she's up, she can't fall back asleep for hours (high wake after sleep onset). Even though she's in bed for what seems like *plenty* of time, her sleep efficiency is low, and she wakes up exhausted and struggling to function the next day.

If this sounds familiar, it's a sign your sleep quality needs attention—because more hours in bed won't fix poor-quality rest.

Sleep Consistency: The Importance of a Regular Sleep Schedule

It's not just about how much or how well you sleep—*when* you sleep matters too. Sleep experts emphasize that keeping a *consistent sleep-wake schedule*—also called "sleep regularity"—is just as important as getting enough hours of rest. That means going to bed and waking up at the same time every day, including weekends. Sound familiar? You've probably seen this in sleep hygiene advice before—but what makes sleep regularity so essential?

At its core, a consistent sleep schedule keeps your body's internal clock—your circadian rhythm—running smoothly. This rhythm controls everything from hormone levels to metabolism and brain function. When your sleep is all over the place, it can throw off these natural processes, leading to grogginess, mood swings, weight gain, and even long-term health issues.

Why Sleep Regularity Could Be More Important Than Sleep Duration

Surprisingly, research suggests that sticking to a regular sleep schedule may be even more important than total sleep duration for long-term health. A groundbreaking study by Windred et al. found that people with irregular sleep patterns had a significantly higher risk of mortality—even if they were getting enough total sleep. In contrast, those with consistent bedtimes and wake-up times saw a 20% reduction in mortality risk.[33]

This study, based on data from 60,977 participants aged 40–69 in the UK Biobank, showed that erratic sleep patterns don't just make you feel groggy—they have been linked to heart disease, metabolic issues, mood disorders, reduced quality of life, and even faster biological aging. The UK Biobank is a large-scale research project that tracks the health, genetics, and lifestyle of around 500,000 people across the UK. With its rich and detailed data, it's become one of the most valuable resources for uncovering how everyday habits, like sleep, impact long-term health and disease risk.

We'd all love to have a biological age younger than our chronological age—imagine being 50 but having the health and energy of a 30-year-old! But the risks don't stop with aging and chronic illness; it seems that an irregular sleep schedule could actually shorten your lifespan.[34]

These effects stem from a disrupted circadian rhythm, caused by inconsistent exposure to light, irregular mealtimes, and fluctuating activity levels. It just goes to show that when your body's internal clock gets thrown off, it can have serious long-term effects on your health, energy levels, and even lifespan.

The Weekend Sleep Trap: Social Jet Lag

Let's say you usually go to bed at 10 p.m. and wake up at 6 a.m. during the workweek. But on Friday and Saturday, you stay up until 1 a.m., then sleep in until 10 a.m. That's a three-hour shift in your schedule—and when Monday rolls around, your body feels like it's been hit with jet lag, and the "Monday blues" creep in.

This is what sleep scientists call "social jet lag." Just like real jet lag, your body needs time to adjust—roughly a day for every hour of shift. So, by Wednesday, you finally feel normal again . . . just in time for another weekend of late nights.[35] The cycle repeats, throwing off your circadian rhythm and leaving you feeling exhausted all week.

A Simple Habit That Can Improve—and Even Prolong—Your Life
The good news? Simply sticking to consistent sleep and wake times—
even on weekends—can break this cycle. By keeping your body in
sync, you'll fall asleep faster, wake up feeling refreshed, and protect
your long-term health.

It's a simple but powerful strategy: prioritizing sleep regularity
could be one of the easiest ways to boost energy, improve mood, and
even add years to your life.

Is There a "Perfect" Bedtime?

It turns out there may be an ideal window for falling asleep—one
that supports both better sleep and heart health. Interestingly, not
all sleep cycles are the same. Deep sleep occurs primarily in the first
few cycles of sleep (usually in the first half of the night—between
approximately 10 p.m. and 2 a.m.). As the night progresses, the
balance shifts and the later cycles are more focused on REM sleep,
with less deep sleep.

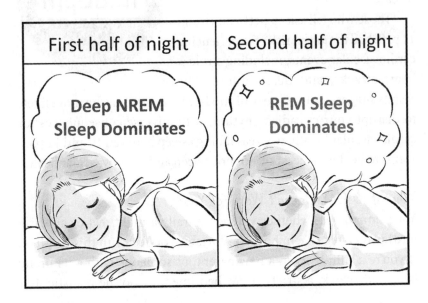

So, if you go to bed late (after 2 a.m.), even if you achieve the same total sleep duration as usual, you may miss out on the early cycles dominated by deep sleep. As a result, you may lose a significant amount of your typical portion of deep, restorative sleep—and will likely waken feeling drained, groggy, and unrefreshed, no matter how many hours you spent in bed.

This cycle happens at roughly the same time every night, no matter what time you go to bed. That means if you push your bedtime too late, you might be missing out on the most restorative deep sleep your body needs to heal, recharge, and function at its best. But going to bed earlier isn't just about sleep quality—it could also protect your heart.[36]

The Science Behind the "Golden Hour" for Sleep

Researchers have found that the best bedtime for heart health and quality sleep falls between *10 and 11 p.m.* This conclusion comes from a six-year study of 88,026 adults conducted through the UK Biobank, which found a clear link between sleep onset timing and risk of cardiovascular disease.[37]

Those who fell asleep between 10 and 11 p.m. had the *lowest* risk of experiencing cardiovascular events, including strokes, heart attacks, and heart failure. The results suggest that too early or too late bedtimes may be more likely to disrupt your circadian rhythm, with adverse consequences for cardiovascular health, whereas falling asleep between 10 and 11 p.m. seems to be the "sweet spot" for both sleep and cardiovascular health.

What if 10 P.M. Doesn't Work for You?

Your *chronotype* (whether you're naturally a night owl or an early bird) plays a big role in how comfortable you feel with this bedtime. If you're a shift worker, a new parent, or someone with a naturally later body clock, a strict 10 PM bedtime may not be realistic. But if you are someone who sometimes chooses to stay up late binge-watching TV or scrolling social media and sacrificing precious deep, restorative sleep in the process, opting for an earlier bedtime could bring many benefits.

Ultimately, it's worth experimenting with different bedtimes until you find what works best for you and leaves you feeling refreshed, energized, and well rested. Once you find your own bedtime sweet spot, it's crucial to make sure you maintain consistency, falling asleep and rising at roughly the same time every day.

Putting It All Together: The Recipe for Your Best Night's Sleep

If you want to wake up feeling truly refreshed, aim for the following:

- **Quantity** → *7–9 hours* of sleep each night.
- **Quality** → Fall asleep quickly, stay asleep with minimal disruptions, and maintain smooth, easy breathing all night.
- **Consistency** → Stick to a regular sleep schedule, going to bed and waking up at the same time every day (yes, even on weekends!).
- **Timing** → The sweet spot for bedtime? Between 10 and 11 p.m. for the best balance of deep sleep and heart health.
- **Nasal breathing** → Your daytime and nighttime breathing can impact everything from how quickly you fall asleep to how deeply you rest, and even how refreshed you feel in the morning.

When you get these elements right, you set yourself up for deeper, more restorative sleep—and better energy, mood, and health overall.

ASSESSING YOUR SLEEP

Now that we've covered what makes for optimal sleep, how can you know if you're actually getting enough high-quality, consistent rest?

Let's be honest—everyone has the occasional restless night. Tossing and turning now and then is completely normal. But there's a big difference between a bad night here and there and an ongoing sleep issue that's impacting your health.

In the next section, I'll outline how to assess your sleep health, plus key signs that might indicate a sleep disorder—and when it might be time to check in with a healthcare professional.

Figuring out whether you're consistently hitting the recommended seven to nine hours of sleep per night is pretty straightforward—but how well you're sleeping is just as important. While some people can tell just by how they feel in the morning, others turn to wearable devices, like sleep trackers, for extra insight into monitoring sleep duration and quality.

Simple Tools to Assess Your Sleep Health

If you're wondering whether your sleep is as good as it should be, there are several sleep assessment tools that can help you evaluate how well you're sleeping and identify areas for improvement. Some of the most widely used include:

- *The Insomnia Severity Index.*[38] Measures the severity of insomnia symptoms.
- *The Pittsburgh Sleep Quality Index.*[39] Assesses overall sleep quality.
- *The Epworth Sleepiness Scale.*[40] Evaluates daytime sleepiness levels.
- *The STOP-Bang Questionnaire.*[41] Screens for obstructive sleep apnea.

Most of these assessments are easily accessible online, so if you're curious about your sleep health, a quick search can help you gain valuable insights into what might be affecting your rest.

The US National Sleep Foundation has also developed a *Sleep Quality Checklist*[42] which is a quick and easy way to assess your sleep quality.

National Sleep Foundation Self-Rated Sleep Quality Checklist
Adults (18–64 years old):
• Did you fall asleep in 30 minutes or less?
• Did you wake up 1 time or less during the night?
• In total, were you awake for 20 minutes or less after falling asleep?
• Were you mostly asleep while in bed (i.e., 7 out of 8 hours)?
Older Adults (65 years old or more):
• Did you fall asleep in 30 minutes or less?
• Did you wake up 2 times or less during the night?
• In total, were you awake 30 minutes or less after falling asleep?
• Were you mostly asleep while in bed (i.e., 7 out of 8 hours)?
If you answer "yes" to most of the questions above, congratulations! You likely have good sleep quality.

If you're still unsure if you're getting the deep, refreshing sleep your body needs, take a moment to reflect on these questions:

- Do you wake up feeling groggy instead of well rested?
- If you didn't set an alarm, would you oversleep?
- Do you often feel like you could take a nap just a few hours after waking up?
- Do you struggle with daytime sleepiness or excessive fatigue?
- Does your focus and concentration fade as the day goes on?

If you answered "yes" to any of these, don't worry—it doesn't necessarily indicate that you have a sleep disorder. But it *does* suggest there's room for improvement in your sleep. The good news? Small changes to your sleep habits can make a big difference. Throughout this book, you'll find simple yet effective strategies to help you sleep better, wake up refreshed, and feel more energized throughout the day.

Sleep Struggles Versus Sleep Disorders: What's the Difference?

So, when does the occasional sleep challenge become a diagnosable sleep disorder? The key lies in how *often* it happens, how *severe* it is, and how *long* it lasts. Plus, sleep disorders don't just interfere with your nights—they spill over into your days, often leading to significant challenges with daytime functioning, particularly in the form of excessive daytime sleepiness.

Occasional Sleep Problems

- Temporary and short-lived
- Often triggered by stress, travel, or illness
- May cause mild or temporary impact on your daily functioning

Sleep Disorders

- Are persistent and long term
- Meet specific clinical criteria for diagnosis
- Can take a serious toll on your health, energy levels, ability to focus, and general daily functioning

If sleep troubles are becoming a regular part of your life and are taking a significant toll, it might be time to consult a healthcare professional.

How Do Doctors Evaluate Sleep Issues?

In an ideal world, every visit to the doctor for insomnia or sleep difficulties would involve a deep dive into the root causes what's really driving the sleeplessness. And while many doctors genuinely want to help, the reality is that most primary care appointments are short and often focused on managing symptoms rather than exploring the full picture. This isn't a reflection of a lack of care; it's often a matter of time, training, or access to sleep-focused resources. That's why understanding the broader picture yourself can be so valuable. When you're informed, you're in a better position to advocate for the kind of support that truly addresses the root of the problem. Here's what you can expect:

- **A prescription for sleep medication.**
- **Sleep assessment tools.** Your doctor may ask you to complete questionnaires, like *The Insomnia Severity Index,*[43] *The Epworth Sleep Scale,*[44] *The Pittsburgh Sleep Quality Index,*[45] or the *STOP-Bang Questionnaire,*[46] to help provide deeper insight into your sleep health.
- **Sleep study (polysomnography).** If needed, you might be referred for a sleep study, where sensors track your brain waves, heart rate, breathing, and more while you sleep. This can help diagnose conditions like sleep apnea.

Curious about what a sleep study entails? More details can be found in the section on obstructive sleep apnea (see Chapter 10D).

A Quick Guide to Common Sleep Disorders

Sleep problems aren't rare—an *estimated 50 to 70 million Americans* struggle with chronic (or long-term) sleep disorders.[47] But not all sleep issues are the same. According to the International Classification of Sleep Disorders (ICSD-3-TR),[48] sleep disorders fall into six main categories and one more category that comprises the rest:

- **Insomnia disorders.** Trouble falling or staying asleep, often leading to fatigue and frustration
- **Sleep-related breathing disorders.** Conditions like sleep apnea, where breathing repeatedly stops and starts during sleep
- **Central disorders of hypersomnolence.** Excessive daytime sleepiness, even after a full night's sleep (e.g., narcolepsy)

- **Circadian rhythm sleep-wake disorders.** When your body's internal clock is out of sync, causing sleep timing issues (e.g., shift work disorder, jet lag)
- **Parasomnias.** Unusual behaviors during sleep, like sleepwalking, having nightmares, or acting out dreams
- **Sleep-related movement disorders.** Conditions that cause unwanted movements during sleep, like restless legs syndrome or periodic limb movement disorder
- **Other sleep disorders.** A catch-all category for less common sleep issues

You'll see these sleep disorders mentioned throughout the book, and you may even recognize some symptoms from your own experience. For a more detailed exploration of sleep disorders, with a particular focus on insomnia disorder and sleep-related breathing disorders, see Chapter 10.

CHAPTER 3

THE EVOLUTION OF SLEEP AND BREATHING

HOW DID OUR ANCESTORS SLEEP?

Modern life has without a doubt distorted our sleep patterns. In most developed nations today, we sleep (or aim to sleep) in a single bout of sleep. Yet historical records, archaeological findings, and studies of traditional societies suggest that our ancestors didn't sleep in one long stretch. Instead, they followed a *biphasic* or even *polyphasic sleep pattern*, breaking their rest into multiple phases over 24 hours. Many cultures had a "first sleep" in the early night, followed by a period of wakefulness, and then a "second sleep" that lasted until dawn.

During this nighttime wakeful period, people might have tended to the fire, checked on livestock, engaged in spiritual practices, or even socialized before returning to sleep. My own ancestors, the Celts, are believed to have embraced this pattern, sleeping in two or more blocks of time rather than one long, uninterrupted period.

Hunter-gatherer societies also followed a biphasic sleep pattern, sleeping in two distinct phases—a longer core sleep at night and a shorter nap during the day. This natural rhythm was common in preindustrial societies, where people typically went to bed shortly after sunset and woke up with the first light of day.

Even today, we see echoes of this ancient sleep pattern in cultures untouched by modern technology, where biphasic sleep remains the norm. The first sleep period resembles the long stretch we aim for at night, but it's complemented by a second, shorter sleep—usually a 30- to 60-minute nap in the afternoon. This tradition is still practiced in some Mediterranean and Latin cultures, where the siesta was once a daily ritual, allowing people to rest and recharge in the afternoon—though this practice is gradually fading with modern work schedules.

Our ancestors' sleep patterns were far more in sync with the sunset and sunrise than ours are today. The advent of electricity and artificial light has extended our waking hours well beyond what nature intended, delaying bedtime but not extending sleep duration to make up for it. Instead of waking naturally, we are usually wakened by our alarm clocks, rousing us from our slumber, often before our bodies are truly ready.

Naps

Do you ever experience a dip in alertness and energy mid-afternoon? That post-lunch dip in energy isn't just a result of a heavy meal—it's actually biologically programmed. Based on how our ancestors slept, it seems our bodies are wired for biphasic sleep, meaning we're naturally inclined to take two bouts of rest: a long sleep at night and a shorter nap during the day. This afternoon lull, known as the "postprandial dip," is a genetic feature of human sleep patterns, not just a sign of needing another coffee.

Naps can be incredibly restorative, providing a much-needed boost in energy, focus, and memory while helping reset the brain for the rest of the day. Research even suggests that regular napping can lower the risk of heart disease[1] (see Chapter 4, under the "Sleep and Heart Health" section).

So, should we all embrace daily naps? It might be a tough sell in a traditional office setting, but if you have the opportunity, a well-timed nap can do wonders. Sleep experts recommend keeping it short—ideally 20 to 40 minutes—to avoid post-nap grogginess, and ensuring it's before 3 p.m. so it doesn't interfere with nighttime sleep.

Personally, I make a point of taking a 20-minute "rest and reset" during the day, typically after lunch. During training sessions, we always include a daily rest and refresh break for everyone attending the instructor certification courses. It makes a lot of sense; participants are absorbing a huge amount of information, and to retain it, focus and mental clarity need to be at their best.

I usually take this time to listen to the *Breathe Light by Relaxation* guided audio, available on the free ButeykoClinic app or by scanning the QR code.

I find it very effective. Just twenty minutes is enough to recharge, leaving me with more energy, sharper concentration, and a calmer mind to carry me through the rest of the day. It's a small habit with a big impact.

Perhaps it's time for workplaces to rethink their approach to productivity. Imagine how much more focused, energized, and less stressed employees would be if they had a dedicated space for a quick recharge. Maybe the secret to a better afternoon isn't another coffee, but a well-timed nap!

EDISON VERSUS EINSTEIN

This natural inclination toward napping and segmented sleep patterns isn't just a relic of our ancestors—it also shaped the sleep habits of some of history's most brilliant minds. Interestingly, two of the most well-known figures in science and innovation, Thomas Edison and Albert Einstein, had dramatically different views on sleep. While Edison saw sleep as a hindrance to productivity, Einstein embraced it as a tool for intellectual and creative breakthroughs. Their contrasting approaches highlight the ongoing debate about sleep's role in performance, efficiency, and innovation—a debate that continues to this day.

Edison

Edison was openly critical of sleep, claiming that it was a waste of time! He reportedly slept only about three to four hours a night and even invented the carbon filament light bulb to extend waking hours. Edison's disdain for sleep shaped public attitudes toward it during the Industrial Revolution, with people being encouraged to "do more" and sleep less.

Edison was famous for practicing *polyphasic sleep*, a method in which he took short naps throughout the day instead of sleeping for a long, uninterrupted period at night. Ironically, many accounts suggest Edison took more naps than he admitted, despite his public comments.

Certainly, his invention of the light bulb did much to divorce us from our innate sleeping patterns and extend our potential hours for work and productivity.

Einstein

Conversely, the influential scientist Albert Einstein had a very different relationship with sleep. Einstein was known to value sleep and believed it played an important role in his cognitive function and creativity. He reportedly slept for about 10 hours a night, which is much more than the average person, and he often supplemented this with daytime naps.

The Hidden Link Between Sleep and Breathing: A Journey Through Time

Edison's and Einstein's contrasting views on sleep highlight how our attitudes toward rest have evolved over time. But beyond the number of hours we sleep or whether we take naps, one fundamental factor has been overlooked for centuries, perhaps even millennia.

Sleep has become a booming billion-dollar industry, packed with gadgets, apps, and supplements all claiming to be the key to better rest. Researchers have also been diving deep into the science of sleep in recent years. But despite all the innovation and attention, one crucial factor has only recently started getting the recognition it truly deserves.

Any guesses?

It is, of course, breathing. Here's the fascinating part—this isn't a new discovery. People have understood the intrinsic link between breathing and sleep for thousands of years.

Let's take a journey through history to see how our understanding has evolved—and why this might just be the missing piece in your sleep struggles.

Ancient Clues: Breathing and Sleep, Long Before Science Knew Best

Surprisingly, some of the earliest observations on the impact of breathing during sleep go all the way back to Ancient Egypt.

- **300 BC–30 BC | Ancient Egypt.** Some Egyptian rulers were described as overweight and heavy snorers—classic signs of obstructive sleep apnea (OSA).
- **Sixteenth century | The mouth-breathing problem.** Dutch physician Levinus Lemnius made a simple but insightful observation: People who breathed through their mouths didn't sleep well.

- **1837 | Sleep apnea in a Dickens novel?** Believe it or not, one of the first descriptions of sleep apnea came from Charles Dickens! In *The Pickwick Papers*, he introduced us to Joe; often referred to as "the fat boy." Joe was overweight, constantly sleepy, and prone to dozing off at the most inappropriate times. In one scene, he nods off while standing and holding a tray of food, only for it to come crashing down. Dickens plays it for laughs, but what he's describing is classic obstructive sleep apnea: loud snoring, excessive daytime sleepiness, and an inability to stay awake even when upright and supposedly alert. Long before sleep studies or CPAP machines, Dickens had already captured the essence of a sleep disorder that wouldn't be medically recognized for more than a century.
- **1869 | What Native Americans knew about sleep and breathing.** American artist and author George Catlin noticed something fascinating while traveling across North America: Native American tribes trained their infants to breathe through their noses, while European settlers tended to mouth breathe. Catlin was so convinced of the benefits of nasal breathing that he wrote a book titled *Shut Your Mouth and Save Your Life*.

The Rise of Sleep Science: What We Got Right— And What We Missed

As technology advanced, so did our ability to study sleep. But while scientists uncovered the mysteries of brain activity during sleep, the role of breathing took longer to be recognized.

- **1879 | Edison's light bulb changes sleep forever.** Before artificial light, people went to bed and woke up with the natural rhythms of the sun. But once Thomas Edison introduced the light bulb, everything changed—people started staying up later, shifting their sleep patterns, and getting less deep rest.
- **1937 | NREM identified.** Loomis in the US first documented the characteristic brain wave patterns of what is now called "NREM sleep."[2]

- **1953 and 1957 | REM sleep and sleep cycles discovered.** Aserinsky, Kleitman, and Dement, pioneers in sleep science, made a major breakthrough with the discovery of REM sleep. They later revealed that sleep isn't just one long, continuous state of rest; rather, we move through cycles that repeat throughout the night.

Breathing Disorders and Sleep: The Missing Puzzle Piece

As the modern world evolved, sleep problems became more common, prompting scientists and doctors to turn their attention to sleep disturbances and disorders.

- **1958 | The first big clue about sleep apnea.** Burwell et al. published a case report linking obesity, extreme daytime sleepiness, and breathing issues, calling it "Pickwickian Syndrome" (a reference to Dickens's novel).[3] This was one of the first scientific connections between breathing and poor sleep.
- **1964 | The first sleep disorders center.** Dr. William Dement, the "Father of Sleep Medicine," opened a narcolepsy clinic at Stanford, which later expanded into a full sleep disorders clinic—marking the beginning of modern sleep medicine.
- **1972 | Breathing finally gets some attention.** Dr. Christian Guilleminault, another key figure in sleep science, joined the Stanford Sleep Disorders Clinic and started emphasizing the need for more focus on breathing-related sleep disorders.
- **1975 | Sleep science gets organized.** The Association of Sleep Disorders Centers, now known as the American Academy of Sleep Medicine, was created by Dr. Dement to maintain professional standards for the evaluation and treatment of sleep disorders.
- **1976 | Sleep apnea publication.** Guilleminault's team published the first major review of sleep apnea syndromes—finally drawing attention to disrupted breathing during sleep.
- **1981 | The CPAP machine is born.** A game-changer in sleep medicine—Dr. Colin Sullivan invented the CPAP (continuous positive airway pressure) machine. This device, which keeps the

airway open by blowing air into it, became the gold standard for sleep apnea treatment.

- **1982 | UARS is identified (but ignored for years).** Guilleminault and colleagues first recognized upper-airway resistance syndrome (UARS) in children,[4] but it wasn't until 1993 that doctors applied the term to adults too.[5] Unlike sleep apnea, UARS causes partial airway closure, fragmented sleep, and exhaustion without such obvious oxygen drops, making it harder to diagnose.
- **1986 and 1990s | Sleep medicine gains more professional recognition**
  - The Association of Professional Sleep Societies was formed.
  - The National Sleep Foundation was launched to educate people about sleep health.
  - The Academy of Dental Sleep Medicine was founded (as the Sleep Disorders Dental Society)—acknowledging that dentists play a key role in treating sleep-related breathing problems. It had only a small number of members to begin with.
  - The American Medical Association finally recognized sleep medicine as a specialty.

Modern Sleep Challenges: Are We Sleeping Worse Than Ever?
- **1997 | The blue light problem begins.** Scientists developed blue LED lights, which are great for saving energy but detrimental to sleep. LED lights suppress melatonin—the hormone that helps us sleep—much more so than old-school incandescent bulbs. Today's light bulbs and screens—phones, tablets, and laptops—expose us to blue light, impacting our sleep.
- **Early 2000s | Sleep clinics boom.** Sleep disorder clinics became more common, making sleep studies easier to access.
- **Today and beyond | Where sleep science is headed**
  - There are now 2,500+ accredited sleep centers in the United States.

- 3,500+ dentists are specialized in treating sleep-disordered breathing.
- The connection between breathing and sleep is finally gaining attention, though there's still a long way to go.

SO, WHAT DOES THIS MEAN FOR YOU?

Despite decades of research and advancements in sleep medicine, the critical role of breathing is often *still* overlooked. Many people struggling with sleep go through medical evaluations, get diagnoses, and try different treatments—yet they still find themselves tossing and turning at night. Why? Because the connection between nasal breathing, airway health, and sleep quality isn't always given the attention it deserves.

A growing body of doctors, dentists, and other professionals are becoming more aware of how breathing impacts sleep, but there's still a gap in the conversation. If you're struggling with sleep, whether or not you have sought professional advice, it might be time to explore how optimizing your breathing can transform your nights—and your days.

CHAPTER 4

SLEEP—THE FOUNDATION OF HEALTH AND WELL-BEING

Healthy sleep is the foundation of our physical, mental, and emotional well-being. While it might seem like a passive state, sleep is actually an active, essential process where the body repairs itself, the mind rejuvenates, and energy is restored. When we get enough high-quality sleep, the benefits are undeniable—we feel sharper, healthier, and more resilient. But when sleep is disrupted or cut short, the effects can be serious, affecting everything from mood and memory to metabolism and heart health.

Despite decades of research, sleep is still undervalued and overlooked, even in parts of the medical and mental health communities. Too often, we treat exhaustion like a badge of honor and ignore the long-term consequences of sleep deprivation. It's time for a cultural shift in how we think about sleep. We need to stop seeing it as optional and start recognizing it as a cornerstone of health—something as important as diet, exercise, and mental well-being. When we prioritize sleep, we don't just feel better—we function at our best.

THE BENEFITS OF SLEEP

Few things are as essential to our health as sleep. Matthew Walker, Professor of Neuroscience and Psychology and author of *Why We Sleep*, captures its importance perfectly:

> "We sleep for a rich litany of reasons, plural—an abundant con-stellation of nighttime benefits that service both our brains and our bodies. There does not seem to be one major organ within the body, or process within the brain, that isn't optimally enhanced by sleep (and detrimentally impaired when we don't get enough)."

Simply put, every part of our body and mind benefits from quality sleep—and suffers when we don't get enough. To give you a clearer picture, I've outlined the key benefits of sleep in Table 4.1.

Table 4.1   *Summary of Benefits of Getting Enough Sleep*[1,2]

Restoration and Recovery Benefits	
	Muscle Repair and Growth: Deep sleep is a key time for physical recovery. The body *repairs tissues, regenerates cells, and strengthens muscles,* making sleep especially important for athletes or individuals engaged in physical activity.
	Improved Athletic Performance: Sleep enhances *motor skills, reaction times,* and overall *physical performance.* Athletes who prioritize sleep tend to perform better and *recover more quickly.*

Table 4.1   *Summary of Benefits of Getting Enough Sleep[1,2] (continued)*

Cognitive Function and Memory Benefits	
	**Memory and Learning:** Sleep is essential for consolidating memories and learning. It promotes our *problem-solving, creativity,* and *decision-making* abilities. **Focus and Concentration:** Healthy sleep improves *attention* and *concentration.* Well-rested individuals perform tasks more efficiently and accurately, making fewer mistakes. These cognitive benefits help us perform better in daily activities, including in the workplace or at school.
	Protection Against Cognitive Decline: During deep sleep, the brain's glymphatic system becomes more active, *flushing out toxins,* including beta-amyloid, which is associated with *Alzheimer's disease.* Sleep is vital in maintaining brain health and helping prevent neurodegenerative diseases (more on that in Chapter 4 under the "Brain Health" section).
	Prevention of Accidents: Sleep helps maintain *attention, alertness,* and *coordination.* Getting enough quality sleep lessens the likelihood of *accidents,* both at work and on the road, and related injury or death.
Physical Health Benefits	
	Cardiovascular Health: Sleep helps regulate *blood pressure* and reduces the risk of *heart disease, stroke,* and *hypertension.* **Lower Risk of Chronic Diseases:** Sleep deprivation has been linked to a higher risk of developing chronic conditions, such as *diabetes, Alzheimer's disease,* and *cancer,* due to impaired metabolic and cellular repair processes.
	Immune System Boost: During sleep, the immune system strengthens and produces essential proteins, like cytokines, which help *fight infections* and *inflammation.* Lack of sleep weakens immune defenses, increasing susceptibility to illness.

(continued on next page)

Table 4.1   *Summary of Benefits of Getting Enough Sleep*[1,2] *(continued)*

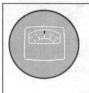	**Helps Prevent Weight Gain and Regulates Metabolic Health:** Sufficient sleep is key to maintaining a healthy metabolism, *regulating hormones* like ghrelin and leptin that *control your appetite*. This helps prevent weight gain and lowers your risk of developing type 2 diabetes. *Sleep deprivation*, by contrast, leads to an imbalance in hunger regulation, contributing to **overeating** and **obesity**.
Mental Health and Emotional Regulation Benefits	
	Sleep Helps Lower Stress Hormone Levels and Regulates Mood and Emotional Resilience: Lack of sleep can lead to irritability, mood swings, and, longer term, *anxiety* and mood disorders like *depression*. Sleep problems are more common in individuals with mental health conditions, and many of these conditions are exacerbated by poor sleep, creating a cyclical pattern that can be difficult to break.
Longevity and Mortality Risk Benefits	
	Increased Lifespan: Research shows that people who consistently get sufficient sleep live longer and have *lower mortality risks* compared with those who experience chronic sleep deprivation.

It's clear our brains and bodies have much to gain from getting sufficient sleep. Getting good sleep should be our biological imperative as humans; yet sleep problems are rife and bring many unwelcome consequences.

If you struggle with sleep, I completely understand if you'd rather skip ahead than dwell on the effects of sleep deprivation. But if you're curious about how sleep disruptions impact your body and mind, let's take a closer look at why sleep is so essential—and how missing out on it can have far-reaching effects.

CONSEQUENCES OF SLEEP DISRUPTION AND SLEEP DISORDERS

Sleep is often regarded as the body's most natural healer, a time when everything from cell repair to hormone balance happens behind the scenes. But in today's fast-paced world, quality sleep is slipping away for many of us, often without us even realizing it. Late-night screen time, stress, and packed schedules have made good sleep harder to come by, and the effects go far beyond just feeling tired the next day.

Sleep research has revealed a disconcerting truth: poor sleep isn't just an inconvenience—it's a serious health risk. It can set the stage for chronic illnesses, weaken the immune system, and even shorten lifespan. The burden of sleep disorders is significant, both for the individual and for society at large, in terms of work absenteeism, accidents, disability, and healthcare costs.

The good news? Understanding the problem is the first step to fixing it.

Short-Term Sleep Disruption

To illustrate the impact of even a small loss of sleep, consider the effects of Daylight Saving Time (DST), which occurs in the Northern Hemisphere. Each March, clocks are turned forward by an hour, potentially resulting in an hour of lost sleep for more than 1.5 billion people worldwide.[3] The transition back to Standard Time in autumn reverses this, adding an hour of sleep.

The spring DST transition has been linked to a significant increase in motor vehicle accidents, primarily due to sleep deprivation and disruptions to the body's internal clock, also known as "circadian misalignment."

By shifting clocks forward, mornings become darker, and evenings brighter, altering lighting conditions during peak traffic times. A large study analyzing 732,835 fatal motor vehicle accidents in the United States from 1996 to 2017 found that the risk of fatal accidents increased by 6% in the week following the spring DST transition.[4] This risk was most pronounced in the mornings and gradually decreased over the following week.

Researchers have also observed a spike in heart attacks the day after the spring DST transition.[5] The most likely explanation is the adverse effect of sleep deprivation on cardiovascular health, including increased sympathetic nervous system activity and higher levels of proinflammatory cytokines. These findings suggest that individuals who are vulnerable to such disruptions might benefit from avoiding sudden changes to their biological rhythms. Conversely, in the autumn, when people potentially gain an hour of sleep, rates of heart attacks and traffic accidents drop significantly.

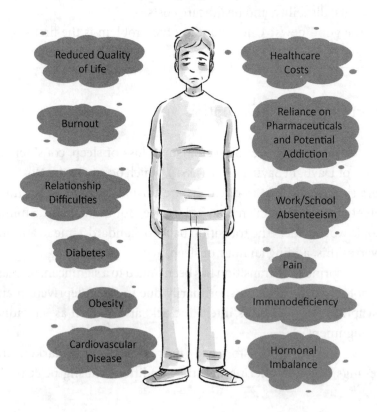

These findings underscore the importance of sleep consistency. Maintaining a stable schedule of waking up and going to bed—even on weekends—might prevent some of the negative effects associated with sleep disruptions, including heart attacks. Future studies could explore whether slightly later wake-up times on Mondays or a more consistent weekly sleep pattern might help mitigate these risks.

Even short-term sleep disruption has been linked to a wide range of negative effects in otherwise healthy adults. These include increased stress responses, somatic pain (such as muscle aches or headaches), emotional distress, anxiety, mood disorders, cognitive impairments, memory issues, performance deficits, and a noticeable decline in overall quality of life.[6–10] Please see Table 4.2 for an overview.

Table 4.2 *Potential Consequences of Disrupted Sleep and Sleep Disorders*[11–19]

Short Term	Long Term	General
• Increased stress response • Increased appetite • Pain • Headache and migraine • Psychological distress • Impaired cognitive processes such as planning, coping, problem-solving, concentration, and memory • Poor work/school concentration and performance deficits, e.g., exam performance • Changes to physical appearance, e.g., eye bags.	• High blood pressure • High cholesterol • Cardiovascular disease • Weight gain • Metabolic syndrome • Diabetes • Kidney disease • Gastrointestinal disorders • Reduced immunity • Anxiety and mood disorders • Depression • Cancer • Mortality	• Reduced quality of life • Burnout • Relationship difficulties • Healthcare costs • Reliance on pharmaceuticals and potential addiction • Work/school absenteeism • Accidents • Increased risk of injury, e.g., falls in the elderly and industrial accidents • Fatigue-related accidents, including car, train, and plane crashes • Medical errors

Long-Term Sleep Disruption

In the long term, sleep disruption is associated with a range of serious health issues, including high blood pressure, elevated cholesterol, cardiovascular disease, weight-related problems, metabolic syndrome, diabetes, gastrointestinal disorders, cancer, and an increased risk of mortality in otherwise healthy people.[20-26]

Focusing on the topic of high cholesterol—a condition affecting millions of people—I was curious to see what the health service in Ireland advises. Unsurprisingly, it lists the usual suspects:

- Eating a healthy, balanced diet low in saturated fat
- Exercising regularly
- Not smoking
- Cutting down on alcohol

In case you're wondering if this is just an Irish approach, the Mayo Clinic offers similar advice, with the notable addition of recommending statins and other medications to help manage high cholesterol.[27]

Many readers with high cholesterol may not have been advised about the link between poor sleep and elevated cholesterol levels. Yet we know that disrupted sleep affects the body's internal chemistry, particularly hormone regulation. When you do not sleep well, your stress hormone cortisol rises, and this signals the liver to produce more cholesterol and triglycerides. It is the kind of shift that can quietly drive up LDL (the "bad" cholesterol) while lowering HDL (the "good" kind), all without changing your diet or lifestyle. In other words, you could be eating well and exercising, but if your sleep quality is poor, your cholesterol numbers may still be heading in the wrong direction.

Let's take a closer look at some of the most surprising ways poor sleep can affect us, so we can better understand why prioritizing good sleep is one of the best things we can do for our overall well-being.

Brain Health

Imagine your brain as a busy city—during the day, it's full of activity, processing information, making decisions, and keeping everything running. But at night, when you sleep, something remarkable happens: the city's "clean-up crew" comes out to clear away the waste left behind. In 2013, researchers at the University of Rochester made a groundbreaking discovery about this process, revealing the brain's built-in waste removal system, known as the "glymphatic system."[28]

This system becomes highly active during deep sleep (NREM 3), when brain cells shrink to create space between neurons, allowing cerebrospinal fluid to flow through and wash away waste—including toxic proteins that could be harmful if they build up.[29] Dr. Maiken Nedergaard, one of the lead researchers, put it simply: "Think of it like a house party. You can either entertain guests or clean up, but you can't do 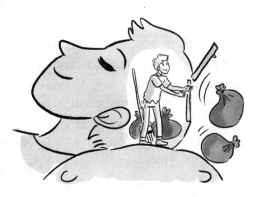 both at the same time."[30] In other words, your brain can either stay awake and alert or focus on cleaning up—it can't do both efficiently.

So, what happens if you don't get enough deep sleep? Well, ever struggled with brain fog, forgetfulness, or difficulty focusing? That could be because your brain didn't get the chance to clear out its "mental clutter" the night before. Over time, this can have serious consequences. When the glymphatic system isn't able to do its job properly, waste products like amyloid-beta and tau proteins start to build up. These toxic proteins are linked to Alzheimer's disease and other neurodegenerative conditions, making sleep an essential part of long-term brain health.[31,32]

Even more concerning, studies have found that poor sleep can create a vicious cycle: when amyloid plaques accumulate, they can actually degrade the areas of the brain responsible for deep sleep.[33] This makes it harder to get the restorative sleep your brain needs, further reducing its ability to clear out toxins.

In short, sleep isn't just about feeling rested—it's about giving your brain the time it needs to clean up and reset for the next day. By prioritizing good sleep, you're not just improving your focus and mental clarity; you're also helping to protect your brain for years to come.

The Hidden Connection Between Sleep and Weight Loss

It may surprise you to learn that not getting enough sleep can actually contribute to weight gain. Research has shown a strong link between sleep deprivation and obesity, and it all comes down to how sleep (or lack of it) affects our metabolism and appetite.[34,35] When we don't get enough rest, our hunger hormones react—our bodies produce more ghrelin (which makes us feel hungry) and less leptin (which tells us we're full). The result? More cravings, especially for high-calorie foods, and a higher chance of overeating.

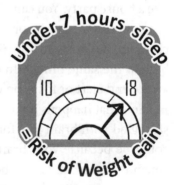

This is especially concerning given the global obesity crisis, which now affects about a billion people worldwide. What's even more alarming is that people who regularly sleep less than the recommended seven to eight hours a night are at a much higher risk of becoming overweight or obese.[36-39] And once the cycle of poor sleep and weight gain begins, it can be tough to break.

The connection between sleep and weight is even more concerning when you consider that obesity raises the risk of serious health issues like heart disease, type 2 diabetes, and even certain cancers. Not getting enough quality sleep doesn't just leave you feeling tired—it can also set the stage for these life-threatening conditions. This is why sleep needs to be a key part of any plan for better health and weight management. It's not just about what you eat or how much you exercise—your sleep habits matter too. Prioritizing good sleep could be a game-changer when it comes to maintaining a healthy weight and lowering the risk of chronic disease.

Now, imagine someone trying to lose weight by waking up at 5 a.m., completely exhausted, to fit in a workout. They're determined to hit the gym, believing that early-morning exercise will help them shed a few pounds and reach their goals. While their dedication is admirable, this approach often backfires. Sacrificing sleep to squeeze in exercise undermines weight-loss efforts and harms overall health. For this person, staying in bed and getting sufficient sleep could be far more effective for their weight-loss journey.

When you sacrifice sleep, your body struggles to regulate energy levels, recover properly, and maintain a balanced metabolism. Inadequate sleep impairs decision-making, making it harder to resist unhealthy food choices and maintain consistency with healthy routines. If you're waking up early to exercise but find it difficult to lose weight despite being disciplined with food and workouts, poor sleep—whether in quantity or quality—may be the root cause.

While morning workouts can be a fantastic way to start the day and build healthy habits, they should never come at the expense of sufficient sleep. Without adequate rest, the body cannot regulate hunger hormones effectively, recover from exercise, or sustain energy throughout the day. This can derail long-term progress and even exacerbate health risks.

Sleep isn't just a complement to a healthy lifestyle—it's the foundation. Prioritizing sleep first can enhance energy, improve hormonal balance, and set the stage for long-term success in weight loss and overall well-being. Sleep is as critical as diet and exercise for managing weight and reducing health risks, and it's an essential part of living a healthier, more balanced life.

So, how exactly can sleep affect weight gain? It's down to an interplay of several biological and behavioral mechanisms that increase appetite, reduce energy expenditure, and make it harder to resist unhealthy foods.[40] Here are some key ways poor sleep contributes to weight gain:

1. **Hormonal imbalance.** Poor sleep disrupts the levels of two key hunger-regulating hormones, *ghrelin* and *leptin*. Ghrelin, the hormone that signals hunger, increases with sleep deprivation, while leptin, which signals fullness, decreases. This imbalance leads to an increased appetite, and an increased calorie intake, particularly via high-carbohydrate or high-fat foods.[41,42] Sleep deprivation makes these foods not just more appealing but also harder to resist. It's as if your brain and body are in survival mode, tricked into craving extra energy to make up for lost rest. High-sugar, high-fat foods become especially tempting—likely because, when fatigued, your body seeks quick fuel to keep going.

2. **Reduced impulse control and increased cravings.** Sleep deprivation alters brain activity in regions responsible for judgment and impulse control, such as the prefrontal cortex. Studies reveal that with poor sleep, activity in the brain's reward center is heightened, making people more drawn to unhealthy food options.[43]

3. **Lower metabolic rate.** A large body of research evidence has linked insufficient sleep duration and quality to the risk of obesity, insulin resistance, and type 2 diabetes.[44] Poor sleep can lead to metabolic dysregulation, meaning the body is less efficient at processing glucose, which is linked to weight gain and increased diabetes risk.

4. **Reduced physical activity.** Lack of sleep generally leads to lower energy levels, resulting in decreased motivation for physical activity.[45] It's completely normal to feel unmotivated to exercise when you're tired—your body is signaling the need for rest and recovery. You've probably been there: skipping a workout because you just didn't have the energy, only to feel guilty about it later.

Poor sleep doesn't just encourage eating more; it also discourages moving, compounding the problem. Conversely, being physically active and exercising is associated with better sleep.[46]

LIAM'S STORY: FROM SNORING AND FATIGUE TO DEEP SLEEP, ENERGY, AND WEIGHT LOSS

Liam, a 41-year-old data analyst from Mullingar, Ireland, struggled with chronic snoring that not only kept him tired but also forced him and his wife to sleep in separate rooms. No matter what he tried—changing sleep positions, using special pillows—nothing worked. Then, he discovered a simple but powerful solution: mandibular advancement device (MAD), nasal breathing, mouth taping, and breathing exercises. The results? Restful sleep, more energy, and even weight loss!

"Apparently, I snore like a hog."

Liam's snoring was so loud that he and his wife had to sleep in different rooms at times. He tried various tricks, but nothing truly worked—until he started mouth taping at night.

"Mouth taping makes everything quieter."

"Nasal breathing makes my sleep more settled."

"I genuinely find sleep more restful."

While snoring still showed up occasionally—especially if he was overtired or had a drink—he discovered the game-changing fix: a custom mouthpiece to position his jaw correctly and mouth taping. Together, they eliminated his snoring, and he and his wife could finally enjoy peaceful sleep again.

More Energy, Less Coffee, and Stronger Workouts

Better sleep didn't just stop at quieter nights—Liam woke up refreshed, had more energy during the day, and even found he no longer needed as much coffee to stay alert.

Even more surprisingly, when he started using nasal breathing during workouts, he noticed his endurance improved. With deeper sleep and better recovery, he had more motivation and energy to stay active.

Unexpected Bonus: Weight Loss!

Liam had been trying intermittent fasting for a while, but it wasn't working. However, once he combined nasal breathing and slower-paced exercise, and his sleep improved, the weight finally started to come off.

"The weight loss happened with nose breathing, along with intermittent fasting, and slower exercise. It's built a really strong foundation for just overall health. My sleep has never been better; my fitness has never been better. I'm actually in the best shape of my life at 41!"

Sleep and Heart Health

Healthy sleep is key for heart health, and research continues to reveal just how deeply our sleep habits affect cardiovascular well-being. In fact, studies have shown a strong link between sleep disorders and a heightened risk of heart disease.

Between 1994 and 1998, the Sleep Heart Health Study became one of the most comprehensive investigations into sleep and health. Researchers used both questionnaires and at home polysomnography; a portable sleep study that tracks brain waves, breathing, and other vital signs during sleep to assess participants' sleep patterns.[47] The study included 4,994 participants with an average age of 64 years, making it one of the largest and most detailed sleep studies of its time.

Among the participants, 14% reported symptoms of insomnia or poor sleep. Interestingly, half of that group slept less than six hours per night, placing them in the "short sleep duration" category. Poor sleep in this study was defined as having difficulty falling asleep, waking up during the night, rising too early, or depending on sleeping pills for at least 16 to 30 nights each month along with sleeping fewer than six hours a night in total.

These participants were followed for a median of 11.4 years to assess health outcomes, including cardiovascular disease and all-cause mortality. Alarmingly, the study found that people with insomnia or poor sleep, along with short sleep, had a *29% higher risk of developing cardiovascular disease* compared with a reference (control) group.[48] How could this be the case?

Sleep can contribute to cardiovascular disease in a number of ways:

- **Increases cardiovascular risk factors.** Poor sleep is linked to an increased risk of obesity, hypertension, and diabetes, all of which are major contributors to cardiovascular disease.
- **Leads to persistently high blood pressure.** During healthy sleep, blood pressure typically decreases, but inadequate or disrupted sleep can prevent this natural dip, leading to persistently elevated blood pressure, a major cardiovascular risk factor.[49]
- **Raises heart rate.** Chronic sleep deprivation also raises heart rate, further straining the cardiovascular system.
- **Triggers the body's stress response.** Chronic sleep loss and sleep disorders, such as insomnia or obstructive sleep apnea, also activate the sympathetic nervous system, leading to increased stress hormones (such as cortisol) and inflammation, both of which are harmful to cardiovascular health.[50]

Midday napping, or siestas, is a common practice in regions with low rates of heart disease, and it may not just be the Mediterranean diet contributing to their long-term cardiovascular health. A Harvard School of Public Health study followed 23,000 Greek adults for an average of six years and found that regular napping significantly reduces the risk of death from heart disease.[51] Specifically, occasional nappers had a 12% lower risk of coronary mortality, while those who napped regularly saw a 37% reduction. The researchers suggested that the stress-reducing effects of naps might explain this protective benefit, as stress is a well-known contributor to heart disease. Please see Chapter 3 for more on naps.

Mental Health

Poor sleep doesn't just take a toll on your physical health—it can have a huge impact on your mental well-being too. Yet, surprisingly, the connection between sleep and mental health is often overlooked, even by professionals in the field. This is concerning when you consider that sleep problems are linked to a wide range of mental health issues, including depression, anxiety, psychiatric disorders, and even an increased risk of suicide.[52-56]

The overlap between sleep disorders and mental health conditions is well documented, with studies showing that 40 to 80% of people with mental health challenges also experience significant sleep disturbances. When someone seeks treatment for a mental health issue, whether from a doctor or therapist, poor sleep is often overlooked. Overlooking sleep can make treatment less effective and slow progress, adding complexity to both diagnosis and recovery.[57,58]

> "I suffered from snoring since I was a little kid. In adulthood I was always tired, had bouts of depression (I'm sure related to non-restful sleep). All aspects of my life were negatively affected by it.
>
> I heard Patrick talking about mouth taping, so I tried doing it. Immediately I noticed a difference. I felt more rested, had more energy during the day! I've been taping my mouth at night for a couple of years now. I can't go without it. If for some reason I fall asleep without taping my mouth at night, I feel very crappy the next day."

Sleep loss contributes to emotional dysregulation, making it harder for individuals to process and manage their emotions effectively. Research indicates that insufficient sleep increases negative mood states like anxiety and depression, intensifies emotional reactivity, leads to social withdrawal and conflicts in personal and professional relationships, and lowers resilience to stress.[59]

What makes this even more challenging is that the relationship between sleep and mental health is a two-way street. Poor sleep worsens stress, anxiety, and depression, which in turn makes sleep even harder to come by, creating a vicious cycle that can feel impossible to break. In a way, it's surprising that the connection between sleep and mental health is still so often overlooked. Perhaps part of the reason is that there's an overlap of symptoms. People living with depression may feel tired, flat, irritable, or have trouble concentrating, and those same symptoms are also common in sleep disorders like insomnia and sleep apnea. It becomes tricky to untangle which came first, or which is driving which.

But most of us don't need a research paper to know the basics. We feel better when we sleep well. And when we don't, our mood, focus, and tolerance take a hit. The science is catching up to what we've known all along: a good night's sleep is not just a luxury; it's essential for mental and emotional balance.

Fortunately, simple breathing techniques can help regulate the nervous system and switch the body from a stress state to a calm state. For example, there is a wealth of research showing that slow breathing can result in increased comfort, relaxation, heart rate variability, pleasantness, and reduced symptoms of arousal, anxiety, panic, depression, and anger.[60-64] (See Chapter 7 for more on how breathing influences the autonomic nervous system.)

Improving sleep doesn't always require drastic changes. Learning to regulate breathing and the nervous system, incorporating sleep hygiene practices, and maintaining a consistent sleep schedule can be a game-changer for mental well-being. With better sleep, you'll feel not only more rested but also more emotionally balanced, resilient, and ready to take on life's challenges.

Please check out Alina's story in Chapter 10A for a real-world example of how these practices can regulate the nervous system and promote sleep, even in the most stressful and traumatic circumstances.

Accidents

When it comes to transportation and operating heavy machinery, a lack of sleep or an undiagnosed sleep disorder can cross the line between safety and disaster. Take the tragic case of the Metro-North commuter train derailment in New York on December 1, 2013. The train was approaching a sharp curve in the Bronx, where the speed limit was 30 miles per hour. At the time of the derailment, it was traveling at 82. Moments later, it left the tracks, resulting in the deaths of four people and injuries to more than 70 others.

Investigators later confirmed the cause: the train engineer had fallen asleep at the controls. He wasn't drunk or distracted. He was exhausted. He suffered from undiagnosed sleep apnea and had recently undergone a drastic change in his shift schedule. His body, unadjusted and poorly rested, simply shut down.

The derailment shook the country and drew national attention to sleep health in safety-critical jobs. In the wake of the accident, the railroad introduced mandatory sleep apnea screening for engineers. But the truth is, this wasn't an isolated case. Sleep-related accidents have occurred across industries, from trucking and aviation to healthcare and construction and they're often brushed off as "human error" when the real issue is sleep-related impairment.

What makes this even more sobering is that it was preventable. A simple diagnosis, a treatment plan, and even awareness of his own condition might have saved lives that day.

Medical Errors

Sleep deprivation among medical professionals continues to be a significant concern, leading to impaired cognitive function and increased risk of medical errors. Recent studies have highlighted the impact of extended work hours and insufficient sleep on healthcare providers and their patients.

A 2023 study published in *BMC Public Health* analyzed the relationship between working conditions, sleep, and medical errors among 661 medical residents. They reported sleeping 6.1 ± 1.6 hours per day, with a sleep debt of 94 ± 129 minutes on workdays. The findings indicated that longer work hours and reduced sleep were significantly associated with a higher incidence of self-reported medical errors. The high workload and longer working hours placed on many healthcare professionals affect their sleep opportunities, and circadian rhythms, which in turn impact their and their patients' well-being and safety.

While it's valuable to understand the numerous benefits of quality sleep and the potential downsides of not getting enough, let me emphasize something important: *time and again, I've witnessed people transform their sleep simply by improving how they breathe.* In this book, you'll find practical, straightforward exercises and recommendations designed to help you address any sleep challenges you, your partner, or your child may be facing.

Here are some quotes from our community who have successfully implemented these techniques:

"I . . . started to practice the Buteyko method as well as taping my mouth overnight.

The magic started to happen quite quickly—I was 61 at the time and had suffered asthma since I was around 30 years old . . . but as I learned and trusted my body to respond to the Buteyko method of breathing . . . my confidence grew and also **my sleep improved and my levels of energy during the day** . . .

"I felt amazing—I never think about any inhalers and I never have daytime fatigue and **I sleep wonderfully** . . .

"I am so grateful to this method as it has **transformed my health and life, thank you so much.**"

"[My] problems included waking up with a dry mouth, mild snoring, feeling tired during the day, and then most alarming, receiving a diagnosis of pre-hypertension.

Once I began a daily breathwork practice and started *religiously* taping my mouth, I began to sleep very soundly for at least 6 hours and then I can easily fall back to sleep, I wake rested with a moist mouth, and I find I never need a 'catnap' during the day and my blood pressure is well within a normal range.

I feel worlds better."

Julia, 51, USA

"I used to have terrible daytime fatigue. **I would wake up and feel like I didn't sleep at all.**

After starting breathing exercises and using mouth tape at night (and sometimes during the day), my fatigue completely went away.

I noticed the difference immediately after my first night of sleeping with mouth tape. As a physical therapist, I discuss breathing issues with many of my patients, and it has made a **huge impact on many of their lives."**

Karl, 34, USA

"For years, **poor sleep quality and frequent snoring left me feeling drained and unable to focus. . . .** That's when I began exploring specific breathing exercises, like reduced breathing techniques, and switched to MyoTape for mouth taping.

MyoTape provided a safer, more comfortable fit. . . . This switch, combined with breathing exercises, reduced my snoring even further and brought me back to a consistent, deep sleep.

Now, I wake up feeling genuinely refreshed, and I have a more balanced energy throughout the day. **Mouth taping with MyoTape and incorporating breathing practices have been transformative for my sleep health and daily well-being."**

Stephan, 31, Germany

CHAPTER 5

BREATHING FOR BETTER SLEEP

BREATHING AND SLEEP: AN INTRICATE CONNECTION

Now that we've covered the benefits of healthy sleep, and the consequences of poor sleep, let's talk in more detail about something hugely important—but often neglected: *how you breathe.* Your breathing patterns—both day and night—play a powerful role in how well you sleep. In fact, the way you breathe can determine whether you glide into deep, restorative sleep or spend the night tossing, turning, and waking up exhausted.

When you sleep, your breathing should naturally slow and deepen, helping your body relax and move through the different sleep stages. This effortless breathing rhythm delivers oxygen efficiently, supports deep rest, and allows your body to repair itself overnight.

But when your breathing is disrupted—whether through shallow, irregular patterns or pauses in breathing that occur in conditions like sleep apnea—it can trigger repeated awakenings. These interruptions keep your body in a state of survival mode, preventing it from entering the restorative deep stage of sleep essential for recovery and repair. Over time, the consequences of these disruptions can extend far beyond fatigue, significantly increasing the risks associated with cardiovascular issues, mood disorders, and even mortality.

Breathing patterns also play a significant role in insomnia. When your breathing is irregular or shallow, it can fuel your body's stress response, increasing your heart rate and causing micro-arousals that keep your brain active and alert—making it very difficult to fall asleep or stay asleep. By improving how you breathe, you can calm your nervous system, reduce nighttime wake-ups, and create the perfect conditions for deep, uninterrupted sleep.

In this chapter, we'll explore the differences between dysfunctional and functional breathing, uncover how poor breathing habits can disrupt your sleep, and introduce practical exercises that you can start using right away to transform your breathing, improve your sleep, and wake up feeling truly refreshed.

WHAT IS DYSFUNCTIONAL BREATHING?

Most babies enter the world breathing perfectly—effortlessly and through the nose. But as we go through life, many of us unknowingly develop less-than-optimal breathing patterns. This shift can happen gradually over time or as a response to stress, illness, anxiety, or even digestive issues. While the term "dysfunctional breathing" may sound concerning, don't worry—this book is filled with practical exercises to help restore healthier breathing habits.

The modern world is vastly different from the environment our bodies evolved to thrive in, and one consequence is that breathing disorders have become surprisingly common. Chronic stress, for example, is at an all-time high, and it directly affects the way we breathe. Other factors—like poor posture, anxiety, illness, trauma, and digestive issues—can also subtly alter breathing patterns without us even realizing it.

You're not alone if you struggle with inefficient breathing. Studies suggest that 9.5% of adults in primary care in the UK experience dysfunctional breathing,[1] while other research estimates that between 50 and 80% of adults have some form of dysfunctional breathing pattern.[2]

Fortunately, with awareness and practice, you can retrain your body to breathe more efficiently and restore optimal, healthy breathing patterns—both during the day and while you sleep.

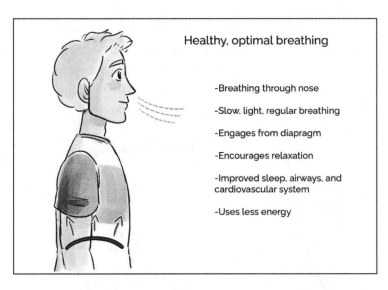

Healthy, optimal breathing

-Breathing through nose

-Slow, light, regular breathing

-Engages from diapragm

-Encourages relaxation

-Improved sleep, airways, and cardiovascular system

-Uses less energy

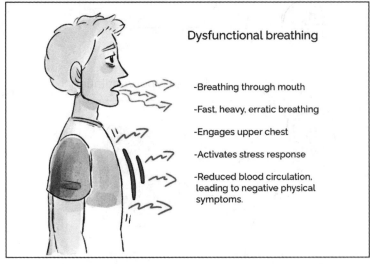

Dysfunctional breathing

-Breathing through mouth

-Fast, heavy, erratic breathing

-Engages upper chest

-Activates stress response

-Reduced blood circulation, leading to negative physical symptoms.

How Much Air Should You Breathe?

So many of us are taught to believe that more is better when it comes to breathing; yet there is simply *no* evidence to support this belief. On the contrary, there is an *optimal* breathing volume, and anything that deviates from it is considered pathological—the cause or effect of illness. The volume of air we breathe is so crucial that it is detailed in every book about the physical processes and disease states of breathing.

The volume of air you need is determined primarily by your metabolic state. When your body needs more energy, for instance during exercise (or more long term, when you're pregnant), your demand for O_2 increases. When you sit still, you need less O_2.

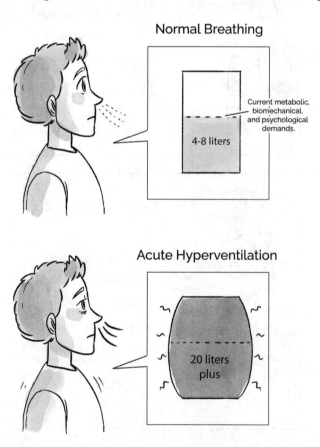

Normal Breathing

Current metabolic, biomechanical, and psychological demands.

4-8 liters

Acute Hyperventilation

20 liters plus

During normal breathing, you take in just enough air to meet your body's needs. But if you're regularly breathing more air than necessary, especially when you're at rest, it can lower the levels of carbon dioxide in your lungs and blood. This is called hyperventilation.

A lot of people think hyperventilating means fast, panicked breathing into a paper bag. But it's not always that obvious. It can happen quietly, as a habit, and most people don't realize they're doing it. When this becomes your normal way of breathing, it may be a sign of chronic hyperventilation. We'll go into more detail on that in the next section.

Minute Volume

Medical textbooks describe normal ventilation for a resting adult as between 4 and 8 liters per minute. Tidal volumes can vary from 500 ml to 600 ml, with respiratory rates of 12 to 14 breaths per minute. As a reminder, minute volume is the volume of air that is inhaled and exhaled from the lungs during the span of 1 minute. This is calculated by multiplying the respiratory rate (RR: the number of breaths per minute) by the tidal volume (TV: the volume of air drawn into the lungs during one breath).

For example:

RR * TV = MV
12 * 500 = 6 liters
14 * 600 = 8.4 liters

The human lungs are remarkably adaptable. At rest, your breathing is quiet and efficient, just enough to meet your body's basic needs. But once you begin to move, especially during physical activity, the demand for oxygen rises quickly and the lungs respond without you even having to think about it.

During light physical exercise, your minute ventilation, the total volume of air you breathe in and out each minute can double. During intense physical effort, it can rise sharply. In well-conditioned athletes, it can exceed 150 liters per minute, and in some cases even reach 200 liters or more.

What is striking is how smoothly the body shifts from the calm rhythm of rest to the powerful drive of movement. The lungs, diaphragm, and breathing muscles all work together to deliver oxygen and remove carbon dioxide at the rate your body needs. This increase in breathing during exercise is appropriate because your muscles are producing large amounts of carbon dioxide as a byproduct of movement. Your breathing matches your metabolic needs.

This is very different from what happens during a panic attack, where breathing also becomes fast and deep but without the same physical demand. In that case, you are breathing more than your body requires, which lowers carbon dioxide levels and can trigger symptoms like dizziness, tingling, or chest tightness. The body reacts as if something is wrong, even though there is no real physical reason for that level of breathing.

So while fast breathing during exercise serves a clear purpose, the same breathing pattern during rest, especially in the absence of actual need, can end up making you feel worse.

Chronic Hyperventilation

Over-breathing, or chronic hyperventilation, is one of the most common forms of dysfunctional breathing, yet many people don't even realize they're doing it. It often goes unnoticed because it can be quiet, habitual, and easily mistaken for normal breathing.

Research suggests that around 10% of the general population experience chronic hyperventilation. That number jumps to about 30% in people with asthma and as high as 75% in those with anxiety. In other words, it is not rare. It is a pattern that shows up across many health conditions, quietly contributing to symptoms like fatigue, breathlessness, brain fog, poor sleep, and emotional instability.[3]

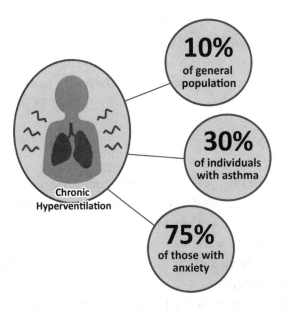

When you breathe more than your body actually needs, you exhale too much carbon dioxide (CO_2) and your levels drop too low, throwing off your body's delicate biochemical balance. Many people assume that CO_2 is a waste gas, but it plays a crucial role in oxygen delivery. When CO_2 levels fall, oxygen remains bound to hemoglobin in the blood instead of being efficiently released to the body's tissues. This means that even though oxygen is present, it's not reaching the cells and organs that need it most—leaving you feeling fatigued and stressed.

People who over-breathe often experience symptoms such as shortness of breath, cold hands and feet, feelings of panic or anxiety, and disrupted sleep. Over time, chronic hyperventilation can be made worse by factors like stress, hormonal changes, overeating, and alcohol consumption. Left unchecked, it can contribute to high blood pressure, heart disease, and sleep-disordered breathing.[4]

Fortunately, you can train yourself to breathe more efficiently using the *Breathe Light Exercise* (see Chapter 1). This technique involves reducing the volume of each breath by breathing lightly, slowly, and through the nose, creating a gentle air hunger. With regular practice, this helps restore the correct balance of oxygen and CO_2, improving circulation, oxygen delivery, and overall health. By retraining yourself to breathe properly, you can enhance sleep quality, energy levels, and resilience to stress, setting the stage for a healthier, more balanced life.

Mouth Breathing

Another common yet overlooked breathing issue is mouth breathing. Many people develop the habit—both during the day and while sleeping—without even realizing it. While occasional mouth breathing, like when you have a cold, is harmless, habitual mouth breathing can have serious consequences for sleep, health, and overall well-being.

Research suggests that between 7 and 60% of children regularly breathe through their mouths.[5-8] Although fewer studies focus on adults, estimates indicate that around 17% of adults are habitual mouth breathers.[9] Mouth breathing during sleep becomes more common with age, and although it remains under-studied, the available research suggests an increased risk of mouth breathing as we get older.[10] If you frequently wake up with a dry mouth, there's a good chance that you breathe through your mouth while you sleep.

Nasal Obstruction

I'd like to focus on nasal obstruction for a moment, as it can have a significant impact on sleep. Dr. Wynne, a Professor of Medicine and Anesthesiology, discussed the impact of nasal obstruction on sleep in an editorial for *Chest* journal.[11] He noted that nasal blockage, whether due to infections, allergies, or structural issues like a deviated septum, can lead to a range of problems during sleep, from serious conditions like heart complications and arrhythmias to milder issues such as daytime sleepiness and restless sleep. He emphasized the importance of considering the wide-ranging adverse effects that nasal obstruction can have on health.

Nasal breathing isn't just preferred—it's how the body is designed to function. The nose filters, humidifies, and slows down incoming air, helping to optimize oxygen exchange and keep the diaphragm strong.[12] It also supports the muscles in the throat, reducing the risk of airway collapse during sleep. When nasal obstruction forces mouth breathing, it disrupts the body's natural respiratory process, leading to a cascade of negative effects.

The Consequences of Mouth Breathing

As journalist and author James Nestor points out in his bestselling book *Breath: The New Science of a Lost Art*, breathing through the mouth, whether it's an everyday habit or something you do without realizing can have more consequences than you might think.

I have already touched on the impact of mouth breathing during sleep, but here are a few more reasons to avoid it during the day too.

When you breathe through your mouth, especially over long periods, it dries out your saliva. That might not seem important at first, but saliva plays a vital role in protecting your teeth and keeping the bacteria in your mouth in balance. Without it, the mouth becomes dry and acidic, conditions that encourage tooth decay, bad breath, and bacterial overgrowth. And here is where it gets even more interesting: changes in oral bacteria can also affect the gut microbiome, since some of those microbes travel downstream when you swallow.

The gut microbiome is the vast community of bacteria living in your digestive tract. These microbes help with digestion, produce important vitamins, support the immune system, and even influence your brain through what is called the gut-brain axis. So something as simple as breathing through your mouth may influence far more than just your teeth. It could be shaping your mood, mental clarity, and even emotional resilience.

For children, the effects can be even more significant. Chronic mouth breathing can influence how the face and jaw develop, often leading to a narrow palate, long face, and crooked teeth. These changes don't happen overnight, but they happen quietly and gradually, which is why they're often missed.[13]

During sleep, breathing through the mouth requires 2.5 times more effort than nasal breathing.[14] In other words, the mouth actually creates more resistance to airflow than the nose does, even though it feels like the easier option. The tongue drops from the roof of the mouth, the lower jaw hinges downward, and the throat narrows—all of which increase the likelihood of snoring, apnea, and other sleep-disordered breathing issues. Studies have found that even partial nasal obstruction can cause or worsen apnea, hypopnea, and periodic breathing disturbances. In some cases, nasal blockage has been shown to increase apnea episodes more than fourfold.[15]

Additionally, mouth breathing worsens nasal congestion, creating a vicious cycle. Increased heat and moisture loss from breathing through the mouth can cause nasal obstruction, making it even harder to switch back to nasal breathing. The counterintuitive solution? Start breathing through your nose—even if it feels difficult at first.

If nasal obstruction is due to structural defects, corrective procedures can improve sleep quality—often significantly reducing symptoms of sleep apnea—though restoring functional, nasal breathing is also important.

How to Shift to Nasal Breathing

Fortunately, you can retrain yourself to breathe through your nose—even if you've been mouth breathing for years. The exercises and breath-holding techniques introduced at the start of this book (see Chapter 1) can help clear nasal congestion, improve breathing efficiency, and support better sleep.

How Can You Assess Your Breathing?

Dysfunctional breathing—whether it's over-breathing, mouth breathing, or rapid, upper chest breathing—isn't always obvious.

But it often comes with signs and symptoms that it can help to be aware of. The consequences of dysfunctional breathing range from subtle discomforts, like frequent sighing, breathlessness, or tension in the chest, to more serious issues, such as anxiety, fatigue, and sleep disturbances. See Table 5.1 for a breakdown of common symptoms and consequences of dysfunctional breathing patterns, some of which may be familiar to you.

If you'd like to delve even deeper into the subject of dysfunctional breathing, you can find extensive information in my previous book, *The Breathing Cure*. As well as considering how many of these signs and symptoms apply to you, you may also assess your breathing using the Control Pause score (see Chapter 1).

Table 5.1 *Common Signs and Consequences of Dysfunctional Breathing*[16–18]

Signs and Symptoms of Dysfunctional Breathing	Potential Consequences of Dysfunctional Breathing
• Mouth breathing • Faster breathing • Breathing into the upper chest • Audible breathing during rest • Frequent sighing or yawning • Noticeable breaths prior to talking • Snoring • Sleep apnea • Paradoxical breathing (when your diaphragm moves in the opposite direction than it should when you're inhaling and exhaling)	• Reduced oxygen uptake • Respiratory issues • Sleep disruptions • Cardiovascular impact • Muscle tension • Impaired posture • Digestive disturbances • Anxiety • Panic • Energy depletion • Impaired concentration • Menstrual cycle irregularity • Compromised immune system • Chronic pain • Compromised sexual life

The Control Pause Score (for Adults)

The Control Pause (CP) is a simple measurement of breath-hold time after an exhalation. It gives feedback about breathlessness and sensitivity to CO_2. A higher CP score equates to ease of breathing. A low CP score indicates dysfunctional breathing patterns. When the CP score is less than 20 seconds, you are more likely to breathe fast, hard, and into the upper chest, and there is room for improvement.

Measuring the CP can be an interesting challenge, given that people with perfectionist natures often push themselves past their limits. These same people are highly prone to dysfunctional breathing patterns, including hyperventilation, and it's important to emphasize that the CP score should not be forced. It is not a "test" to be done competitively. It simply indicates how functional your breathing is today. If you find yourself getting too focused on the CP score, forget about it for a few weeks.

As you begin to practice the breathing exercises in this book, you will notice an improvement of between three and four seconds in your CP score during the first few weeks. Thereafter, progress slows but with consistent practice, improvement in the CP score does take place. Integrate the breathing techniques into your daily life to increase your CP score above 20 seconds. Work consistently and gently with your breath. Remember, it can take a lifetime for breathing to become dysfunctional. It takes gentle, consistent practice to learn to breathe optimally again.

Note: The CP is only suitable for adults, as it doesn't provide much feedback on children's breathing.

Do You Have a Good Control Pause?

- **Poor.** Less than 15 seconds.
- **Room for improvement.** Between 15 and 20 seconds.
- **Good.** Above 20 seconds.
- **Great.** 40+ seconds.

Now that we've explored dysfunctional breathing patterns and their impact on sleep and overall health, let's shift our focus to what healthy, optimal breathing looks like—and more importantly, how you can restore and strengthen your own breathing habits. By understanding the foundations of functional breathing, you'll be able to make small adjustments that lead to better oxygenation, reduced stress, and deeper, more restorative sleep.

THE FOUNDATION OF HEALTHY BREATHING

Healthy breathing should feel light, quiet, effortless, and soft. It flows through the nose, engages the diaphragm, follows a steady rhythm, and includes a gentle pause after each exhale. This is how humans naturally breathed for thousands of years, until modern comforts, stress, processed foods, and the mistaken belief that breathing more air is better began to take hold. Our ancestors breathed through their noses, moved often, ate whole foods, and lived in tune with the rhythms of nature, all of which supported calm, efficient breathing. Today, many of us sit for long hours, eat soft processed foods, live under constant stimulation, and unconsciously breathe through our mouths. This shift has quietly altered how we breathe, often without us even realizing it making over-breathing, shallow breathing, and mouth breathing the new norm.

The Core Principles of the Buteyko Method

Healthy, functional breathing is built on three key dimensions:

1. **Breathe light (biochemical).** Corrects over-breathing and ensures proper oxygen and carbon dioxide balance in the body.
2. **Breathe slow (psychophysiological).** Activates the parasympathetic nervous system, reducing stress and calming the mind.
3. **Breathe deep (biomechanical).** Engaging the diaphragm supports proper posture, stabilizes the spine, improves gas exchange, and plays a key role in regulating the nervous system.

Each of the three dimensions plays a crucial role in maintaining respiratory efficiency and stability during both wakefulness and sleep.

At the core of all three dimensions is the need for full-time nasal breathing, which is essential for improving oxygen delivery, reducing airway resistance, and stabilizing sleep-related breathing disorders.

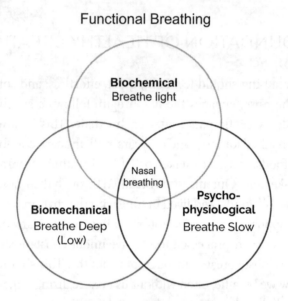

Functional Breathing

Breathe Light, Slow and Deep

Why Nasal Breathing Matters

Breathing through your nose—instead of your mouth—is one of the simplest ways to improve your overall health.

You might be surprised to learn that your nose has at least 30 vital functions that help protect and regulate your body (see Table 5.2 for a breakdown). One of its most important jobs? Optimizing the air you breathe.

The air around us is always shifting, hot and dry one moment, cool and damp the next, often carrying dust, allergens, and pollutants. Nasal breathing serves as your body's built-in air filter and climate control system, warming, humidifying, and purifying the air before it reaches your lungs. This not only reduces irritation but also helps maintain the ideal balance of oxygen and carbon dioxide, supporting relaxation and overall well-being.

Table 5.2   *Summary of Functions of the Nose*

	Function	Detail
	Filtration	Your nose acts as a filter, *trapping dust, allergens,* and *other particles* in the mucus and nasal hair to prevent them from entering your lungs.
	Temperature regulation	Your nose *warms inhaled air* to body temperature before it reaches your lungs.
	Humidification	Your nose adds *moisture* to inhaled air, which is important to *reduce inflammation* and maintain proper lung function.
	Defense mechanism	Your nose is part of the body's defense system against harmful particles and pathogens. The mucus membrane traps potentially harmful substances. Your nose produces *nitric oxide,* which plays a role in maintaining healthy lung function and may help to *protect against certain respiratory infections.*
	Helps to induce relaxation	During wakefulness, nasal breathing provides resistance to slow down the breathing rate. The nasal passages are smaller than the mouth, which means that air has to pass through them more slowly. This creates a natural resistance that helps to *regulate breathing rate* and *promote relaxation.*[23]

(continued on next page)

Table 5.2   *Summary of Functions of the Nose (continued)*

	Function	Detail
	Increases oxygen uptake in the blood	Nose breathing is more effective at *increasing oxygen uptake* in the body than breathing through the mouth.
	Improves cognitive function	Persons with normal function of the nose have *improved cognitive function* and *energy levels* in comparison with persons with chronic nasal issues.
	Sense of smell	The nose contains olfactory receptors that allow us to detect and identify various odors.
	Taste perception	The nose communicates with a part of the brain responsible for taste perception called the "orbitofrontal cortex." This brain center receives taste and smell signals and processes them together, coupling smell and taste.
	Promotes better sleep	The nose is necessary for proper nasal breathing, which has been shown to contribute to *deeper and more restful sleep.*

Nasal breathing also produces nitric oxide, a gas that plays a critical role in improving oxygen delivery, reducing inflammation, and enhancing respiratory efficiency.

In 1998, the Nobel Prize in Physiology or Medicine was awarded to three pharmacologists who discovered the wide-ranging benefits of nitric oxide, often called the "panacea molecule." But here's the catch: your lungs harness the most nitric oxide through nasal breathing—not mouth breathing. This gas helps to:

- Sterilize the air you breathe, killing harmful bacteria and viruses.
- Dilate the airways, making breathing easier.
- Redistribute blood in the lungs, ensuring better oxygen exchange.

When you breathe through your nose, nitric oxide helps direct oxygen deep into the lungs, reaching the alveoli—the tiny air sacs responsible for gas exchange. But when you breathe through your mouth, this process is bypassed, leading to lower nitric oxide levels and less efficient oxygen delivery.

Why Nasal Breathing Improves Energy, Sleep, and Hydration

Beyond its role in oxygenation, nasal breathing provides multiple benefits that impact your breathing efficiency, hydration, and even immune function:

- **Keeps your airway open.** Nitric oxide helps maintain muscle tone in the upper airway, reducing the risk of obstruction (a key issue in sleep disorders like sleep apnea).[19] When the muscles in the throat and upper airway have good tone, they're more likely to stay open during sleep and less likely to collapse or block airflow.
- **Regulates body temperature.** When air enters through the nose, it's warmed by tiny capillaries before reaching the lungs.[20] Nasal nitric oxide dilates these capillaries, increasing air temperature by more than 10°C between the nostrils and the back of the nose.[21]
- **Prevents dehydration.** Mouth breathing causes 42% more moisture loss than nasal breathing.[22] Breathing through your nose preserves humidity in the airways, preventing dry mouth and supporting immune function.
- **Reduces nasal congestion.** While it may seem counterintuitive, breathing through your nose (even when it feels stuffy) can actually help clear nasal passages and improve airflow over time.

The Key to Calm, Controlled Breathing

Nasal breathing naturally leads to slower, lighter, and deeper breaths—reducing airway resistance and promoting a sense of calm.

Practicing nasal breathing during both day and night can enhance sleep quality, focus, energy levels, and overall well-being.

Breathe Light (Biochemical Dimension)

For optimal breathing, your body needs the right balance of oxygen (O_2) and carbon dioxide (CO_2). Although CO_2 is often misunderstood as a "waste gas," it actually plays a crucial role in breathing regulation. Here's how it works:

1. The rhythm, rate, and depth of your breathing are controlled by your brainstem, which monitors blood pH and CO_2 levels (to ensure the proper balance is maintained).
2. As CO_2 builds up, blood pH lowers slightly, triggering the brainstem to signal your diaphragm to take another breath.
3. The trouble is, many people are overly sensitive to carbon dioxide. This sensitivity causes them to breathe more than they need to, even at rest. When CO_2 levels drop too much, oxygen delivery is affected in two important ways. First, blood vessels constrict, which reduces blood flow throughout the body, including to vital organs like the heart and brain. Second, the body struggles to release oxygen from red blood cells to the tissues that need it most. This is known as the "Bohr Effect," a natural process where CO_2 helps oxygen detach from red blood cells so it can reach working muscles and organs. Without enough CO_2, that oxygen stays "stuck" and can't be used efficiently.

This imbalance can lead to a range of common symptoms, including cold hands and feet, anxiety, and poor sleep. (See Chapter 5 to learn more about chronic over-breathing and hyperventilation.)

How Light Breathing Restores Balance
The *Breathe Light Exercise*, described in detail in Chapter 1, is a simple yet powerful technique to retrain your breathing. This

exercise involves reducing the volume of air you breathe through light, nasal breathing—softening and slowing your breath to create a gentle air hunger. With consistent practice, this approach decreases your sensitivity to CO_2 and restores the natural balance of O_2 and CO_2 in the body.

Over time, as your tolerance to CO_2 improves, your breathing becomes lighter, your respiratory rate slows, your breathing becomes lighter, and oxygen delivery to your heart, brain, and other tissues increases. This balance not only enhances circulation and tissue oxygenation but also promotes calmness and a resilience to stress. What's more, light, gentle breathing reduces airway resistance and turbulence, which can minimize snoring, sleep disturbances, and nighttime awakenings. The result? A quieter, deeper, and more restorative night's sleep.

> "Breathing light before bed helps me to sleep better especially when I extend the exhale. I also find when I do it regularly, I have an easier time managing stress and anxiety and just feel better overall."
>
> *Jamie, 48, USA*

By incorporating light breathing into your daily routine, you can unlock a powerful pathway to better health, increased energy, a greater sense of calm, and better sleep.

Breathe Slow (Psychophysiological Dimension)

The term "psychophysiological" refers to the connection between the mind (psyche) and the body (physiology). This idea isn't new; in fact, it goes all the way back to the ancient Greeks, who believed that breath was the bridge between body and soul. The word *psyche* itself meant both soul and breath, showing just how closely they saw the two as connected. Philosophers like Plato and later the Stoics spoke of breath as something that could steady the mind and strengthen character, long before we had names for the nervous system.

Today, science confirms what the ancients observed. Slowing down your breathing does more than just help you relax. It also improves the mechanics of how you breathe. Gentle, slow breaths create smoother airflow through the airways, reduce resistance, and make it less likely that the airway will collapse during sleep. This promotes more stable breathing throughout the night, which helps support uninterrupted, restorative sleep.

Slow breathing also has a profound calming effect on the nervous system, stimulating the vagus nerve and activating the parasympathetic "rest, digest, and repair" state.[24] This shift brings the body into a place of calm, making sleep more accessible and restorative. Studies have shown that slow breathing can help regulate emotions and reduce stress, and can result in increased comfort, relaxation, heart rate variability, pleasantness, vigor, and alertness and reduced symptoms of arousal, anxiety, panic, depression, and anger.[25–30]

To experience the full benefits of slow breathing, it can be helpful to practice breathing at a rate of 4.5 to 6.5 breaths per minute. This gentle pace helps regulate the nervous system, improve emotional balance, and support deeper, more restful sleep. You can try this using the *Breathe Slow Exercise* introduced in Chapter 1.

That said, this isn't about maintaining a perfect breathing rate all day long. You don't need to fixate on hitting six breaths per minute or try to control every breath you take throughout the day. The real purpose of this practice is to help retrain your breathing and reset your nervous system so that, over time, your body finds a rhythm that feels calm, quiet, and natural.

It may not land on exactly six breaths per minute, and that's perfectly fine. What it will do, however, is encourage your breathing to become a little slower and more gentle than it may be right now. And that shift alone can have a meaningful impact on how you feel, especially when it comes to sleep, focus, and recovery.

At different moments throughout the day, it can be useful to pause and simply bring some awareness to your breath. No need to count; just breathe in and out through your nose, keep it silent, and allow the pace to slow. With practice, this becomes less of a technique and more of a habit, quietly supporting your energy and mental clarity throughout the day.

Breathe Deep (Biomechanical Dimension)

By practicing the *Breathe Deep Exercise* and engaging your diaphragm, you can improve your breathing biomechanics. Low, diaphragmatic breathing is key to strengthening the respiratory muscles, stabilizing the airway, and improving oxygen intake. While the diaphragm is the main muscle responsible for breathing, other muscles—including the intercostals, abdominals, and even those in the face, mouth, and throat—also play a role. When any of these muscles become weak or dysfunctional, the airway can narrow, making breathing more difficult. The natural connection between the diaphragm and throat muscles helps prevent airway collapse, reducing issues like snoring and sleep apnea.

Modern lifestyles, however, often interfere with this natural breathing pattern. Hours spent hunched over a computer or smartphone encourage shallow, upper chest breathing instead of deep, diaphragmatic breaths. Poor posture restricts the diaphragm's ability to move freely, forcing the body to rely on smaller, less efficient accessory muscles in the chest, neck, and upper back. Over time, this not only reduces breathing efficiency but also leads to physical strain, muscle tension, and pain in the neck and back.

By consciously shifting to low, diaphragmatic breathing and practicing the *Breathe Nose, Slow, and Deep Exercise* described at the start of the book, you can unlock a range of benefits.

Earlier in the chapter, we looked at the word "psychophysiological," which refers to the connection between the mind (*psyche*) and the body (*physiology*), and how the ancient Greeks believed that breath was the bridge between the two. They saw breathing not just as a physical act, but as something that shaped character, steadied the mind, and reflected the state of the soul.

This understanding becomes even more relevant when we look at the diaphragm, the main muscle involved in breathing. Strengthening and improving the function of the diaphragm doesn't just support better oxygen delivery; it also plays a key role in spinal stability, breathing efficiency, mental calm, and sleep quality.

The Greeks may not have known the anatomy in today's terms, but they were remarkably close in spirit. The phrenic nerve, which sends signals from the brain to the diaphragm, shares its roots with the Greek word *phren*, meaning both diaphragm and mind. This same word appears in terms we still use today, like schizophrenia, which literally translates to "a split in the mind." The term reflects the historical belief that the condition involved a kind of fragmentation or disconnect within one's mental processes; such as thoughts, emotions, or perception. While modern psychiatry understands schizophrenia in more nuanced ways, the language still carries that ancient idea of a disruption between different parts of the self.

Physiologically, when we engage the diaphragm through slow, steady breathing, we stimulate the vagus nerve, which supports relaxation, lowers heart rate, and helps bring the body into a "rest, digest, and repair" state. This shift can also help lower high blood pressure, which is why diaphragmatic breathing is often recommended for stress reduction.

So when you practice breathing nose, slow, and low, you're not just improving lung function. You're tapping into a system that connects mind, body, and breath; something the Greeks understood thousands of years ago, and something science is now beginning to understand. With regular practice, these breathing principles—nose, light, slow, and deep—become second nature, ensuring that the way you breathe during the day extends seamlessly into your nighttime breathing. These simple shifts foster quiet, uninterrupted sleep and can ease snoring, alleviate sleep apnea, and pave the way for truly restful sleep.

BREATHING AND SLEEP DISORDERS

At the beginning of this chapter, I highlighted the intricate connection between breathing and sleep. Dysfunctional breathing is a feature of many sleep disorders, and both sleep disorders and sleep-disordered breathing are on the rise. As we have learned, the way you breathe during the day affects how you breathe at night, which impacts the quality of your sleep, which in turn impacts your overall health and well-being.

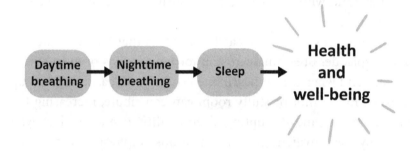

How Can Your Breathing Wake You Up at Night?

Most of us don't give much thought to how we breathe during sleep, but it could be the very thing pulling us out of it. If you've ever woken up suddenly, feeling restless or anxious without a clear reason, your breathing might be the missing link.

There are a few reasons why breathing can become harder or faster during sleep. One common factor is a low CP, which reflects your body's sensitivity to carbon dioxide. When the CP is low, breathing tends to shift into a pattern that is faster, harder, and more in the upper chest. This type of breathing increases the likelihood of waking and makes it harder to stay in deep, steady sleep.

Airway narrowing is another factor. Whether from nasal congestion, a naturally small airway, or sleep-disordered breathing, the respiratory muscles have to work harder to overcome resistance, making sleep feel less restorative even if you don't fully wake up.

If you have asthma, you might already be familiar with this connection. When asthma is not well controlled and symptoms like chest tightness or wheezing are present, breathing often becomes more shallow and rapid. This pattern can make night-time awakenings more common. On the other hand, when asthma is under control, sleep tends to be more continuous and refreshing.

It's worth noting that asthma rarely exists in isolation. Fatigue often tags along. The reason may lie in the combination of poor breathing patterns and inflammation, two things that frequently go hand in hand with asthma. I'll be exploring asthma in more detail in Chapter 5.

Then there's the classic catch-up breath that happens after an apnea episode. Breathing can stop for ten seconds or even over a minute, and when it resumes, it often comes with gasping, catch-up breaths. Even a hot or stuffy room can contribute, increasing the breathing rate and disrupting sleep quality. It may explain why so many sleep hygiene recommendations emphasize keeping the bedroom cool and well ventilated. A cooler, fresher environment supports calmer breathing, which in turn creates the conditions for deeper, more restful sleep.

Scientists at Stanford Medical School, led by researcher Mark Krasnow, uncovered something remarkable that helps explain why disturbed breathing during sleep can trigger wakefulness.[31] They discovered a small group of neurons; the tiny messenger cells your brain uses to send and receive information tucked away in the brainstem, right at the base of your brain. This part of the brain quietly runs all the behind-the-scenes operations, like keeping your heart beating, your blood pressure normal, and your breathing going, even while you sleep. This group of neurons acts like a surveillance system for breathing. It constantly monitors the rhythm, speed, depth, and regularity of each breath, even when you are asleep. When your breathing becomes fast, hard, irregular, or labored, especially during rest, these neurons pick up on it and send signals to other parts of the brain. The message is simple: something isn't right. This often results in a subtle increase in alertness or a full awakening, depending on the severity of the disturbance.

This might help explain why some people wake up during the night without knowing why. The breathing disturbance may be subtle; just a few faster breaths, some upper chest effort, or a blocked nose, but the brain is watching. It's not trying to sabotage your sleep. It's trying to protect you. If your breathing doesn't feel slow and regular, the brain stays on guard.

We know that stress changes breathing patterns. When we're anxious or under pressure, breathing naturally becomes faster, and often moves into the upper chest. That's expected. But if these patterns become habitual and carry over into sleep, the brain's internal monitor doesn't switch off. It notices the shift, and that can keep you from dropping into deeper stages of rest.

Now think back to the person with a low CP, or someone with asthma waking during the night. Could the brain be responding to poor breathing patterns, even before the person is fully aware of it? It's likely. The brain may be receiving subtle distress signals that lead to frequent arousals and broken sleep. In this way, breathing isn't just something that keeps us alive. It's something the brain carefully monitors.

But the brainstem isn't the only part of the brain involved. The amygdala, your brain's built-in threat detector, also plays a role in regulating and monitoring your breathing.[32] If it senses that your breath has become irregular, fast, or hard, it too may register this as a red flag and activate the body's "fight, flight, or freeze" response.[33] If your amygdala perceives your breathing patterns as a sign you could be in danger, it can trigger wakefulness or keep you in a lighter stage of sleep, disrupting the quality of your rest. Essentially, the brain's alarm system is trying to protect you, but in doing so, it prevents deep, restorative sleep.

Knowing that your brain is constantly monitoring your breathing and that how you breathe influences how your brain responds gives you something powerful to work with. It means you can shape your sleep quality by working with your breath.

If your CP is low, improving it will naturally change how you breathe during sleep. A higher CP reflects lighter, slower and deeper breathing, which helps reduce nighttime wake-ups and supports deeper rest.

While you are likely unaware of your nighttime breathing patterns, if you suffer from nasal congestion due to allergies, asthma, or rhinitis, you are almost twice as likely to experience moderate to severe sleep-disordered breathing.[34] Mouth breathing often develops when nasal breathing is impaired. Your body prioritizes respiration, so if breathing through the nose is challenging, mouth breathing will suffice.

Research suggests that for people who habitually breathe through their mouths at night, making changes to support nasal breathing can significantly reduce sleep-disordered breathing, with symptoms like snoring and sleep apnea improving by up to 50%.[35] Small shifts in breathing habits can lead to big improvements.

How Can Breathing Re-education Help Sleep?

To improve your breathing patterns and establish a foundation for better sleep and overall well-being, follow the recommendations and exercises provided in Chapter 1. These exercises not only enhance your breathing patterns and reduce snoring and sleep apnea, but they also regulate your nervous system and promote relaxation, leading to more restorative sleep and better daytime functioning.

Some quotes from our community who have found a range of benefits from adopting the Buteyko Method:

"I used to be a **mouth breather** when sleeping, which caused significant issues with my sleep, including **insomnia**. I also drank a lot of water during the night, which meant **frequent trips to the** toilet, further disrupting my rest. **After using mouth tape . . . I noticed a massive improvement in the quality of my sleep and reduced fatigue** during the day. I completely stopped drinking water at night and felt rested in the morning, which was a break-through for me.

Since then, I've experienced no fatigue, my muscle and joint inflammation disappeared, my sleep improved dramatically, my anxiety vanished, and even my back pain resolved over time."

"I had difficulties with **snoring and waking up during the night.** Because of taping I feel my body gets more rest during the nights.

Even when I still sometimes wake up during the night, it's not a problem to fall asleep again. This is a huge difference for me!

So taping helps me during the night and during the day. Feeling **more energized!** Besides that, because of the Buteyko exercises my breathing is getting better by the day. These results give me so much inner peace."

Jespe, 36, Netherlands

"**I snored and mouth breathed** from a young age. When I started puberty, my daytime energy plummeted and I **needed a nap every day** from 13 years–37 years.

Napping always felt like a source of shame, embarrassment, and anxiety for me (worrying about if I could fit a nap into my day). I hated having less energy than my friends and colleagues, and it made me feel like I was weak and less of a person.

I started taping my mouth at night. . . . Almost straight away my 1 hour naps reduced to 15 minutes. After about 6 weeks I found myself not being able to fall asleep when I went to nap . . . I found myself not even thinking about needing naps.

I felt like I had my life back and so much more time in the day."

Lydia, 40, England

CHAPTER 6

WHAT DETERMINES WHEN AND HOW WELL WE SLEEP?

HOW YOUR BODY, LIFESTYLE, AND BREATHING SHAPE YOUR REST

Have you ever stopped to think about what actually controls your sleep? Your body has a built-in 24-hour clock—known as your "circadian rhythm"—that works alongside a natural sleep drive that builds up throughout the day. These two forces team up to decide when you feel wide awake and when you start to nod off at night.

But there's more to sleep than just feeling tired at bedtime. Light exposure, daily habits, and even your genetics play a huge role in how well (or poorly) you sleep. Ever wonder why some people thrive as early birds while others are night owls struggling to fit into an early-start world? And how does your environment, including morning sunlight or blue light from screens, impact your ability to fall asleep and stay asleep?

Reading this chapter, you might conclude that our modern way of life undermines sleep quality in almost every way. Compared with our ancestors, it seems that today's habits do little to support good sleep. Perhaps it's time to go back to basics and apply common sense to improve our rest.

While this chapter offers practical advice rooted in sleep hygiene, it's important to remember that this book focuses on breathing re-education. There's no doubt that good sleep hygiene can help, but focusing on breathing—and understanding how it overlaps with these strategies—may prove even more impactful in improving your sleep.

In this chapter, we'll explore the fascinating interplay between circadian rhythms, sleep drive, and lifestyle factors that shape your sleep. By understanding these mechanisms, you'll gain insights into how to improve not just the quantity of your sleep but its quality, ultimately supporting better health and well-being.

CIRCADIAN RHYTHMS AND SLEEP DRIVE

When you sleep and how long you sleep for are determined partially by volitional control (e.g., whether you choose to stay up late, or when you set your alarm to wake you) and partially by your genetics. Two key innate processes also regulate your sleep, each playing a distinct but complementary role in managing your sleep-wake cycle:

1. **Circadian rhythms.** Circadian rhythms affect many bodily processes, and the most well-known circadian rhythm is the sleep-wake cycle. This internal clock is influenced by various factors, including light exposure, hormones, and neurotransmitters (chemical messengers) like serotonin. It regulates cycles of sleep and wakefulness over 24 hours, influencing when you feel alert and when you feel sleepy.

2. **Sleep drive.** Sleep drive is the natural buildup of sleepiness the longer you stay awake. It's like an internal pressure that grows stronger throughout the day, making you feel increasingly drowsy as bedtime approaches. However, your circadian rhythm (your body's internal clock) doesn't always align perfectly with your

sleep drive. In the evening, your circadian rhythm can send signals that promote alertness, even if your sleep drive is high. This is why some people experience a "second wind"—a sudden burst of energy or wakefulness in the evening, despite feeling tired earlier in the day. For example, you might feel sluggish in the late afternoon but then get a surge of energy around 9 or 10 p.m., keeping you up later than planned. This happens because your circadian clock is still in "wake mode," even though your sleep pressure is high. This mismatch can lead to delayed sleep onset, especially if you're exposed to bright lights (like screens) in the evening, which further push back your body's natural sleep signals.

How Your Circadian Rhythm Shapes More Than Just Sleep

Your circadian rhythm isn't just in charge of your sleep-wake cycle— it also influences body temperature, hormone levels, brain function, metabolism, and even your immune system. While this internal clock is controlled by your brain, external factors—especially light—play a huge role in keeping it running smoothly. That's why getting morning sunlight helps you feel awake and alert, while late-night screen time can leave you staring at the ceiling when you should be asleep.

Your body produces specific hormones to regulate your circadian rhythm, each with a unique job:

- **Melatonin.** The "sleep hormone" helps signal to your body that it's time to wind down and sleep.
- **Cortisol.** The "stress hormone" helps wake you up and stay alert, but too much at night can interfere with sleep.
- **Ghrelin.** The "hunger hormone" increases appetite and cravings (especially when you don't get enough sleep).
- **Leptin.** The "fullness hormone" tells your body when you've had enough to eat. Poor sleep can throw this off, making it harder to feel satisfied after meals.

When your circadian rhythm is *in sync,* everything runs more smoothly—you sleep better, wake up feeling refreshed, and even maintain a healthier metabolism and immune system. But when it's out of balance? You might feel groggy during the day and wired at night, and struggle with everything from hunger cravings to brain fog.

You can reset and regulate your circadian rhythm with simple lifestyle tweaks—starting with reducing light exposure at night, timing your meals, and managing stress levels. Small changes can have a big impact on how well you sleep and how energized you feel throughout the day!

How Does Light Influence Sleep?

Morning Light

In the morning, sunlight emits blue light, which suppresses melatonin—the hormone that makes you feel sleepy. As exposure to light increases, *melatonin production stops,* body temperature begins to rise, and cortisol is released, increasing your alertness and causing you to wake up. While cortisol is responsible for regulating your body's stress response, it also has other important effects and functions throughout your body such as suppressing inflammation and regulating metabolism.

As the day continues, there is a gradual decline in your cortisol levels. As sleep ensues, there is a continued decrease in cortisol levels which helps promote sleep.

Exposure to natural light by going outdoors early in the day is recommended and is beneficial for regulating the circadian rhythm.

Evening Light

At night, on the other hand, as the sun sets, your brain senses the absence of light and begins *producing melatonin, which induces sleepiness.*

Melatonin levels stay high throughout the night, promoting sleep. Core body temperature also drops, and cortisol levels drop (ideally—more on that later), contributing to decreased alertness.

These changes, driven by circadian rhythms, combine with sleep drive *to cause you to fall asleep at night.*

The presence of *blue light* from artificial lighting such as LED lights in our homes and electronic devices at night *reduces melatonin levels* and can interfere with this process, making it harder to sleep.[1]

Sleep experts recommend dimming lights and avoiding bright blue-light-producing lights and screens (phones, tablets, computers) before bedtime to allow natural melatonin production. Some people choose to wear blue-light-blocking glasses at night, but this is a topic of ongoing research, and the evidence is mixed.[2] You may also buy blue-light-free bulbs for use in bedroom lamps.

Sleep Drive

Sleep drive, also known as "sleep pressure," is a biological process that regulates your need for sleep. The longer you're awake, the *stronger* the sleep pressure becomes. Typically, when you've been awake for about 16 hours, your sleep drive tells you it's time to sleep. Think of it as a reservoir that gradually fills throughout the day, becoming harder to resist as it reaches its peak. You've probably experienced it on a late evening when you're watching a fascinating program on television or reading a captivating book—something so engaging you don't want to stop—but despite your interest, you find yourself struggling to keep your eyes open. That overwhelming need to sleep, even when the mind is occupied, is your sleep drive in action, signaling that your body needs rest.

As you sleep, your sleep drive diminishes. Finally, your need for alertness grows, telling you that it's time to wake up.

The primary mechanism behind sleep drive is the accumulation of a chemical messenger in the brain called "adenosine." Adenosine is involved in storing and releasing energy throughout your body. Once you fall asleep, adenosine is believed to prolong deep sleep (NREM sleep stage 3) where important restorative functions occur.

Caffeine is a stimulant that blocks adenosine receptors in the brain, effectively masking your sleep drive and making you feel more awake. It typically stays in your system for several hours, with an average half-life of 5–6 hours—meaning half of the caffeine consumed remains in your body during that time. While its stimulating effects usually last 4–6 hours, residual caffeine can linger for up to 10–12 hours, potentially disrupting sleep.

Factors like genetics, age, pregnancy, medications, and smoking influence how quickly caffeine is metabolized. Some people process it rapidly, while others experience its effects for much longer. Sensitivity to caffeine varies widely; regular users may build up a tolerance and not feel its effects as strongly, but even habitual consumption can still interfere with sleep quality.[3] To minimize its impact, it's recommended to avoid caffeine at least 6–8 hours before bedtime, or even earlier for those who are more sensitive.

Are You an Early Bird or a Night Owl?

Have you ever wondered why your ideal bedtime is so different from your partner's or your friends'? Although humans all possess a biological circadian rhythm, the precise timing of that 24-hour rhythm differs from person to person.

- **Early birds.** Approximately one-third of people naturally prefer to wake up at or around dawn and function well at this time. Such "early birds," or "larks," prefer an early bedtime.

- **Night owls.** Another third of people prefer to go to bed late at night, earning them the name "night owls." They prefer to wake up later the following day.
- **Neutral.** The remainder of people are neutral and lie somewhere between these two extremes of being "morning types" and "evening types." You may have heard the saying: "Early to bed and early to rise makes a man healthy, wealthy, and wise," which is commonly attributed to Benjamin Franklin. It seems that is not *always* the case.

Your natural inclination towards *morningness* or *eveningness* is genetically determined and is called your "chronotype." If your parents prefer a later bedtime, it's likely you will too. Like your circadian rhythm, your chronotype has an influence on appetite, exercise, and core body temperature. It is responsible for making you feel more alert at certain periods of the day and more tired at others.

Night owls will struggle to function if obliged to wake early, robbing them of their last few precious hours of sleep. And despite the unwelcome early start, they are unlikely to be able to fall asleep until later in the evening, as determined by their genetic programming and circadian rhythm. Over time, this will have a cumulative effect and has an obvious impact on daytime functioning and concentration. The typical early start time imposed in most schools and places of work is not at all ideal for evening types.

For adolescents, the importance of sleep highlights how societal structures often work against natural circadian rhythms. Teens naturally fall asleep and wake up later due to shifts in their biological clocks; yet the average US high schools start is 8 a.m.,[4] cutting into the nine hours of sleep they need. Research shows that delaying school start times allows teens to sleep longer, leading to better academic performance, fewer car crashes, and reduced depression. Experts like Kyla Wahlstrom advocate for start times of 9:00 or later, though 8:30 is often seen as a compromise.[5] Backed by organizations like the CDC and the American Academy of Pediatrics, hundreds of schools have adopted later start times.[6,7] However, early schedules remain the norm, leaving many teens sleep-deprived.

What's a Sleep Divorce?

In recent years, the term "sleep divorce" has gained popularity as more couples choose to sleep in separate bedrooms to prioritize better rest. While it might sound like the end of romance, this trend is helping many couples strengthen their relationships. According to Tamara Green, a New York couple's therapist, sleeping separately can improve communication and intimacy, "They get enough rest and feel like they are able to hear each other out and get their needs met," she explained to TODAY.com.[8]

The primary reason for sleep divorce is sleep loss. Snoring, tossing and turning, differing schedules, or even bed-sharing with children can lead to poor-quality sleep for one or both partners. Over time, this lack of sleep causes irritability, conflicts, and diminished patience, putting strain on the relationship. By sleeping in separate rooms, couples can enjoy uninterrupted rest, and feel more energized, emotionally balanced, and better equipped to engage with each other during waking hours.

Differences in chronotypes—where one partner is a lark and the other a night owl—can also impact a relationship. A study published in *Frontiers in Psychology* found that couples with similar chronotypes reported higher relationship satisfaction, likely because their daily routines and preferred times for activities, including intimacy, were more aligned. However, for those with mismatched chronotypes, there is no strong evidence linking these differences to higher divorce rates. Instead, understanding and adapting to your natural chronotype can help improve sleep quality, energy, and mood. Tools like the *Morningness-Eveningness Questionnaire*[9] can help couples identify their chronotypes and navigate these differences, fostering greater harmony and balance in their relationships.

One woman shared her experience during an Instagram Q&A, explaining how she and her partner maintain connection despite sleeping apart: "We juggle the household and kids, and if there's any time at night, we'll watch something, give each other a massage, have a bath, or get frisky. Other nights, we just want to do our own thing. It's a wild ride, but we're doing it together."[10] This open communication and shared understanding can preserve emotional and physical closeness, even when sleeping in separate rooms.

The broader lesson here is that sleep isn't just a personal matter—it has societal and relational implications. For couples, sleeping apart can reduce stress and improve relationship satisfaction by addressing sleep-related conflicts. Similarly, acknowledging and adapting to differences in chronotypes or aligning societal schedules to natural rhythms can create better outcomes for individuals and relationships alike. Whether it's managing sleep disruptions, parenting demands, or differing schedules, prioritizing quality rest can help everyone—from couples to teens—rest well and live better.

How Can I Regulate My Sleep-Wake Cycle?

Your *circadian rhythm* and *sleep drive* work together like a built-in sleep system, keeping you on a natural cycle of wakefulness and rest. When they're in sync, you feel energized during the day and ready for deep, refreshing sleep at night. But when they're off balance? You might struggle with falling asleep, waking up groggy, or feeling tired at the wrong times.

You can take control of your sleep-wake cycle by making small, science-backed changes to your daily habits. Many sleep hygiene tips are rooted in how these two systems function—so by understanding what influences your sleep drive and circadian rhythm, you can fine-tune your routine to promote quality sleep.

The core components of good sleep hygiene include:

	Early Natural Light Exposure to natural light, especially in the morning for just 5–10 minutes, helps regulate melatonin and strengthens the circadian rhythm. If stepping outside isn't an option, sitting near a window or using a bright light can still provide benefits. While windows aren't as effective as being outdoors—because glass filters out some wavelengths of natural light, including portions of blue light—daylight exposure remains crucial. A study investigating workplace environments found that workers in windowless spaces reported poorer overall sleep quality, as measured by their global *Pittsburgh Sleep Quality Index* scores and the sleep disturbances component.[11] In contrast, workers with access to windows experienced greater light exposure during the workweek, engaged in more physical activity, and had longer sleep durations compared with those without windows. These findings emphasize the importance of daylight exposure, even if it's through a window.
	Keep Regular Sleep Hours Make a habit of going to bed and getting up at roughly the same times each day (including weekends).
	Avoid or Minimize Naps Some sleep experts say that naps should ideally be avoided for those who have trouble sleeping at night. Long naps or naps taken later in the afternoon may reduce sleep drive, making it harder to fall asleep at night. As noted earlier, naps can bring many benefits and act as a rest and reset. If you do nap, keep it short (around 20–40 minutes) to reduce grogginess and avoid napping late in the day to prevent interference with nighttime sleep.
	Create a Restful Environment Dark, quiet, and cool environments generally make it easier to fall asleep and stay asleep.

	Move More, Sleep Better Regular exercise is good for your physical health and the mind too—and being active during the day can help you sleep better. Aim for 30 minutes a day, 5 days a week, at a moderate intensity—enough to increase your heart rate and make you breathe a little harder, like brisk walking, cycling, or swimming.
	Limit Caffeine Caffeine is a stimulant that can negatively impact your sleep drive. Limit caffeine consumption to 1-3 cups maximum per day, preferably in the morning. Avoid consuming caffeine at least 8 hours (some sources advise 10-12 hours) before bedtime.[12] Be careful about energy drinks, as these are particularly popular with teenagers, and can have a high caffeine content.
	Limit Alcohol Intake Alcohol can prevent deep, restorative sleep. It suppresses melatonin production, disrupting the body's natural sleep-wake cycle. For optimal sleep, it's recommended to abstain from alcohol entirely or limit consumption to 1-2 drinks maximum, earlier in the evening.[13] Although alcohol can help some people fall asleep faster initially due to its sedative effects, it ultimately causes more frequent awakenings, especially in the second half of the night as blood alcohol levels drop. Overall, alcohol consumption leads to more fragmented and disrupted sleep and can worsen sleep apnea by relaxing throat muscles and increasing airway resistance.
	Limit Fluid Intake Before Bed Limit fluid intake before bed to reduce nighttime bathroom trips. While it's true that breathing through your nose promotes deeper sleep and can help reduce the need for nighttime trips to the bathroom, it's also important to note that mouth breathing increases the risk of dehydration, which may lead to greater fluid intake. Nasal breathing helps conserve moisture by recovering it from each breath on the exhaled air, making it a more efficient and hydrating way to breathe.

(continued on next page)

Avoid Eating Too Close to Bedtime

Dining late in the evening can negatively impact sleep as well. Sleep experts advise not eating for at least 2 hours before bed.

Limit Exposure to Artificial Light Before Bed

Exposure to artificial light at night can hinder the production of melatonin and disrupt your circadian rhythm. Experts recommend dimming the lights before bed. Some people switch their regular bedroom lighting LED bulbs to red-light spectrum bulbs, which can be purchased relatively inexpensively (approx. $22).

Electronic devices such as phones that emit blue light should be avoided before bed and ideally kept out of your bedroom. You may use a "nighttime" setting on your phone to automatically come on at a particular time, e.g., 8 p.m. each evening, to reduce phone-related exposure to blue light.

For those who do make nighttime bathroom visits, motion-sensor red-light spectrum night lights may be used, and these too can be bought for (approx. $26).

Confront Sleeplessness

Being awake during the night can lead to rumination on problems or daily sources of stress. It's important to calm the mind before those thoughts become overwhelming. Meditation and breathing exercises are effective at removing focus from one's thoughts.

Listen to my free 20-minute audio *Insomnia—How to Fall Back Asleep* (download to your device using the QR code). If listening to guided meditations using your phone at night, put your phone in flight mode to avoid notifications and have your phone on a dim nighttime setting.

Avoid Overstimulating the Mind and Exposure to Stressors Before Bed

It's best to avoid anything that may increase your stress levels and consequently your cortisol levels before bedtime. This may include avoiding watching news and scrolling online in the hours before bed. We've all been guilty of mindlessly scrolling, only to realize that a considerable amount of time has passed with little to show for it. Most of the information consumed is unimportant, yet it grabs our attention and can leave us feeling agitated or overstimulated. Higher levels of cortisol in the evening disrupt the sleep-wake cycle and can contribute to problems falling or staying asleep.

Above all the recommendations in this book regarding sleep hygiene, I strongly emphasize the importance of addressing dysfunctional breathing patterns and incorporating light, slow, deep nasal breathing. These techniques help reduce breathing resistance that contributes to sleep-disordered breathing and reduce sympathetic nervous system activity, promoting relaxation and better sleep. These practices not only are supported by scientific evidence but are also simple to adopt, cost-free, and free from side effects.

Life Events, Lifestyle, and Health Factors That Disrupt Sleep

Sleep is influenced by so many factors, and while some are within your control, others simply aren't. Sometimes, life throws curveballs that turn your sleep upside down—whether it's the joy (and exhaustion) of a new baby, the stress of grief or trauma, or the demands of night shift work, caregiving, or jet lag. These situations can knock you out of sync with your natural sleep-wake cycle, making restful sleep feel like a distant memory.

But even when your sleep schedule is out of your hands, you can still take steps to protect your sleep quality. This book offers practical strategies that can help you optimize your rest, even during life's most challenging moments. While you may not always be able to control when or how long you sleep, you can still make choices that support deeper, more restorative rest—helping you feel more resilient, even in tough times.

> "Our sleep issues began after our child was born. Frequent night-time wake-ups led to insomnia—despite being tired, we found it difficult to fall back asleep. This significantly impacted our concentration and energy levels during the day.
>
> Initially, the thought of taping our mouths seemed stressful, but to our surprise, it brings an additional sense of calmness during sleep. Our sleep quality has improved considerably—we wake up less and find it easier to fall back asleep after any wake-ups.
>
> Additionally, we practice breathing techniques before bed. . . . We have more energy during the day and cope better with stress."
>
> *Anna, 40, Poland*

Leaving these less predictable and controllable circumstances aside, many lifestyle-related sleep-disrupting factors may be more within our power to address.

CHAPTER 7

BREATHING TO BALANCE STRESS, MENTAL HEALTH, AND MODERN-DAY LIVING

We live in a world where chronic stress has become the norm. Consider, for a moment, our ancestors. When they finished work, they didn't just rest their *bodies*; they gave their *minds* a rest, too. Fast-forward to today, and the opportunity to have a still mind and enjoy quiet time, maybe even experience boredom, is in short supply. We are distracted, busy, stressed, wired, tired, and overwhelmed. No wonder our sleep suffers.

Stress is all too common in today's modern world. At its core, stress is the body's response to demands or challenges, triggering a cascade of physical, emotional, and mental reactions. You might recognize stress if you find yourself cutting corners on tasks, losing your temper more easily, or struggling to focus because the mind is preoccupied with worries or ruminations. Stress can also manifest physically, such as tension in your body or difficulty sleeping, with insomnia often being a telltale sign that stress is interfering with your ability to relax and recharge.

According to a poll carried out by the American Psychological Association in 2022, about 55% of adults in the United States said they had experienced stress during "a lot of the day" prior. Alarmingly, around a third of adults in the poll (34%) reported that stress is completely overwhelming most days.[1]

Most of us feel stressed at times—it is our body's natural reaction to a specific event or stressor; and from an evolutionary point of view, this short-term response is essential for survival purposes. However, when the body experiences stressors with such frequency or intensity that *chronic* stress occurs, the "fight, flight, or freeze" response stays turned on and the body remains in a constant state of physiological arousal (see the section on the autonomic nervous system later in this chapter).

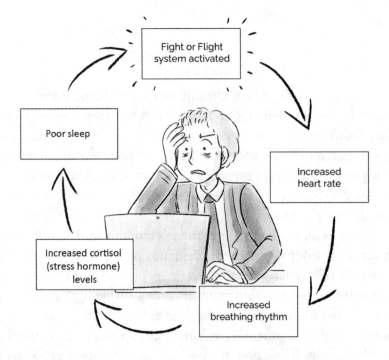

When symptoms of stress become persistent and affect daily functioning, it can have a detrimental impact on your health and well-being. Long-term activation of this stress response results in overexposure to cortisol and other stress hormones, affecting virtually every system in the body, either directly or indirectly. It increases inflammation, lowers immune defenses, and makes us more susceptible to a range of illnesses. Stress makes it hard for us to relax and can come with a range of emotions, including anxiety and irritability. What's more, prolonged exposure to stress results in elevated cortisol levels, disrupting the circadian rhythm and interrupting sleep onset and sleep duration.

Prolonged stress can also cause or exacerbate mental health conditions, most commonly anxiety and depression.[2] These conditions are very difficult to manage and address if sleep quality is poor.

But don't let this stress you out! There is much you can do to down-regulate your nervous system, shifting it away from stress and into a more relaxed state that is beneficial to sleep.

MODERN-DAY CULTURE AND TECHNOLOGY

Alongside chronic stress, today's culture brings many other barriers to attaining a restful night's sleep. The modern workday has increased time pressures. There's more shift work. Many businesses, such as supermarkets and airports, now operate 24/7. In Western society, sleep is often seen as non-essential, even perceived as a weakness.

Technological advancements, like computers, tablets, and smartphones, have brought undeniable benefits, enabling constant connectivity and information access around the clock. These tools have become indispensable for many. However, modern-day technology, particularly smartphones, has stolen our attention span and our time, often to the detriment of our well-being.

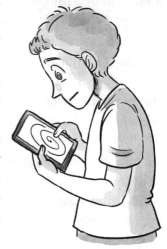

Fifty years ago, the information people consumed was limited, local, and curated by editors or broadcasters. A typical day might involve reading a single newspaper, watching a concise 30-minute evening news broadcast, or listening to the radio for updates. This information was finite, focused on key events or community news, and didn't demand constant engagement.

In contrast, today's information landscape is vast, global, and relentless. Within just one day, a person might scroll through hundreds of social media posts, receive breaking news alerts, watch countless YouTube videos, and engage with algorithm-driven content feeds pushing personalized updates. This deluge includes not only critical world events but also memes, opinion pieces, clickbait headlines, and ads—much of it engineered to provoke emotional reactions and keep users endlessly scrolling. The shift is not only in volume but also in intensity and immediacy. Where natural breaks once allowed the mind to rest, the endless stream of content now creates constant stimulation, leaving the brain hyper-engaged and unable to reset.

For many, checking their phone is the first and last action of the day, a habit that reflects how deeply digital engagement has become ingrained in daily life. Social media platforms, fueled by profit motives, invest heavily in capturing and holding our attention, leading to overstimulation, heightened stress, and disrupted sleep patterns. When we're tired, our ability to focus and make intentional decisions diminishes, making it easier to fall into the habit of mindless scrolling. Platforms offer quick dopamine hits that temporarily stimulate, which can feel especially appealing when energy is low. However, this overstimulation makes it harder to relax and fall asleep, creating a cycle of exhaustion.

This cycle often continues the next day, as tiredness further weakens self-control, making it more likely to reach for the phone again for mental escape. Over time, this loop disrupts sleep patterns even further, leaving many feeling trapped in a cycle of poor rest and overstimulation. Breaking this cycle starts with recognizing it and adopting intentional habits, such as setting boundaries for screen time and practicing relaxation techniques like breathing exercises. These small steps can help regain control, improve sleep, and reduce the stress caused by information overload.

Don't feel guilty about the time you've spent scrolling—we're all navigating an entirely new digital environment. None of us were prepared for the speed and intensity of today's digital world, and as parents, it's even harder to guide our children when we never experienced this ourselves. However, taking ownership of our attention is essential. It's a finite resource, and it's vital to focus on what truly matters—achieving goals, building relationships, and living a fulfilling life. Reflect on how you feel after scrolling: do you feel tense, tired, irritable, or guilty about wasted time?

THE AUTONOMIC NERVOUS SYSTEM

To understand the relationship between stress, sleep, and breathing, it helps to first get familiar with the autonomic nervous system, or ANS. This is the part of your nervous system that runs quietly in the background, taking care of all the things your body does automatically, like keeping your heart beating, your blood pressure steady, your temperature regulated, and of course, keeping you breathing.

Let's pause for a moment on the word "nervous." We use it all the time: "I'm nervous," "That gave me nerves," but it actually comes from the Latin word *nervus*, meaning sinew or tendon, something that binds or connects. Over time, it came to refer to the system of wiring that links the brain to the rest of the body. In modern use, we associate "nervous" with anxiety or tension, which makes perfect sense. When this system gets thrown out of balance, we feel it as restlessness, tension, or that familiar flutter in the stomach.

In this context, your nervous system is your body's internal communication network. It tells your body what to do in any situation, whether you're facing a real threat, dealing with stress, or lying in bed trying to fall asleep.

Breathing is one of the few bodily functions controlled by the autonomic nervous system that you can also influence voluntarily. That's what makes it such a powerful tool. By working with your breath, you can influence your internal state, calm the mind, and guide your body out of stress and into rest.

The autonomic nervous system has two main branches that are constantly working to maintain balance: the sympathetic and parasympathetic nervous systems. You can think of the sympathetic system as the gas pedal. It speeds things up. The parasympathetic system, on the other hand, is like the brake. It slows things down.

Sympathetic Nervous System: "Fight, Flight, or Freeze"

The sympathetic nervous system is associated with the "fight, flight, or freeze" stress response, which is activated when we are facing danger or feeling threatened, triggered, or stressed. This causes an instant, carefully orchestrated series of physiological and hormonal responses. It causes our hearts to beat faster, our breathing rate to increase, our muscles to contract, and our pupils to dilate; we begin to sweat, and we are more alert.

Triggered by hormones like epinephrine and cortisol, the sympathetic nervous system bolsters your ability to either fight your way out of a dangerous situation or run away from it. It is part of an ancient, innate survival mechanism. It gives you the necessary physical resources to keep you safe.

When the sympathetic nervous system is activated, the body also shuts down functions such as digestion to conserve energy and direct available resources for your body to use. Historically, our sympathetic response was typically only activated short term in the presence of predators, or other immediate danger.

Unfortunately, the accelerated pace of modern life and stressors like the endless news cycle, worries about climate change, war, finances, or maybe even unresolved trauma have caused many to live in a chronically elevated sympathetic "fight, flight, or freeze" state.[3] This has widespread consequences, not least for our sleep.

Sympathetic Nervous System Stress Response

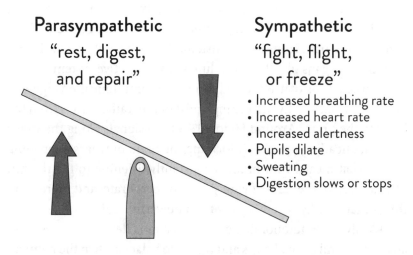

Parasympathetic "rest, digest, and repair"

Sympathetic "fight, flight, or freeze"
- Increased breathing rate
- Increased heart rate
- Increased alertness
- Pupils dilate
- Sweating
- Digestion slows or stops

Parasympathetic Nervous System: "Rest, Digest, and Repair"

The parasympathetic nervous system acts like the braking system and is associated with "rest, digest, and repair" responses. It counterbalances the "fight, flight, or freeze" response, causing our breathing and heart rates to slow and inducing more gentle and calm states, like relaxation, rest, recovery, and digestion.

Many of us find ourselves feeling stressed all too often, with our bodies always on high alert. That's why it's so important to learn how to apply the brakes and activate our built-in relaxation mode—the "rest, digest, and repair" state. One of the fastest and most effective ways to tap into this calming system? Your breath.

The Vagus Nerve and Heart Rate Variability

The *vagus nerve* plays a key role in your ability to relax by activating the parasympathetic nervous system, which helps bring the body into a calm, restful state. Today, the vagus nerve is widely recognized and often mentioned in healthcare and wellness conversations, but its story goes much further back. The word *vagus* comes from Latin, meaning "wandering," a fitting name for a nerve that travels a long and winding path from the brainstem, down through the neck, and into major organs like the heart, lungs, and digestive system.

You can think of it as the body's internal communication highway. But here's what's really interesting: most of the traffic travels from the body to the brain. Around 80 to 90% of the signals along the vagus nerve are heading upward, informing the brain of what's happening inside. That means your brain is constantly listening to the rhythm of your breath, the state of your gut, your heart rate, and more. And this is exactly why breathing is such a powerful tool.

Ideally, your autonomic nervous system is flexible and resilient, able to respond to challenges and return to balance when the moment has passed. Take a common situation; maybe you've had a disagreement with your boss. Your heart rate goes up, your breath quickens, and your body shifts into alert mode. That's your sympathetic nervous system stepping in to help you deal with the stress.

But what happens afterward is just as important. Can you recover quickly? Can you ramp down once the situation is over? This ability to bounce back and return to calm after stress is a sign of nervous system resilience.

In the corporate world, researchers often talk about grit; the ability to stay focused, handle setbacks, and keep going under pressure. But grit isn't just about pushing through. It's also about knowing how to reset, how to regulate yourself so you don't stay stuck in that heightened state for hours. That's where your breath comes in.

Over time, with experience and maybe a bit of age, we do tend to take things a little less personally. But breathing gives us a practical tool we can use right now. Do that for a minute or two, and you are basically telling your body, "Hey, it is okay now. The danger has passed." You give your nervous system permission to stand down. And that's real resilience; not just staying strong in the moment but knowing how to return to balance afterward.

These days, many people are wearing smartwatches and fitness trackers to keep an eye on their sleep, steps, and stress. One number that often pops up is heart rate variability, or HRV. It might sound technical, but it's actually a really useful window into how adaptable your nervous system is.

You've probably heard that a healthy resting heart rate is around sixty beats per minute, but that doesn't mean your heart is ticking along like a metronome, beating once every single second. In a healthy, resilient system, the time between each heartbeat varies slightly. One beat might land a fraction earlier, the next a bit later. That subtle flexibility is a good thing. It's a sign that your body can shift gears easily, speeding up when it needs to focus or deal with stress and slowing down when it's time to rest.

A high HRV is generally associated with better recovery, stronger emotional regulation, and improved sleep. It's one of the key indicators of a nervous system that is not stuck in high alert but rather able to adapt, respond, and reset. And just like with breath, you don't need to track every number to benefit from it.

You could even try this for yourself, even if you don't have a wearable device. Simply locate your pulse near your wrist crease. Now pay attention to your breathing and the speed of your heartbeat at the same time. What do you notice? As you breathe in, does your heart rate seem to pick up slightly? As you breathe out, does it slow down? This gentle rise and fall in rhythm is a good thing. It's your heart responding to the breath.

Now take it one step further. Begin slowing down the pace of your exhalation. Take a soft breath in through your nose, and then allow a long, relaxed breath out. As you do this, notice if your heartbeat slows even more on the exhale. That slowing is your vagus nerve kicking into gear. When stimulated, the vagus nerve releases acetylcholine, a chemical messenger that tells the heart to take it easy.

And the beautiful thing is, it doesn't take long. With specific breathing techniques, especially light, slow, and nasal breathing, you can begin to stimulate the vagus nerve in as little as 30 to 60 seconds. The effects might feel subtle at first; a softer heartbeat, a slight release of tension in the muscles, a gentle quieting of the mind, but they are real, and they build with regular practice.

This has been known since the early 1900s, when researchers stimulated a frog's vagus nerve and observed the heart rate slow down. They even gave it a name, vagusstuff.

So next time you have a run in with your boss or something else puts you on edge, you don't have to stay in that heightened state all day. Instead of overthinking what just happened, bring your attention to your breath. Slow down the exhalation. Let the body know the crisis has passed. This is how you ramp down. You'll feel better for it. Carrying that tension around with you all day doesn't help, and while it's not always easy to let go, it's still worth it. And here is something else to think about; why hand over so much of your emotional energy to your boss, or to anyone for that matter? Are they really worth that much of your headspace?

The vagus nerve plays a crucial role in promoting relaxation, deep sleep, and emotional balance by reducing the production of stress hormones like norepinephrine and cortisol (too much of which are detrimental to sleep) and boosting key neurotransmitters that regulate mood, stress, and sleep quality. By stimulating the vagus nerve, we can naturally increase the production of these neurotransmitters and improve overall mental and physical health.

Here are some examples of how key neurotransmitters influence well-being and sleep:

- **GABA: The brain's calming neurotransmitter.** You may think of GABA (gamma-aminobutyric acid) as your brain's built-in brake pedal—it helps slow things down when the mind is racing.[4] As the brain's primary calming neurotransmitter, GABA plays a key role in reducing stress, easing anxiety, and promoting deep sleep.[5]

When GABA levels are low, it's like your brain is stuck in overdrive—leading to stress, anxiety, and sleep problems like insomnia. Research indicates that individuals with insomnia often exhibit reduced GABA levels. One way to naturally boost GABA is by stimulating the vagus nerve,[6] helping to reduce overthinking, anxiety, and restlessness. Higher GABA levels make it easier to unwind, relax, and get deep, restorative sleep—in fact, many prescribed sleep medications work by enhancing GABA activity.

- **Acetylcholine: The relaxation booster.** Acetylcholine is a neurotransmitter that slows heart rate, reduces stress, and promotes relaxation. When the vagus nerve is activated, it releases acetylcholine, which signals the body to relax and recover.[7]
- **Serotonin: The happiness and sleep regulator.** Serotonin is essential for mood stability, relaxation, and sleep. During the day, your body produces serotonin, which boosts mood, energy, and alertness. As it gets dark, serotonin is converted into *melatonin*, the "sleep hormone," signaling the body that it's time to sleep.[8] This delicate balance between serotonin and melatonin is crucial for maintaining a healthy sleep-wake cycle. Individuals with insomnia tend to have lower levels of serotonin. It is also thought that serotonin is involved in the development and progression of obstructive sleep apnea.[9]

Exposure to natural sunlight during the day can help *increase* serotonin production and regulate the sleep-wake cycle, as can practicing stress-reduction techniques such as deep breathing exercises (like the *Breathe Deep Exercise*), meditation, or yoga.[10] Around 90% of serotonin is produced in the gut, and the vagus nerve helps regulate its production and transport to the brain.

The best part? By stimulating the vagus nerve through practices like the breathing exercises and relaxation techniques in Chapter 1, you can enhance HRV and improve both sleep and overall well-being.

A Framework to Gauge Your Stress Levels

Even if you don't have a wearable device, you can still get a good sense of how your body is doing. Just pay attention to how you sleep and how you feel during the day. Are you waking up feeling rested, or do you feel like you've barely slept? Do you feel calm and clear-headed, or tense and wired for no reason? These are simple but powerful clues. Using a framework inspired by the Combat and Operational Stress Code (COSC)—green, yellow, orange, and red—you can identify where you stand in terms of stress and its impact on your sleep.[11]

Originally developed by the US military, the COSC framework was designed to help soldiers recognize and manage stress in high pressure environments. What's striking about this is that it was created for people who are specifically trained for stress. These are individuals who are physically fit, mentally prepared, and conditioned for extreme situations. And yet, even in that world, there was a clear need for a system to help them identify when stress was beginning to take a toll.

It makes you pause and reflect. If highly trained soldiers need a framework to understand whether or not they're under stress, what about the rest of us? Stress isn't always obvious. We might be living with constant tension, struggling to sleep, feeling irritable, or stuck in brain fog and assume that's just how life is. But is it?

That's the strength of a framework like COSC. It gives us a way to step back and ask, "Where am I right now?" instead of blindly pushing through or waiting for something to break. Pushing through might be common, but it's not always wise. Often, we don't realize how much we're carrying until we pause and check in.

What stood out to me most about the COSC model is the quiet reminder that none of us are invincible. We're human. And with that comes vulnerability; not as a weakness, but as a truth. Stress builds up in all of us, no matter how strong, young, or resilient we may appear.

The COSC framework helps service members recognize their stress levels, ranging from "green" (ready and well) to "red" (high stress or crisis), and implement strategies to maintain readiness and mental health. This color-coded system is widely used in military and high-stress operational contexts to promote resilience and prevent long-term psychological harm. Adapting this framework to everyday life, especially in the context of sleep, can help individuals better understand their stress levels and take actionable steps to improve both sleep quality and overall well-being.

Combat and Operational Stress Code Framework	
Green Zone: Rest and Recovery	In the green zone, your autonomic nervous system is balanced, with the parasympathetic branch ("rest, digest, and repair") dominating. This state is characterized by restful, restorative sleep. You wake up feeling refreshed, energized, and ready to face the day. Breathing during sleep is quiet and rhythmic, without snoring or interruptions. Falling asleep and staying asleep comes naturally, and you experience little-to-no tension in your body.
Yellow Zone: Mild Stress	The yellow zone indicates mild activation of the sympathetic nervous system, which can interfere with sleep quality. Symptoms might include occasional difficulty falling asleep or waking up during the night. You may notice light snoring or a feeling of tension in your jaw or shoulders upon waking. Sleep might feel less restorative, leaving you slightly groggy or irritable during the day. These signs suggest that stress is starting to affect your sleep, even if it hasn't yet caused significant disruption.
Orange Zone: Moderate Stress	In the orange zone, the sympathetic nervous system ("fight, flight, or freeze") is in overdrive, leading to noticeable sleep disturbances. Insomnia—difficulty falling asleep, staying asleep, or waking too early—is common at this stage. Snoring may intensify, and you might experience symptoms of obstructive sleep apnea, such as gasping for air or waking up with a dry mouth. You could also find yourself feeling fatigued throughout the day, struggling to concentrate, or experiencing heightened emotional sensitivity. These symptoms indicate that stress is significantly impacting your sleep and overall health.

(continued on next page)

Combat and Operational Stress Code Framework	
Red Zone: High Stress or Crisis	The red zone signals a state of high stress or crisis, where the sympathetic nervous system dominates entirely. This level of stress often manifests as chronic insomnia, severe sleep apnea, or restless nights punctuated by frequent awakenings. You may feel perpetually exhausted, even after spending hours in bed, and experience significant daytime impairments, such as extreme fatigue, brain fog, or emotional instability. Physical symptoms like increased heart rate, chest tightness, or persistent headaches may also accompany disrupted sleep. At this stage, stress is taking a serious toll on your sleep and well-being, and immediate action is needed.

Recognizing and Responding to Your Stress Level

Understanding where you are in this framework can help you take proactive steps to restore balance. If you're in the green or yellow zones, simple lifestyle changes like mindfulness practices, regular exercise, or nasal breathing may help you return to restorative sleep. For those in the orange or red zones, addressing stress with targeted interventions—such as cognitive behavioral therapy, breathing exercises to activate the parasympathetic system, or medical evaluation for sleep apnea—is crucial.

By tuning into your symptoms and how your body responds during sleep, you can identify and address stress before it escalates, promoting better sleep and overall health.

It almost goes without saying that the "rest, digest, and repair" mode is more conducive to achieving a restful night's sleep. *Slow breathing* is one of the most studied breath practices, and various studies have emphasized the importance of slow breathing as an effective tool in stimulating the vagus nerve and regulating the autonomic nervous system.[12]

For example, a 2023 systematic review (a summary of existing high-quality research) of 12 randomized controlled studies concluded that breathwork may be effective for improving stress and mental health by managing several psychophysiological functions.[13] Studies included in the review found that participants who had engaged in breathwork (including slow, paced breathing) had significantly *lower levels of stress* than control participants, along with *lower self-reported anxiety and depressive symptoms*. The authors noted that people with stress and anxiety disorders tend to chronically breathe faster and more erratically; yet with increased breathwork practice, respiration rate can become gradually slower, translating into better health and mood, along with less autonomic activity.

> "[I am] **sleeping much better** and waking up rested with mouth tape. I used to wake up feeling physically tense and anxious. **The first time I used mouth tape I woke up feeling like a puddle of relaxation.** I've been hooked ever since!
>
> These exercises have almost completely **stopped my snoring** . . . I have archived this in around 3–4 weeks of daily breathing exercises; I feel more **relaxed and less stressed** during the day, and I noticed I can stay calmer if I focus on nasal breathing."
>
> *Stefano, 52, UK*

Association Between Dysfunctional Breathing, Poor Sleep, and Mental Health

Sleep, mental health, and breathing are intrinsically connected, and dysfunctional breathing is common to both sleep disorders and many mental health conditions.

There is a bidirectional relationship between breathing and emotions. When we feel stressed or anxious, breathing becomes faster, harder, irregular, and predominantly limited to the upper chest. When breathing is dysfunctional, you're more likely to experience anxiety, panic attacks, and chronic stress.[14-16]

There is also a bidirectional relationship between breathing and sleep. When breathing is a little faster, harder, into the upper chest, or through an open mouth, sleep quality and quantity will suffer, while a bad night's sleep will leave you anxious, stressed, and dehydrated, perpetuating dysfunctional breathing.[17]

Sleep problems are more common in individuals with mental health conditions such as depression and anxiety, while many mental health conditions are exacerbated by poor sleep. The co-occurrence of sleep disorders and mental health disorders is well documented, with studies showing prevalence rates ranging from *40–80%*, depending on the specific mental health issue, population, and diagnostic criteria.[18,19] It's important that mental health professionals consider the often-overlooked association between sleep, breathing, and mental health, given their role in perpetuating mental health conditions and their therapeutic potential.

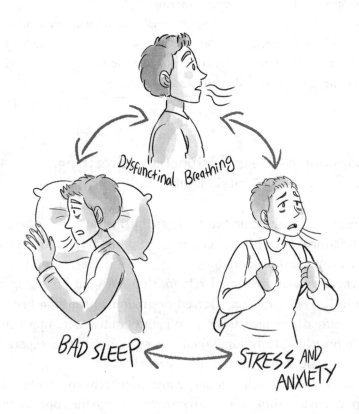

The autonomic nervous system is integral to mood and emotional regulation and also sleep initiation, maintenance, and disruption.[20] "Hyperarousal" is a term that refers to a state of heightened physiological and psychological alertness, where the body's stress response is activated even in the absence of immediate danger. It is often characterized by an overactive sympathetic nervous system, which is responsible for the "fight, flight, or freeze" response. In hyperarousal, the body remains in a state of increased vigilance, with elevated levels of stress hormones like norepinephrine and cortisol, even during periods when relaxation or rest should occur, such as sleep.

> "Since I started Buteyko breathing, life became much easier and effortless. Using techniques during exercise, during the day, and at night has been great for my health. Anxiety is now super low, stress management is great. Digestion became much better. Having the tools to be able to let my body rest changed my life.
>
> I was stressed my whole life, but I did not notice. My sleep was giving me the sign of that. Then I discovered breathing and took the time to work on nervous system balance and show my body what is resting. Buteyko Breathing was my entry point to start restoring my body's health."
>
> *André, 24, Portugal*

Hyperarousal is common in individuals with sleep disorders like *insomnia*, as well as post-traumatic stress disorder (PTSD), anxiety disorders, and other stress-related conditions. Hyperarousal is often linked to sleep disorders because it prevents the body from achieving the relaxed state needed for deep, restorative sleep. Research shows that slow, controlled breathing is linked to reduced respiratory rates along with reduced autonomic reactivity, distress, and pain.[21-23]

Practices to Regulate the Nervous System, Manage Stress, and Promote Relaxation

As we have learned, disrupted sleep is linked to *heightened activity of the sympathetic nervous system and underactivity of the parasympathetic nervous system.*[24] Your breath serves as a direct gateway to your nervous system, allowing you to influence internal states by maintaining a balance between the parasympathetic and sympathetic systems.[25] Light, slow, diaphragmatic breathing stimulates the vagus nerve, which regulates vital functions like digestion, heart rate, and respiration. During exhalation, the vagus nerve releases acetylcholine, a neurotransmitter that dilates blood vessels and slows the heart rate. Research shows that slow breathing activates the parasympathetic nervous system and enhances comfort, relaxation, and HRV, while reducing symptoms of stress, anxiety, panic, depression, and anger.[26–29]

I have compiled a library of guided audios for breathing exercises you can use to help regulate your nervous system and promote a sense of calm and relaxation:

- *Practice Breathing to Activate Relaxation* (Chapter 1).
- Practice *Breathe Slow* (Chapter 1).
- Practice *Breathe Light* by listening to the 20-minute *Relaxation and Recovery Guided Audio* spoken by Patrick McKeown (download using the QR code).
- *Hum* for one-to-two minutes, five times throughout the day. A great place to hum is in the shower! Humming promotes slower breathing and extended exhalations, stimulating the vagus nerve and shifting us into a parasympathetic "rest, digest, and repair" state.

SIMON'S STORY: FROM INSOMNIA, STRESS, AND ANXIETY TO RESTFUL SLEEP AND NERVOUS SYSTEM REGULATION

Simon, a 53-year-old from Wellington, New Zealand, spent decades grappling with chronic insomnia, anxiety, and panic attacks. He was a lawyer and the high-stress environment of his job exacerbated his struggles, ultimately forcing him to leave his full-time career over a decade ago.

Simon's challenges with sleep began over 20 years ago. Chronic mouth breathing and waking multiple times a night, often with a racing mind, left him exhausted. His anxiety about sleep itself created a vicious cycle: sleepless nights led to heightened anxiety, and heightened anxiety fueled sleepless nights. The effects seeped into his days, manifesting as fatigue, reduced focus, and, eventually, severe anxiety and panic attacks.

"With fatigue, I think you just push through. You're so busy at work. I was in high levels of urgency. . . . It's not until you actually stop that the wheels come off. And eventually, your brain says 'I'm not doing this anymore.'"

This breaking point led to a forced pause—a retreat from his demanding career.

It wasn't until late 2024 that Simon began to seriously explore how breathing could transform his sleep and regulate his nervous system. A chance encounter at a yoga retreat introduced him to James Nestor's book *Breathe*, which opened the door to Patrick McKeown's Oxygen Advantage® techniques. Intrigued, Simon started using tools like mouth taping and breathing exercises. He noticed immediate and significant changes in his sleep and overall well-being.

"I started using MyoTape and a nasal dilator at nighttime. There was a big change. I was going to sleep more quickly and stopped waking up in the night. My sleep became deeper, and I felt more rested in the morning. I also noticed my daytime fatigue disappearing—I wasn't needing afternoon naps anymore."

Simon began tracking his progress using a Fitbit, which confirmed the improvements. *His sleep scores jumped from the low 70s to the mid-to-high 80s within weeks.*

Simon's scores also revealed longer sleep duration (more overall time spent sleeping each night). And another benefit— more time spent in deep and REM sleep translated to waking up feeling more refreshed and emotionally balanced.

Simon's Sleep Data Before and After Mouth Taping and Breathing

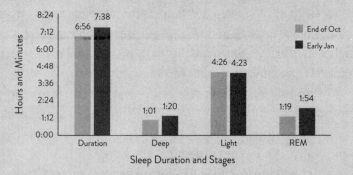

The Breath: A Gateway to a Regulated Nervous System

By practicing nasal breathing, slowing down his breath to breathe less air, and incorporating light breath holds, Simon had the tools to calm his mind, reduce anxiety and reactivity in stressful situations, and shift into parasympathetic "rest, digest, and repair" mode.

"I've learned to recognize when stress creeps in," Simon explains. "Instead of letting it take over, I pause and focus on my breathing. I ask myself, 'What can I adjust? Do I need to slow my breath? Should I do a recovery breath? Maybe light breathing?'"

"I'm now thinking I can take on a little bit more work because I'm able to self-regulate more efficiently than I did. My partner says I'm much more focused and calm than I used to be."

Simon has also encouraged his 17-year-old twins to adopt better breathing habits. His daughter, who has autism and experiences high levels of anxiety, has found relief through breathing exercises.

"When she's really on edge, or teary, I encourage her to focus on nasal breathing or do recovery breaths," Simon says. "She does chill out. Breathing exercises just down-regulate her nervous system quite well. It's amazing how quickly it helps her calm down."

Spreading the Message

Simon's experience has inspired him to help others, particularly young people, navigate the pressures of modern life.

"I've got a real interest in breathing and mental health because of what I've been through. Who would want to grow up in the world at the moment with technology and all the political stuff that's going down, you know? It's no wonder young people are stressed out of their trees!"

As a certified Oxygen Advantage® Instructor, he's now passionate about teaching children and teens how breathing can bring balance to their nervous systems and transform their mental health.

"We never learned these tools growing up, but they're life-changing."

CHAPTER 8

A PERSONAL REFLECTION ON MANAGING AN OVERSTIMULATED MIND

Ever find yourself waking up at 3 a.m. with your mind running in circles? You're not quite awake enough to get up and start your day, but you're also not sleepy enough to drift back to sleep. It's almost as if you're stuck in limbo—just lying there while your brain decides it's the perfect time to go over every little detail of your life.

So many people struggle with sleep, whether it's trouble falling asleep, waking up in the middle of the night, or rising too early. But we rarely stop to consider what's actually keeping us awake. More often than not, the real culprit isn't the body—it's the mind.

You're lying in bed, wrapped up in a cozy duvet. It's dark, quiet, and safe. Everything *should* be perfect for sleep. And yet the mind won't switch off. Nighttime—when there are no distractions—is when the brain loves to replay every conversation, worry about things that haven't happened yet, or remind you of something embarrassing you did 10 years ago.

Of course, poor sleep doesn't just affect the night—it spills over into the next day. We wake up feeling groggy, more stressed, and less focused. We're more likely to overthink during the day, and that same restless thinking follows us right back to bed at night. And so, the cycle continues.

If you see your doctor because you're struggling to sleep, there's a good chance you'll leave with a prescription for sleeping pills. In 2020, the National Center for Health Statistics found that 8.4% of adults in the United States took sleep medication most nights to help them fall or stay asleep.[1] Women were more likely than men to rely on sleep aids—10.2% compared with 6.6%. And as people got older, their use of sleep medication increased. Interestingly, among men, those with the highest incomes were the least likely to take sleep meds compared with those in middle- or lower-income groups.

These numbers paint a clear picture: millions of people are struggling with sleep, and for many, the solution is a pill rather than addressing the root cause. But what if there was another way?

Many sleeping pills, like Xanax, Valium, and Ambien, work by boosting GABA (gamma-aminobutyric acid), a calming neurotransmitter. GABA *slows brain activity*, reduces stress and anxiety, and promotes relaxation, making it easier to drift off to sleep. Essentially, these pills work by slowing down thinking and calming the mind. No matter how you look at it, the inability to switch off the mind seems to be at the core of sleep struggles.

So, wouldn't it make sense to learn how to quiet the mind and slow down thinking *without* relying on pills or anything else? Once you develop these skills, they don't just help you sleep—they improve your entire day. These tools have no side effects, they are completely free, and they don't leave you feeling groggy the next day. In fact, they do the opposite. They sharpen focus, enhance concentration, and help you stay present in whatever you're doing.

Thinking is a lot like breathing or even eating. It's essential, but too much of it can become a problem. A busy mind during the day doesn't suddenly switch off when it's time to sleep. If we spend our waking hours caught up in thought, it's no surprise that our brains keep racing at night.

We've all been there, lying in bed, staring at the ceiling, wishing we could just *turn off* our thoughts. But is it possible to choose *when to think* and *when to quiet the mind*? Can we actually learn how to stop overthinking? And if so, what steps can we take to make that happen?

The good news is, we *can* train the mind to slow down. We can reduce thought activity and create more space between thoughts. This isn't about trying to force thinking to stop; that's not possible. Instead, it's about allowing the mind to settle. And the more we integrate this into our daily life, the more natural it becomes until quieting the mind feels just as effortless as thinking.

Overthinking doesn't just keep our minds busy—it creates a cycle where our thoughts fuel our emotions, and our emotions fuel our thoughts. This loop can spill into every part of our lives, making it nearly impossible to switch off and truly rest.

Your brain doesn't distinguish between real and imagined threats. It reacts to stressful thoughts the same way it would to actual danger. If you're constantly playing out "what if" scenarios or going over past conversations in your head, your nervous system stays on high alert, as if something urgent is always just around the corner. Stress and overthinking don't just affect the mind—they subtly change the way we *breathe*. Without realizing it, our breath becomes faster and shallower and moves into the upper chest. Sometimes, we even hold our breath or sigh more often. You might notice this while reading emails, scrolling through your phone, or trying to get through a long to-do list. Holding our breath could be linked to an evolutionary trait. It would make sense that if a predator were lurking nearby, we'd instinctively stop breathing to avoid making a sound that could give us away. In that context, holding our breath was a survival mechanism—one that might have saved our ancestors' lives.

But in today's world, there are no predators hiding in the bushes while we type. The threats we react to are often just deadlines, notifications, or an overwhelming to-do list. Yet our body still responds the same way, momentarily pausing our breath as if danger were near. And when this becomes our default pattern, repeated in small moments throughout the day, it builds tension in the body and tells the brain to stay on edge.

When this pattern happens over and over throughout the day, it sends a signal to the brain that something is wrong. And when the brain gets that message, it shifts into high alert—activating the "fight, flight, or freeze" response. On the surface, the solution seems obvious—just stop overthinking. But the real challenge is that most of us don't even *realize* how much time we spend lost in thought. The mind wanders automatically, pulling us into worries, past regrets, and imagined scenarios.

So, how do we break this cycle? How do we stop overthinking and quiet the mind?

It starts with paying attention to both our thoughts and our breath. Noticing when we've slipped into overthinking. Recognizing when our breathing has become shallow or tense. You don't need to control your thoughts; you just need to notice when you're caught in them. The moment we catch ourselves in that pattern, we have a choice: stay stuck in it or shift out of it.

We'll explore this in more detail later, but for now, a simple way to signal to the brain that the body is safe is by slowing the breath, especially the exhale. This sends a clear message: *everything is okay.* And when the brain gets that signal, it stops sounding the alarm. The body relaxes, the mind settles, and sleep comes much more easily.

THE EDUCATION OF THE FUTURE

For a species as intelligent as we claim to be, it is surprising and maybe even a little baffling that we are not able to stop thinking. We have sent people to the moon, mapped the human genome, and created artificial intelligence. Yet when it comes to something as personal and fundamental as quieting the mind, we still haven't quite figured it out. Yes, mindfulness and breathing are becoming more common in certain circles, but they're far from mainstream. For most people, they're still unfamiliar or feel out of reach, more like something "other people do" than everyday tools for managing stress and settling the mind.

The ability to manage the mind, to consciously direct our attention rather than being hijacked by an endless stream of thoughts, is one of the most valuable skills we could ever develop. It shapes everything— our creativity, productivity, success, and, most importantly, our happiness. If our minds are always somewhere else, how can we give our full attention to what matters most? How can we do our best work, enjoy an experience, or really connect with the people around us when we're caught up in thoughts that have nothing to do with the moment we're in?

We train our bodies, pursue careers, and acquire knowledge, but we rarely take the time to develop the one ability that affects every aspect of our life experience: the ability to control what goes on in the head.

From an early age, we are taught to plan ahead, focus on the future, and keep moving forward. There is pressure to get good grades, choose the right career, find a partner, buy a house, and settle down. Life becomes a checklist of milestones we are expected to reach. And while having goals is important, constantly chasing what's next can trap us in a loop of thinking, worrying, planning, and predicting, without much space to just be where we are.

When we are young, the mind is locked onto the future. But as we grow older and realize there is less future ahead, our focus shifts. Instead of looking forward, we start looking back, replaying old events, analyzing what was, what could have been, and what we might have done differently.

Setting goals and working toward something meaningful is an essential part of life. There is something deeply fulfilling about developing our skills, using our natural talents, and making progress toward something that excites us. But here's the catch; it only really works when our attention is in the doing, not just fixated on the outcome. If we are too focused on the finish line, we miss the process. And the process is where life actually unfolds. It's like the saying commonly attributed to philosopher and transcendentalist Ralph Waldo Emerson, "Life is a journey, not a destination."

Like many people who went through Western education, I have often wondered why there was so little discussion about what was actually happening in the mind. Of course, thinking is what makes us uniquely human. The front part of the brain, the prefrontal cortex is where conscious thought, decision making, and planning take place. Thinking is essential. It helps us choose a direction, solve problems, and reflect. But in reality, productive thinking only occupies a small portion of our day.

There's a time to think but there's also a time to stop thinking.

Why weren't we taught how to recognize when thinking becomes unhelpful? Or given tools to slow it down? These are the very skills that shape our ability to concentrate. Our capacity to direct and sustain attention—whether on a task, an event, or a conversation—is what allows real learning to take place. Beyond learning, having control over the mind helps us make better decisions. Trying to solve a problem while the mind is racing from thought to thought is far from easy. We cannot focus when the mind is overloaded with thoughts. To really concentrate, to stay present, work through a challenge, or connect with another person, we need space in the mind. Not more noise. Not more thinking. Just space. Either we are fully immersed in what we are doing, or the mind is elsewhere. When the mind drifts away and loses touch with the task at hand, that is the essence of poor concentration.

Yet instead of being taught how to regulate our thoughts so we could focus, think clearly, and engage fully with the present, we were mostly taught to memorize, recite, and regurgitate information. Of course, I do not blame teachers. They have a curriculum to follow, and I am sure any teacher who tried to incorporate breathing re-education, mindfulness, or self-regulation techniques would likely be seen as unconventional, maybe even brushed off by their peers. But isn't that the very conversation we should be having? Is our current education system truly serving children, teenagers, and young adults? Is it equipping them with the life skills they need to reach their full potential and lead happy, fulfilling lives?

It is hard to argue that we are preparing young people well when mental health issues among them are at an all-time high. At its core, a lot of this comes down to one simple challenge: not knowing how to quieten the mind. Even if the goal were purely productivity, we're still missing the mark. Because concentration depends on managing your mind; on being able to place your attention where you want it, instead of being pulled into the same loops of worry, regret, and distraction. And here's the ripple effect, when we build the capacity to concentrate, we're also building the capacity to take charge of our mental health. To me, that seems obvious. Why wouldn't we be teaching that from the start?

And I get it. Teaching these techniques to teenagers might be met with some serious eye rolls and dramatic sighs. But isn't that the case with most things we learn in school? How many of us sat through algebra wondering, "When will I ever use this?"—only to later find ourselves trying to split a dinner bill or figure out a mortgage payment. Or dismissed history, only to realize later that understanding the past might actually help us make sense of the present. Some lessons don't seem important until years down the line. It's not just what we teach, it's how we teach it. If breathing, focus, and emotional regulation were just another part of the school day, like math or history, imagine the difference that could make. If these tools were introduced in a way that made sense to students, something that actually clicked with their experience, they might not just listen. They might use them.

A simple breathing practice might not seem like a big deal at first, but over time, it could become a tool for life; something a young person turns to in moments of stress, panic, or overwhelm. Imagine a life where everything feels a little softer, a little less overwhelming, where sleeping pills and other coping mechanisms aren't the default solution. That's a return on investment that's hard to ignore. And even if the message doesn't land the first time, I don't believe it's wasted. Sometimes a lesson has to be heard a few times, from different angles, before it really sinks in. But when it does, it can change everything.

Awareness is growing. More and more people are realizing that we don't have to live stuck in our heads. And once these ideas get repeated often enough, they stop feeling new. They start to feel normal. I spent thirteen years in formal education, and in all that time, only one teacher ever led us through a short meditation session. His nickname was "Hippy," which pretty much sums up how we saw him. He had a scruffy gray beard, had long hair tied back in a ponytail, and wore the same oversized woolen jumper every day—complete with holes in the elbows.

I went to a school run by the Christian Brothers, and beneath the surface, they couldn't stand him. Hippy didn't exactly fit their standards. He was a constant thorn in their side. They couldn't fire him because he was employed by the state, but if they had their way, he'd have been marched straight out the front gates, jumper and all.

I still remember that session clearly. He guided us to shift our focus away from our thoughts and onto our breath. It was so different from anything else we had ever been taught. Like most teenagers, I thought it was a bit "out there." We all did. But the fact that I still remember it all these years later says something. Maybe, without realizing it, he planted a seed. One that took years to grow but, in some way, shaped the path that led me here today.

And now I wonder. Did he have any idea of the impact that one session might have had?

In my late teens and early twenties, I was really into self-help books. I read all the big names at the time, Richard Branson, Tony Robbins, and the classics like Napoleon Hill. They all preached the same message: if you want to be successful, you need to write down your goals. Have a clear vision of where you want to go in life and go after it with everything you have.

So, like a good student of self-improvement, I made my own list. I wrote down everything I wanted to achieve over the next five years.

That list? I have no idea where it is now. It is probably scribbled on the back page of an old self-help book. But if I had to guess, my goals were probably the same as yours—getting into university, finding work I loved, meeting a wonderful partner, having a comfortable home, being financially secure, and living without the constant stress of not having enough.

One of my biggest goals was to go to university. This meant even more to me because I had originally left school for good at 14, right after my Inter Certificate state exam (now the Junior Certificate). Earning a degree felt like such an important milestone that I sacrificed three years to get to university and another four years at university to achieve that one goal.

And by sacrifice, I don't just mean the hours spent studying. No, what I really mean is that I was always racing toward the future. My attention was almost entirely fixed on what was ahead. The present moment barely got a look in, except for the odd moment when I was pulled back briefly, before drifting off again. I was here, but I wanted to be there—at the finish line, holding that piece of paper in my hand. I had reduced my entire time to getting to the future, as if happiness and success only existed at the end of those four years. And yet, when I finally got the piece of paper, I wasn't sure I felt the happiness I had expected. I remember feeling strangely empty. This was something I had worked so hard for, something that had felt so important to me, and yet it didn't bring the joy or celebration I had imagined. I didn't even feel relief.

In truth, I'm not sure what I felt. Maybe it was the result of spending four years with my attention fixed entirely on the end goal—caught up in the pressure, the anticipation, the belief that once I got *there*, everything would fall into place. And when I finally arrived, I was left wondering, "Is this it?"

So, I set my next goal—get a job. I sent out my CV and landed a position with a multinational car rental company. And if I'm being completely honest, I hated working there. There were monthly targets. Managers were constantly compared with each other.

And my job? I was a branch manager of the branch in Galway, Ireland, where part of our role was upselling collision damage waiver insurance to customers, even though most of them already had coverage through their own insurance. In other words, we were selling peace of mind . . . twice.

But that didn't matter. It was good for the company. I don't place all the blame on the job, though. What about me? I was running on poor sleep. I couldn't handle stress well. On the outside, I might have looked calm, but inside, my mind was constantly churning. I was stuck in my head, trapped in an endless cycle of overthinking.

Life feels so much harder when you have no control over the mind, especially when you don't realize how much your own thoughts are making things worse. Overthinking amplifies problems, drains your energy, and turns everyday challenges into something far more overwhelming than they need to be. And at the time, I had no idea how to stop it.

Ironically, when I stopped fixating on the future, when I brought my attention to my breath and started paying attention to the present moment instead of getting lost in thought, everything started to fall into place, with much less effort. I became more successful, more productive, and, strangely enough, I ended up achieving every goal I had set for myself in my early twenties.

Even finding a job that I loved was unexpected, especially considering that my degree had absolutely nothing to do with breathing or experiencing how to get out of my own head. But here I am, enjoying a topic that fascinates me so much that I read about it in my free time—not because I *have* to, but because I *genuinely* want to.

And lucky for me, it also happens to fit my skill set. Lucky for *you*, well . . . you're now reading this book about sleep, so I hope that works out for both of us.

It felt like the more I stopped forcing things and started paying attention to my breath, to my thoughts, to how I actually felt, the more things started to click into place. Or maybe there is something bigger at play. When the struggle in the mind stops, life itself seems to step in and help. I do not know for sure. But here is what I do know: if you want to achieve your goals, do not spend all your time living in your head.

I hope this chapter does not come across as being all about me. I just find it easier to talk about overthinking through my own experience. I was lucky to discover the power of breathing in my mid-twenties. Before that, I spent the first 20-plus years of my life completely stuck in my head, lost in constant thinking. But over the past 25 years, something changed. My thought activity has reduced by about 30 to 40%. And it is not just about learning to direct my attention more effectively. The sheer volume of thoughts running through my mind has significantly decreased. I am no longer trapped in a cycle of analyzing everything or overthinking every little detail. And that shift has made all the difference.

Now, I check in with my thoughts regularly. Throughout the day, I make a habit of shifting my attention out of my head and onto my breath, into my body, or simply into what is happening around me. And I can honestly say this one shift has had the biggest impact on my life. If I had to choose between this ability to influence my own state of mind or the master's degree I worked so hard for, I would choose this without hesitation.

That is why I want to share these tools with you. These are the same practices I use every day, the same ones I bring into my talks and client sessions. Breathing, sleep, and the state of mind are deeply connected, and you cannot separate one from the other. If the mind is unsettled, sleep suffers. If sleep is disrupted, the mind is affected. That is why this chapter belongs in this book—because sleep and the mind go hand in hand.

Step One: Check In with Your Thinking

The first step is simply checking in with what's going on in your head. It means taking a step back and observing your thoughts. Take a moment, pause, and ask yourself: "What am I thinking about right now? Is it useful, or is it just mental noise?"

So much of our thinking happens on autopilot. We don't even realize how much unnecessary thought is running in the background, shaping our emotions, stress levels, and even our ability to rest. Getting lost in thought is a habit, and the real problem is *overthinking*.

Maybe you recognize some of these patterns:

- **Worrying about the future.** "What if this goes wrong? What if I fail?"
- **Replaying the past.** "I should have said this. Why did I do that?"
- **Self-criticism.** "I'm not good enough. I should be doing more."
- **Imaginary arguments.** "If they say this, I'll say that."
- **Comparing yourself with others.** "They have it all figured out. Why am I behind?"

Most of the time, we don't even *choose* these thoughts—they just show up. They pull us in, keeping the mind busy with things that often don't matter or don't need our attention. The problem isn't that we think; it's that we think too much. Thoughts that don't help, don't solve anything, and often just make us feel worse.

And here's the thing: overthinking can't be solved by more thinking. How could it?

You don't need to analyze your thoughts or figure out why they're there. This isn't about thinking about your thinking or piling more thoughts on top of thoughts. Instead, it's about simply noticing what's happening in the mind. Even when your thoughts feel heavy and you're feeling low, just checking in with what you're thinking can be helpful. That simple act gives you a choice. Now, you can see the source of how you feel, step back, disengage from unhelpful thoughts, and begin shifting toward a quieter, clearer state of mind.

The Mind as a Garden
A few years ago, I bought an old house in Connemara, a breathtaking yet wild part of the West of Ireland. The house had been abandoned for decades, and when I arrived, the garden was completely overgrown.

The weeds had taken over to the point where I couldn't even tell where the garden began or ended.

I can only imagine how beautiful it must have been, tall trees, lush green lawns, and patches of colorful roses, all framed by old stone walls and little winding paths inviting you to wander through it all. My neighbors told me that for over 70 years, the garden had been lovingly cared for. But when the last owner grew old and passed away, no one was left to tend to it. The house was abandoned, and the garden was left to grow wild. No one pulled the weeds, watered the flowers, or planted anything new. It didn't take long for nature to take over completely. That's why a gardener must check in regularly—to spot the weeds as soon as they appear, pull them out before they spread, and tend to the soil to make space for new growth.

After all, when the weeds take over, there's no room for the flowers to bloom. And the mind works in much the same way. We need to be gardeners of the mind.

Our thoughts shape our happiness, our stress, and our entire experience of life. If we let negative, anxious, or repetitive thoughts run wild, how can we expect to feel at peace? How can we be happy if we are constantly in a state of worry? Even reducing worrying thoughts by just 10% creates space for more contentment. Just like a garden, the mind needs tending.

We need to notice when the weeds start creeping in, when our thoughts become unhelpful or overwhelming. Instead of feeding them with more stress and worry, we can shift our attention away from the mind and into the body, breaking the cycle before those thoughts take root.

And here is the thing. When weeds are not fed, they die. And when they die, the flowers have room to grow again. But if we don't take the time to check in with what's going on in the mind, negativity and worry can quietly take over. And before we realize it, the weeds have spread so much that we forget there was ever a garden underneath.

Step Two: What Effect Does Your Thinking Have on You?

Paying attention to what we are thinking about is one thing, but recognizing how those thoughts are affecting us takes it to the next level. Noticing the impact of our thought activity gives us a deeper awareness and, in many ways, the motivation to make a change.

Overthinking can leave you feeling tense, drained, or even physically exhausted. It is easy to forget that thinking is hard work. It drains mental energy, often without solving anything. When your head feels heavy, it is usually a sign that your thoughts have spiraled out of control. And it is not the productive, useful thoughts that do this—it is the repetitive, pointless ones that serve no real purpose. Simply understanding this gives us an incentive to do something about it.

How you think affects how you feel. How you feel affects how you think. You've probably had those moments when you suddenly catch yourself, realizing just how much your mind has been weighing you down. When that happens, you have no choice but to begin taming it. By simply observing your thoughts throughout the day, even for brief moments, you begin to notice their effect. You may realize that instead of helping you solve problems, your thoughts might actually be making things worse.

Step Three: Get Out of Your Head

At any given moment, you have two choices: you're either lost in your thoughts or fully present. When you're stuck in your head, that becomes your world; a constant loop of worry, distraction, or replaying moments that have already passed. But when your attention shifts to your breath, your body, or the world around you, you step out of that mental fog and into the present moment. The key isn't just catching brief glimpses of presence; it's learning to expand those moments so they happen more often and more intentionally.

The old story of wanting to see the bottom of a bucket filled with muddy water perfectly illustrates the problem with overthinking. The more you stir, the murkier the water becomes. No matter how hard you try, the cloudiness remains, keeping the bottom out of sight.

But if you stop stirring and give it time to settle, the mud sinks on its own, and the water clears—revealing what was there all along. It's the same with the mind. When we stop overthinking, even briefly, the noise quietens and a kind of natural clarity begins to surface.

Alan Watts was a British philosopher, writer, and speaker best known for popularizing Eastern philosophy in the West. Born in England, he moved to the United States in his twenties, where he became a leading interpreter of Zen Buddhism, Taoism, and Hinduism for a Western audience. In *The Way of Zen*, Alan Watts challenges the idea that stillness is unproductive, offering a perspective that runs counter to the modern obsession with constant action. He writes:[2]

"Muddy water clears when left alone, just as those who sit quietly and do nothing may be making one of the best possible contributions to a world in turmoil."

Watts reminds us that clarity often comes not from forcing solutions, but from allowing things to settle on their own. When Watts speaks of "doing nothing," he's not just referring to sitting still. He's also pointing to the stillness of the mind, a quiet inner space where thought doesn't dominate. Doing nothing means not only pausing movement, but also releasing the need to mentally analyze, or fix. And that's the space where true insight can rise to the surface on its own.

Being stuck in the head isn't a great place to be. And if we're not really present to life as it's happening, it's easy to feel like we're missing out, even when we're right in the middle of it. We need to move beyond the belief that presence is about setting aside an hour to meditate in complete silence. What really makes a difference is how often, throughout the day, we bring ourselves back—to the breath, into the body, and into the present moment. Those small moments of stillness add up, creating calm in everyday life.

If we spend half our waking hours lost in thought, and most of those thoughts are repetitive or unhelpful, it's no wonder we feel stressed, overwhelmed, or disconnected. And if the mind is cluttered, how can we expect to feel happy or even get things done efficiently?

So, how do you actually quiet the endless mental chatter?

That search for inner silence is universal. It crosses age, background, gender; we're all looking for a way to feel more at ease. People look for it in all sorts of ways: a glass of wine to take the edge off, cannabis to slow the thoughts, or pills to mute the noise.

Even the "junkie" on the street whom others often look down on is searching for the same thing: a moment of peace, a break from the mind, some kind of silence inside. We might walk very different paths, but the need is deeply human: to get out of the head and find some stillness, even if only for a little while.

But there is a better way, one that is healthier, sustainable, and completely within your control. You do not have to force the mind to be silent. You just have to create the right conditions for stillness to emerge. That quietness is already inside you—it is just buried under layers of non-stop thinking.

Since childhood, we've been surrounded by advice, information, customs, and practices—absorbed from family, friends, religion, government, society, education, and the people around us. Much of it was well-intentioned. But not all of it. Human beings, especially when operating through powerful structures can be highly manipulative. And that hasn't changed. It's just evolved. Today, we see it in the constant noise and influence of social media platforms. Every voice, every influence, every message has shaped the way we think. And most of us don't even realize how much of what we believe is simply inherited from others.

Take the word "money," for example. A child growing up in a household where there was constant talk of *lack* is likely to develop a fearful relationship with money. Another child may have been taught that *money is the root of all evil*, seeing wealth as something negative or even corrupting. Meanwhile, a third child might have been raised in a family that openly spoke about money in a positive way—understanding it as a tool for freedom, a reward for providing value to others, and something that can be used wisely. Each of these children sees money in a completely different way, and each will grow into adulthood believing their perspective is the *truth*, even though their views were simply shaped by their environment.

But which perspective is actually true? Is money something to be feared? Is it the root of all evil? Or is it simply a tool—neutral on its own, but shaped by how we choose to use it? The answer isn't as clear-cut as we might think, and that's exactly the point. So much of what we believe to be *true* is just conditioning—passed down from those around us.

We take our thoughts so seriously, but how do we *really* know they're true? As Dr. Daniel G. Amen, a psychiatrist and brain health expert, says, "Don't believe every stupid thing you think." I'm not sure how you might take this. I know I was confused when I first came across it. After all, I had spent years investing energy in reinforcing inherited thinking, thoughts and beliefs passed down by others that I'd never truly examined. Letting go of that isn't easy. It takes a brave step and often, what sparks it is a quiet inner realization that the way you've been thinking just isn't working anymore. A sense that something needs to change. Or that, deep down, there might be another way.

When you start paying attention to the breath, bringing awareness into the body, and fully experiencing the present moment as life unfolds, something shifts. The layers of conditioning begin to dissolve. The noise of other people's beliefs and expectations fades into the background, making space for a clearer, more authentic way of seeing the world—one that isn't shaped by programming but by direct experience.

And in that space, you begin to experience something far more valuable—*your own life*, lived with less influence from others and more freedom to simply *be*.

And while there are many ways to quiet excessive thinking, my preference is to use three approaches:

1. Focusing on my breathing.
2. Bringing attention to my body and holding it there.
3. Shifting my awareness to the present moment.

Each of these techniques helps to create space between you and the thoughts, making it easier to step out of the mind's constant chatter. When the mind slows down, even for a few seconds, that stillness has a chance to surface. It is always there, waiting beneath the noise, ready to be noticed.

In the first few weeks and months, I found it much easier to focus on my breath (being aware of the inhale and exhale) or my body (noticing physical sensations like warmth, tension, or relaxation) rather than fully engaging with the present moment (shifting attention to my five senses and actively noticing what was happening around me).

But like anything else, it gets easier with practice. The brain takes time to adapt, but with consistency, it does change.

This ability of the brain to change, adapt, and rewire itself is known as "neuroplasticity." Research has shown that bringing attention to your breathing and similar practices can physically reshape the brain, strengthening areas associated with attention, emotional regulation, and self-awareness while reducing activity in regions linked to stress and overthinking. Studies using MRI scans have demonstrated that regular meditation increases the density of gray matter in the prefrontal cortex (which governs decision-making and focus).[3] It also decreases activity in the amygdala (the brain's alarm system that detects potential threats or danger and activates the "fight, flight, or freeze" response).[4] This means that with consistent practice, we can train our brains to be calmer, more present, and less reactive.

So, whether you focus on your breath, tune into your body, practice present moment awareness, or use a mix of all three, the goal remains the same: getting out of the head. And please do not worry about how you are doing. Worries are just more thoughts, and that is exactly what we are looking to bring some silence to. For me, it was important to remember that every time I had my attention on my breath, in my body, or in the present moment, I was already there. In other words, there is nothing to achieve. The achievement happens every time you bring your attention out of your head. That is all there is.

Even now, can you bring your attention to your breath for just a few seconds? In that moment, you're out of the mind, out of thinking. That's it. *Simple as that.* As you go about your day, the more often you practice this, the easier it becomes. And over time, those small moments add up—creating more clarity, calm, and a quieter mind without forcing anything at all.

I wasn't naturally good at this. My mind didn't just slow down because I wanted it to. But I stuck with it because I had reached a point where I was done with the constant mental noise. That alone gave me the push I needed to keep going. I also knew there had to be another way. I had this feeling that something was missing, but I couldn't quite put my finger on it. And then, when I experienced my first real glimpse of a quiet mind, I *knew*—this was the missing piece.

Life is challenging. It always has been, for every person, every animal, and all of nature. But when the mind fuels those challenges with endless worries and anxieties, life becomes *so much harder*. And in my own life, I had finally found a way to quiet that unnecessary inner struggle.

Bringing Attention to the Breath and Practicing *Breathe Light*

Breathing practices generally fall into two categories: paying attention to the breath and actively changing it. Many mindfulness and meditation traditions focus on simply *noticing* the breath—feeling the cool air enter the nose and the warmer air leave. This can be a powerful way to calm the mind, and I've found it helpful to check in with my breath throughout the day. Irrespective of the tasks of that day, bringing my attention to my breath for a few seconds here and a few seconds there can be very helpful, a small act that brings a sense of calm, almost like daily maintenance for stillness of the mind, but not in a formal way. But there's also great value in taking it a step further—not just observing the breath but *adjusting* it. Specifically, *Breathe Light* involves gently slowing down the flow of air as it enters and leaves the nose, allowing about 30% less air into the body. This naturally creates a slight feeling of air hunger—a subtle sensation of wanting more air. And that's actually a *good* sign.

That mild breathlessness indicates a small rise in carbon dioxide (CO_2) levels in the blood, which sets off a series of physiological benefits. As I said at the beginning of the book, many people still think of CO_2 as just a waste gas, something the body needs to eliminate. But in reality, it plays an essential role in human physiology.

If you've ever been told to take big, deep breaths to "oxygenate" your body, you might be surprised to learn that this advice, while well meaning, contradicts basic respiratory science. In fact, the opposite is true. Practicing *Breathe Light* increases CO_2, slightly lowers blood pH, enhances blood flow, improves oxygen delivery to the brain and muscles, and promotes a state of calm in both the body and mind. It's a small, simple shift in breathing that can have a surprisingly powerful impact.

In the first few weeks, I noticed my mind didn't go completely quiet right away. As I inhaled, I'd think, "There's my breath coming in." As I breathed out, "There's my breath going out." It was as if the mind didn't want to let go, still running a commentary, still needing to narrate everything, even the stillness.

If this happens to you, don't worry—it's completely normal. Over time, the thinking mind settles. Eventually, it's just you and your breath, no internal narration, no overanalyzing—just a quiet, steady rhythm.

Breathing less air helped me feel calmer, and the more I practiced, the clearer it became that this simple technique had far-reaching effects. By focusing on the breath, attention is naturally redirected away from mental chatter. The mind will still wander because that's what minds do—but every time you bring your focus back to your breath, you strengthen your ability to hold your attention.

Carbon dioxide is a natural vasodilator, meaning it relaxes and widens blood vessels. When CO_2 levels rise, blood vessels in the brain expand, improving oxygen delivery. Considering that the brain consumes 20% of the body's oxygen, this is a big deal. Better blood flow means better cognitive function, improved emotional regulation, and a calmer nervous system.

A 1988 paper by researchers Balestrino and Somjen at Duke University described how "the brain, by regulating breathing, controls its own excitability."[5] More recently, Dr. Andrew Huberman discussed this in his podcast, explaining how increasing CO_2 levels through controlled breathing can help regulate brain activity.

Dr. Michael Binder, a neurologist and researcher, has explored this connection further. His paper, "The Multi-Circuit Neuronal Hyperexcitability Hypothesis of Psychiatric Disorders" suggests that excessive electrical activity in the brain may be a key factor in conditions like anxiety, depression, and bipolar disorder.[6] When certain brain circuits become overly excitable, specific thoughts, emotions, or behaviors can take over, leading to persistent mental health challenges.

Brain circuits are networks of interconnected neurons (nerve cells) that communicate with each other to control thoughts, emotions, and behaviors. These circuits act like highways in the brain, transmitting electrical and chemical signals that help regulate everything from decision-making to mood, memory, and movement.

Different circuits control different functions. For example:

- The fear circuit processes threats and triggers anxiety or a "fight, flight, or freeze" response.
- The reward circuit is linked to motivation and pleasure.
- The attention circuit helps us focus and filter out distractions.

When brain circuits are working well, thoughts and emotions flow smoothly. But when they become overly excitable—meaning the neurons fire too much or too easily—certain thoughts, feelings, or behaviors can take over. This can lead to racing thoughts, anxiety, overthinking, or emotional instability.

When carbon dioxide levels rise, even just a little for example, when you *Breathe Light*, it causes a gentle drop in blood pH, making the blood slightly more acidic.

Brain cells, which behave like tiny electrical sparks, are highly sensitive to these changes. They like their environment to be just right. When the blood becomes a little more acidic, it dampens their excitability.

In plain English, the brain cells become less jumpy, less likely to fire off signals without good reason. They settle down. They become more selective about when they light up, allowing the nervous system to shift into a calmer, more balanced state.

This makes it all the more ironic that some yoga instructors are still telling students to take full, deep breaths to "detox" and "oxygenate" their bodies. Meanwhile, the very gas they're trying to "flush out" is *helping* their heart and brain. So, next time you're in a yoga class and your instructor passionately cues you to take full, deep breaths, go ahead and follow along—but do it your way. Breathe lightly, in and out through your nose, with nothing for anyone to notice. In fact, the less you do, the better. Meanwhile, you'll be the one quietly optimizing your oxygen delivery.

Breathing light also stimulates the vagus nerve, which signals to the brain that the body is safe. When you inhale, your heart rate speeds up slightly. When you exhale, especially if the exhale is slow and relaxed, your heart rate slows down. This natural rhythm is part of what's known as respiratory sinus arrhythmia, and it plays a crucial role in regulating stress. *Breathe Light* stimulates the vagus nerve in two key ways: the increase in CO_2 itself has a *vagotropic effect*, meaning it activates the vagus nerve, and slowing the breath down, particularly the exhale, reinforces the body's relaxation response.

One of the most important aspects of the *Breathe Light Exercise* is getting the air hunger just right. If it's too strong, it can feel stressful. If it's too mild, you won't get much benefit. The key is to gently soften the breath so that the air hunger is noticeable but still comfortable. For those prone to panic attacks or anxiety, it's best to ease in gradually. Shorter sessions of 30 seconds at a time can be a good way to start.

What I found was that everything connects. *Breathe Light* improves sleep quality. Better sleep quality leads to a calmer mind. A calmer mind maintains light, slow breathing. Light, slow breathing reinforces good sleep. It's a positive cycle.

And once you experience it, you start to wonder—why didn't anyone teach me this sooner?

In the first few weeks, focusing on my breath was my main practice for quieting the mind. It was the easiest entry point—keeping my attention on the inhale and exhale gave me something steady to anchor to.

At that stage, my awareness was in the body, but only in a limited way—directed solely at my breathing. Over time, I began expanding that focus, shifting my attention beyond the breath to different body parts and physical sensations. This is what I mean by bringing my attention into the body—moving beyond just breathing to fully experience what is happening internally. I'll describe this next.

Bringing Attention into the Body

One of the best ways to quiet the mind is to bring attention into the body. I really like this approach. In fact, I think I stumbled across it completely by accident when I was about 15 or 16 years old.

At the time, I was working in a small food market, and the owner, Vivian, was *not* in a good mood. She was telling me off about something—probably stacking the bread the wrong way, not lining up the cans properly, or some other mistake. And for some reason, instead of just absorbing it all in my head, I brought my attention into my body.

It wasn't intentional, and I had no idea what I was doing. I just shifted my focus inward and *felt* my body. I could still hear every word Vivian was saying. I understood the message. But somehow, it didn't *get* to me. Vivian, on the other hand, thought I wasn't listening at all. At one point, she actually stopped and asked, "Are you even listening to me?!"

I was listening. I just wasn't *absorbing* the stress of it. The words were there, but they weren't sinking in and affecting me. Looking back, I can still remember that moment. But unfortunately, I didn't fully understand or apply what I had stumbled upon until about 10 years later. And let me tell you, this is a brilliant trick to try the next time someone is in a bad mood or has something negative to say. Listen, yes, but not from your head. Listen from your body. You'll still hear their words, and you can still take whatever useful advice they have to offer, but it won't drag you down emotionally.

Bringing awareness into the body is one of the most effective ways to quiet the mind. If you want to give it a try, start small. Focus on one part of the body—maybe your hand. It helps to close your eyes and bring your attention to your hand. Can you feel the inner sensations of your hand? The temperature of the air against your skin? Does it *feel* alive? Once you've got that, move your attention to your arm. Same thing—notice the sensations, the air, the feeling of your skin, the bodily sensations. Then, slowly work your way across the body—to your shoulders, chest, abdomen, legs, and feet. Notice how your body is supported by the chair beneath you. Feel your feet on the ground. Feel the fabric of your clothes against your skin. Just *be there*.

There's something incredibly grounding about this. The human body has an intelligence of its own, and when you connect with it, the mind naturally settles.

I use this technique all the time now, especially before giving a presentation. If I have to speak in front of a group, of course, I want to do my best. And the best preparation? A solid night's sleep with my mouth closed so I wake up feeling refreshed—that's the foundation. If I'm jetlagged or just not feeling my best, I'll take a moment to rest and reset by listening to a guided audio I recorded about 15 years ago. It still works just as well today, and you can try it too. It's free on the ButeykoClinic app. Before a talk, I'll hide away in my hotel room, avoiding conversation. It's not that I'm being rude, I just want to save all my energy for the talk itself. Instead of getting caught up in small talk or distractions, I bring my attention inward, into my body. Because honestly, when it comes to public speaking, the *last* thing I want is to be trapped in my own head. The topic of breathing, quieting the mind, and sleep is something I've worked with for years. And like anyone who's spent a long time immersed in their work, the knowledge, the experience—it's all there. It's already stored in the brain, just waiting to come out. The key is simply to quiet the mind and get out of my own way, so the information already there can flow. There's a term for this—"flow state," or what people call "being in the zone."

It's that peak-performance state where everything just clicks. It's effortless. Time slows down, and yet, somehow, it also flies by. You're fully immersed in what you're doing, and for that moment, nothing else exists. Athletes, musicians, artists, and people who excel in any field can access this state. Some people seem to enter it naturally. For me, I had to learn how to get there.

To reach a flow state, a few key elements need to be in place. First, you have to know your subject inside out—there's no faking it. But knowledge alone isn't enough. You also need the right balance of stress and concentration.

Too much stress, and your brain switches into survival mode, shutting down creativity, problem-solving, and deep focus. Too little stress, and there's no drive—no urgency to stay engaged. The sweet spot lies in between: enough activation to stay alert and focused, but not so much that tension takes over.

Concentration is the next piece. To enter flow, the mind needs to be fully absorbed in the task, not split between the work and the constant background noise of overthinking. Flow doesn't happen if your thoughts are somewhere else. The thinking mind isn't just too slow for flow—it can also be unhelpful.

Imagine standing in front of an audience, about to give a talk, and your brain decides *this* is the perfect time to say:

- "What if I mess this up?"
- "Did I prepare enough?"
- "Oh no, there are some important people in the audience—what will they think?"
- "If I bomb this, I'll never get asked to speak again."

Yeah, *no thanks*. I don't need that running in the background. And I certainly don't need my mind throwing extra obstacles at me when I'm trying to do my job. So, for me, it's simple, I want to give my full energy to the talk. I want to talk with every cell in my body. No distractions, no safety nets, and no backup slides filled with bullet points that I read off a screen.

But here's the real question: can we access flow if poor sleep is driving stress, draining energy, and dulling focus? Can we find flow if we're stuck in a state of anxiety or hyperarousal? That alone is enough to block the flow state for most people. Flow states shouldn't be reserved for the lucky few who stumble into them naturally. Yes, some people access flow effortlessly—but I wasn't one of them. I had to work on it.

And what made the difference? Breathing, sleep, and learning how to get out of my own head. These aren't just minor details; they're the foundation for creating the right physiological and mental state to enter flow—not just once in a while, but consistently.

Bringing Attention to the Present Moment

We're either stuck in our heads, lost in thought, or actually *living*—connected to what's happening around us, without all the mental noise.

After a few weeks of focusing on my breath and body, something shifted. My mind got a little quieter, and it became easier to notice what was happening *outside* of me. I wasn't just thinking about life—I was actually *experiencing* it.

I started paying attention to my surroundings—looking, listening, feeling, but without that constant inner commentary. I wasn't mentally labeling everything I saw or trying to analyze what it all meant. If I went for a walk, I didn't need to think, "That's an oak tree," "Those are daffodils," "I wonder what species of bird that is?" Instead, I just *saw* the tree. I *heard* the bird. I *felt* the wind.

Have you ever gone for a walk and suddenly realized you weren't really there at all? Your body was moving, but your mind was somewhere else entirely. That's the habit we're trying to shift. Can you go for a walk and just *be there*? Can you see a tree without immediately slapping a label on it? Can you listen to the sounds around you? Can you feel the warmth of the sun or the chill of the wind without mentally reviewing how you *feel* about it?

It doesn't have to be out in nature. Sometimes I visit an art museum like the Van Gogh Museum in Amsterdam, not to analyze the brushstrokes or wonder what Van Gogh was thinking when he painted *The Bedroom*, but just to look. No commentary, no critique. Just noticing.

And that experience of simply being there with the art feels much more fulfilling than overanalyzing it.

Even now, as you read this, ask yourself: "Am I really here with this sentence?" Or are you catching only bits and pieces, grabbing a few words here and there, while the mind drifts? You might finish a page and not remember a word of it. I've done that plenty of times, my eyes were staring at the page while my mind wandered off.

This is what mind-wandering looks like. It happens all the time, and it's often why we feel unfocused or disconnected. The truth is, we *can't* multitask. We can only do one thing well at a time. And wouldn't it be easier if reading actually meant *reading*—taking it all in, moving with time, absorbing every word?

In my early twenties, someone suggested I go to the seaside, sit for 10 or 15 minutes, and just look out at the water. They said it would help to reduce stress. So, one Sunday, I drove down to the coast, found a spot on the stones, and sat there, staring out at the water for a solid 10 to 15 minutes. And when it was over? I walked away thinking it was a load of crap. Why didn't it work for me? I had done exactly what they suggested. I was by the coast. The weather was actually pretty decent for the West Coast of Ireland. And yet I got *nothing* from it.

Now, the reason is obvious. Yes, my body was at the seaside. But my mind? It was somewhere else entirely.

I missed out on the sights and sounds around me: the waves rolling into shore, children laughing and playing on the sand and in the water, dogs barking with excitement. The sun was warm on my skin, the salty air carried the smell of the ocean and I missed all of it. I caught only glimpses of the water, but in truth, I barely registered it. I hardly saw the waves, barely heard them. My mind just wouldn't switch off.

Sitting by the sea isn't relaxing if you can't switch off in the first place. I didn't have the knowledge or experience to quiet my mind and direct my energy to what was happening around me. Instead of being present, my attention was stuck in my head.

I was surrounded by a beautiful environment, yet I didn't have the capacity to truly notice it. To do that, I would have needed to quiet my mind. What was I thinking about at the time? I have no idea. And does it even matter? I can say with certainty that my thoughts had nothing to do with the moment I was in. I was either lost in the future or stuck in the past, anywhere but there.

And that raises a big question: how can we *appreciate* anything if we're not even paying attention?

The funny thing is, I never thought of myself as an anxious person. Even now, I wouldn't say I had anxiety back then. But my mind was racing. My stress levels were high. My concentration wasn't great.

These days, nature helps me connect again. That's one of the reasons I moved to the countryside. My walks are no longer just about movement; they're a practice in presence, in training both my mind and my breath.

Here's how I do it, and how you can too:

- When you see something, just *see* it. Let your eyes rest gently. There is no need to label what you see. Just take it in.
- When you listen, just *listen.* Bring your attention to the sounds that you hear—the wind in the trees, the birds, but without turning it into a mental commentary.
- When you feel something—your feet on the ground, the movement of your legs, the warmth of the sun, the coolness of the breeze—just *feel it.*
- When you breathe, actually notice it—the slightly cooler air as it enters your nose and the slightly warmer air as it leaves.

Even if you can only do this for five seconds before the mind kicks in again, that's still a win. Five seconds is better than nothing. Five seconds is *way* more than I managed back when I was sitting at the beach, lost in my thoughts.

And let's be real, humans have been trying to figure out how to stop overthinking for *thousands* of years. But there are a few simple steps that make a real difference:

1. First, start with your breath. Just spend a week or two bringing your attention to it.
2. Then, shift your focus into your body. Get comfortable tuning into different parts of yourself and actually *feeling* what's happening.
3. Finally, engage with your senses. Train yourself to experience life *without* immediately turning it into words and thoughts.

It really helps to find someone—a teacher, a book, a video, or a lecture that resonates with you. For me, that book was *The Power of Now* by Eckhart Tolle. I stumbled upon it in a bookstore in Canada back in 2000, and from the moment I picked it up, something about it struck a chord.

I loved *The Power of Now* so much that I actually recorded myself reading the entire book onto cassette tapes so I could listen to it in my car, over and over again. I must have played it hundreds of times, to the point where it felt like the words had become part of my DNA.

I had plenty of motivation to practice because my mind was constantly *on*. But I was also lucky enough to catch glimpses of what it felt like to have a quieter mind. And those glimpses kept me going.

Looking back, I can say without hesitation that three things— each interconnected, with one feeding into the next—changed my life:

1. **The Buteyko Method.** Learning how to breathe properly, which in turn reduced stress levels and improved sleep quality.
2. **Getting good sleep.** Breathing through my nose during sleep, ensuring deeper rest and better recovery.
3. **Listening to the Eckhart Tolle book.** With optimal sleep and a more balanced autonomic nervous system, my mind became calmer, allowing stillness to emerge naturally.

Each step built upon the last, creating a foundation for better health, mental clarity, and presence. The goal wasn't to eliminate thoughts completely. But by improving my physiology and training my attention, the noise in the mind began to settle. I had fewer thoughts and more space between them. And in that space, I found greater clarity, calm, and a true sense of mental quiet.

Helping Children and Teenagers Quiet the Mind

Helping a child find quietness in their mind starts with the way we live as parents. Children learn more from what we do than what we say. And today, more than ever, children are feeling anxious. Is it because we are diagnosing anxiety more, or is anxiety actually increasing? It seems like the latter, especially with the rise of smartphones and constant distractions. Even young children now live in a world that rarely slows down; constant notifications, background noise, and fewer opportunities for quiet, calm focus.

So, how do we help a child calm their mind? The steps are the same as they are for adults. When a child feels anxious, their mind is often busy, full of thoughts bouncing around, creating a kind of mental noise. Breathing, sleep, and state of mind are all connected, so we start by asking: "How is the child breathing?" "How is the child sleeping?"

One simple way to check is to listen to how they breathe during sleep. We should never *hear* a child breathing at night, not because they've stopped breathing, of course, but because their breathing should be so smooth and free that it makes no sound. Silent breathing means their airways are open and their body is relaxed.

If you hear loud breathing, frequent sighs, or snoring, these are cues that something might need attention.

When I talk to a child with anxiety, like a 14-year-old, I always share my own experience. I keep things simple, explaining what worked for me. I let them know that feeling nervous or overwhelmed isn't something to be ashamed of; it's something we all feel sometimes, and there are tools to help.

Every now and then during the day, I suggest they take a moment to check in: "What am I thinking about? Can I observe my thoughts for just a few seconds?" The next step is to ask, "Are these thoughts helpful, or is it just noise?" If it's just noise, we don't need to fight it; we just need to take a little break from the mind. Kids don't need to name every emotion or analyze every thought. Often, just noticing that the mind is busy is enough.

And how do we take a little break from the mind? We focus on the breath.

I explain that they can feel the slightly cooler air coming in through the nose and the slightly warmer air as it leaves. The mind will wander—that's normal. But every time it does, we notice it and gently bring attention back to the breath. Each time we do this, we are training the brain to be more focused and calmer.

I also remind them that *there is a time to think*. When they are in class working on a math puzzle, they *need* to think. That kind of thinking is useful and productive. But it's the *other* kind of thinking—the constant noise—that we want to take a break from.

Taking a holiday from the noise means paying attention to your breath. And the best way to tell the brain that everything is okay is to breathe slowly and silently in and out through the nose. A simple way to do this is to breathe in for about three seconds and breathe out for about five seconds. But I also tell them they don't have to count; just let the breath feel easy and soft going in, and slower on the way out. The magic is in the exhale.

Slowing the breath out is like telling your body, "We're safe now. We can calm down." And the body listens.

Once I explain this, I ask the child to repeat it back to me in their own words. This helps them remember the technique and feel confident using it whenever they need a break from the noise in their mind.

The Hierarchy of Needs

You've probably heard of Maslow's Hierarchy of Needs—that famous pyramid that lays out what we, as humans, need to thrive.[7] Psychologist Abraham Maslow introduced this idea back in the 1940s, and at the time, it made a lot of sense. He argued that human needs are built in layers, starting with the basics: food, water, shelter, and safety. Once those are covered, we move up to social belonging, self-esteem, and, at the very top, self-actualization—essentially, reaching our full potential.

Back then, securing basic survival needs was a daily struggle for many. But today, most of us aren't waking up worried about where our next meal is coming from or whether we'll have a roof over our heads. So, if our fundamental needs are already met, why aren't we all thriving at the top of the pyramid—fully engaged, fulfilled, and operating at our highest potential?

Maslow presented self-actualization as the ultimate human drive, the desire to reach one's full potential. But what he didn't emphasize is that achieving our full potential isn't just about external security—it depends on internal balance too. You can have food, shelter, and even financial stability, but if your breathing is off, your sleep is broken, and your nervous system is in a constant state of stress, the pathway to self-actualization becomes much harder to access.

Let's take a closer look at Maslow's key stages through this lens:

- **Physiological needs (food, water, shelter, sleep, and breathing).** Maslow's foundation includes basic survival needs, but we need to go beyond just having a place to sleep; we need to focus on the quality of that sleep. A solid night's rest depends on breathing through the nose, proper airway function, and a balanced autonomic nervous system. Chronic stress, irregular breathing patterns, and mouth breathing at night all disrupt sleep quality, making it harder to recover and function optimally.

- **Safety needs (physical and psychological security).** True safety isn't just about avoiding danger; it's about feeling secure in your own body. If your nervous system is constantly in a state of "fight, flight, or freeze" due to stress, sleep deprivation, or dysfunctional breathing, you'll never feel truly "safe," even if your external environment is stable. Poor breathing habits like breathing too fast, too much, or through the mouth keep the body in a subtle state of stress, preventing real physiological calm.

- **Love and belonging (connection with others and self).** Our relationships thrive when we're present, engaged, and emotionally regulated—all of which depend on how well we breathe and sleep. When we're exhausted or mentally overstimulated, we're more reactive, less patient, and connection becomes harder. Conversations feel more draining, small frustrations become bigger than they need to be, and we lose the capacity to truly *listen* rather than just react.

But love and belonging aren't just about our relationships with others—they also include the relationship we have with *ourselves*. How we breathe, how we manage our emotions, and how much we live in the present moment all shape our ability to give and receive love.

Because here's the thing—how can you fully love your partner if the mind is constantly caught up in negative thoughts about them? And more importantly, how do you *know* those thoughts are even true?

- **Esteem (confidence, self-worth, and achievement).** A strong sense of self-worth is difficult to develop when your energy is depleted from poor sleep, the mind is overstimulated, and your nervous system is constantly on high alert. Confidence doesn't just come from achievement—it comes from how you feel. And how you feel is directly tied to how you breathe, how you sleep, and how balanced your nervous system is.

- **Self-actualization (reaching full potential and living with purpose).** At the top of Maslow's pyramid is self-actualization—the ability to fully express who you are, contribute meaningfully, and operate at your highest level. It's about becoming who you're capable of being. But self-actualization isn't something that simply clicks into place once your basic needs are met. It requires a deeper connection to yourself, the ability to pay attention, stay present, and act in alignment with what matters most. You might have everything in place on the outside, but without internal calm and clarity, you can still feel off-track. Maslow's framework is valuable; we see that self-actualization—becoming the best version of ourselves—doesn't happen without a strong foundation.

And that foundation includes breathing well, sleeping deeply, and keeping the nervous system in balance. Without these, it's difficult to feel safe, connected, or confident—let alone reach our full potential.

And the reality is, we can't expect to sleep well at night if the mind is overstimulated all day. If we're constantly stuck in thought loops, breathing dysfunctionally, or living in a state of chronic stress, our nervous system doesn't just shut off because we've climbed into bed. That's why the practices we've explored—paying attention to the breath, bringing awareness into the body, and stepping into the present moment—aren't just for mindfulness; they're essential for good sleep.

Because sleep isn't just about closing your eyes; it's about allowing the body and mind to shift into a state of restoration. And that starts long before bedtime.

So, if there's one thing to take away from this, it's this: get out of your head. The mind is a powerful and beautiful instrument, capable of incredible things. But when left unchecked, it can also work against us, especially when it interferes with the most basic functions like sleep. And when sleep is affected, everything else begins to unravel. Clarity, energy, mood, focus all depend on a mind that knows when to switch off.

SECTION 2

ADULT SLEEP

CHAPTER 9

HOW GENDER AND AGE SHAPE YOUR REST

Ever wondered why women tend to struggle with insomnia more than men, why men are more likely to snore, or why older adults find themselves waking up multiple times a night to use the bathroom? Sleep is far from a one-size-fits-all experience. Hormones, anatomy, and lifestyle choices all play a role in shaping how well and how long we sleep.

In this chapter, we'll dive into how biology and hormones shape the way we sleep. How do pregnancy, menstruation, and menopause interfere with women's rest? Why do men snore more and face a higher risk of sleep apnea, and how does that impact their health? Does aging affect the way men sleep, and what role do hormones play? And as we get older, what changes in our sleep patterns—and what can we do to sleep better? By understanding these differences, you'll gain valuable insights into adult sleep health and practical ways to improve your own rest.

MEN'S SLEEP

Men's sleep is influenced by a mix of biology, anatomy, and lifestyle habits. These factors make them more prone to certain sleep disorders—especially snoring and obstructive sleep apnea (OSA).

Why Are Men More Likely to Snore and Have OSA?

In the United States, 44% of men between the ages of 30 and 60 snore regularly, compared with just over a quarter (28%) of women.[1] This gap begins to narrow with age, particularly after menopause, as snoring becomes more common in women. Nearly half of people over 60 snore regularly, and in both men and women, snoring can serve as an early warning sign of more serious conditions, such as obstructive sleep apnea (OSA).[2]

One major reason men snore more comes down to anatomy. Men typically have larger necks and more collapsible airway tissue, which makes them more prone to airway obstruction when they sleep. Combined with lifestyle factors such as higher rates of obesity and alcohol consumption, these structural differences significantly increase the likelihood of developing sleep apnea. Research shows that more than half of men over 40 experience at least mild-to-moderate-OSA, while about 12% suffer from a severe form of the condition.[3]

What makes OSA especially concerning is that it often goes unnoticed. Studies estimate that up to 90% of people with sleep apnea have never been diagnosed,[4] leaving their condition untreated and their health at risk. Many men either don't recognize the symptoms, such as daytime grogginess, poor concentration, and loud snoring, or ignore them altogether. But untreated, OSA doesn't just ruin sleep; it can have serious health consequences. Sleep apnea has been strongly linked to an increased risk of heart disease, diabetes, stroke,[5] and even cognitive decline.[6] Recognizing and addressing these symptoms early is critical for maintaining long-term health and quality of life. Please see Chapter 10D on OSA for more information.

Testosterone and Sleep: A Two-Way Relationship

When people think about testosterone, they often associate it with muscle growth, energy levels, and libido. But testosterone also plays a crucial role in sleep. This hormone follows a daily rhythm, peaking at night to promote deep, restorative sleep. However, as men age, testosterone levels naturally decline, starting around age 30 to 40, dropping by about 1% per year.[7] This gradual shift can lead to a range of symptoms, including lower energy, daytime fatigue, difficulty concentrating, reduced libido, and, perhaps surprisingly, poorer sleep.

Lower testosterone levels have been linked to trouble falling and staying asleep, as well as a higher risk of sleep disorders like insomnia and sleep apnea.[8] At the same time, poor sleep itself can significantly lower testosterone production, leading to issues such as reduced sperm quality, erectile dysfunction, and diminished libido.[9-11] This creates a vicious cycle: the less you sleep, the lower your testosterone levels, and the lower your testosterone levels, the worse your sleep becomes.

For men with sleep-disordered breathing, particularly OSA, this cycle becomes even more pronounced. Frequent interruptions in breathing during sleep reduce oxygen levels in the blood, which in turn suppresses testosterone production.[12] In other words, poor sleep and low testosterone reinforce each other, making it even harder to break the pattern and get quality rest.

The good news is that improving sleep can help support healthy testosterone levels, just as maintaining balanced testosterone can enhance sleep quality. Prioritize deep, uninterrupted rest by addressing snoring and sleep apnea (see Chapters 10B and 10D), and follow a consistent sleep schedule and sleep hygiene recommendations.

WOMEN'S SLEEP: THE FORGOTTEN GENDER

For decades, women have been underrepresented in sleep studies, earning them the title of the "forgotten gender" in sleep research.[13] Most sleep disorder studies and criteria for diagnosis were designed around male physiology, overlooking the unique ways sleep issues manifest in women. And that matters, because what often gets missed is that sleep struggles in women don't always show up the same way they do in men.

While a man might present with loud snoring or obvious pauses in breathing, a woman may report fatigue, anxiety, brain fog, or waking frequently during the night. These symptoms can easily be dismissed as stress or hormones, when in reality, there could be an underlying sleep disorder.

As a result, women have been disproportionately underdiagnosed and undertreated, often walking away from medical appointments without answers, let alone solutions. This has left many without the support they need for optimal sleep health.

Why Are Women More Likely to Experience Insomnia?

Insomnia is significantly more common in women than in men. Research shows that women are 1.58 times more likely to develop insomnia,[14] and this gap widens with age. Several biological and psychological factors contribute to this heightened risk.

Hormonal fluctuations play a major role, with shifts during the menstrual cycle, pregnancy, and menopause all disrupting sleep regulation. You might notice you sleep differently right before your period, or that your sleep changed during pregnancy or after entering perimenopause. These changes are very real, and they're happening on a hormonal level.

Additionally, women experience higher rates of anxiety and depression, both of which are strongly linked to insomnia. It becomes a bit of a vicious cycle; poor sleep increases stress and anxiety, and stress and anxiety make it harder to sleep.

On top of that, women tend to have a lower arousal threshold than men, which means they are more likely to wake up in response to subtle changes in their internal environment like slight breathing irregularities, body temperature shifts, or hormonal fluctuations that occur during the night. It's not just about being a light sleeper because of noise or light; this is happening on a deeper physiological level. Even if the room is quiet and dark, the body may still be on higher alert, making it harder to stay in deep, restorative sleep.

Upper Airway Resistance Syndrome: The Underdiagnosed Sleep Disruptor

Women are also more likely to have upper airway resistance syndrome (UARS), a lesser-known sleep disorder that narrows the airway and increases breathing resistance during sleep. Unlike obstructive sleep apnea, UARS doesn't cause complete airway blockages, making it harder to detect in standard sleep studies.

A woman with UARS undergoing a clinical sleep study might receive an apnea-hypopnea index (AHI) score of just 1 or 2 events per hour, which falls below the diagnostic threshold for OSA. On paper, this might seem like no big deal but for many women, those "mild" numbers don't tell the full story. Research reports that women with an AHI of 2–5 experience symptoms just as severe as men with an AHI of 15 or higher, a level that qualifies as moderate sleep apnea.[15] In other words, many women are living with real sleep disruption, but because their numbers aren't high enough, they're often told everything looks fine.

The result? They go home without answers, still exhausted and wondering why they can't get a decent night's sleep.

Greater awareness among healthcare providers is crucial to ensuring that UARS is recognized and properly treated.

Obstructive Sleep Apnea: Why Women Are Often Misdiagnosed

For years, OSA was considered a "men's disease," with early estimates suggesting men were three to five times more likely to have it than women.[16] Because of this, most of the research and diagnostic criteria were developed with men in mind, overlooking the unique ways the condition presents in women.

Although some women experience the classic OSA symptoms of loud snoring, choking, or gasping for air during sleep many don't. Instead, their symptoms are often more subtle and don't match the traditional profile, which makes it easier for their sleep issues to be missed or misdiagnosed.[17] Instead of loud snoring, women with OSA are more likely to report insomnia, restless legs, nightmares, palpitations, morning headaches, feeling wiped out during the day, low mood, muscle aches, or even unexplained weight gain.[18] And because these symptoms overlap with common issues like anxiety, depression, or menopause related sleep changes, it's no surprise that many women get overlooked.

But here's what's concerning: the risks of untreated OSA in women extend to cognitive health. There's growing evidence that sleep disordered breathing in women may raise the risk of cognitive problems later in life, including mild cognitive impairment and dementia. These issues are especially linked to lower oxygen levels and longer periods where breathing is reduced or stopped during sleep.[19] All of this points to a simple truth: we need to start paying closer attention to how OSA shows up in women.

How Hormones Affect Women's Sleep: Menstruation, Pregnancy, and Menopause

Menstruation: How the Monthly Cycle Disrupts Sleep

If you've ever noticed your sleep patterns shifting throughout the month, you're not imagining it; your hormones might be playing a big part. Estrogen and progesterone fluctuate during the menstrual cycle, influencing everything from how easily you fall asleep to how rested you feel in the morning.

The luteal phase—the second half of your cycle, after ovulation—brings a surge in progesterone, a hormone with natural sedative effects that can promote deeper sleep.[20] However, the *rapid increase* in progesterone during the early luteal phase may actually shorten sleep duration, making it harder to stay asleep as comfortably as in the first half of the cycle (the follicular phase).[21-23]

Progesterone acts as a respiratory stimulant, making some women more prone to hyperventilate during this phase, a subtle shift that can disrupt sleep.[24] Progesterone increases core body temperature, which can make it harder for some people to fall and stay asleep, particularly if the sleeping environment is too warm. While progesterone itself is sleep promoting due to its calming effects on the brain, its thermogenic action may partially offset these benefits, especially during the luteal phase of the menstrual cycle.

And just before your period starts, progesterone levels drop sharply. That sudden shift can trigger mood swings, anxiety, or restlessness, all of which can make it harder to wind down at night and get the sleep you need.

> "[My] sleep was poor quality—I was waking several times in the night to go to urinate. Also waking feeling tired/unrefreshed.
>
> Mouth taping and doing breathing exercises I believe have been really helpful (along with some nutrition supplements).
>
> I think the poor sleep was part of a 'sympathetic dominant state' I was living in unaware. **My hormone cycling had stopped. The improved sleep was a big part of getting my [menstrual] cycle back.**"

Pregnancy: Sleep Disruptions from Hormonal and Physical Changes

Pregnancy brings a host of changes that can interfere with sleep, from back pain and frequent urination to hormonal shifts and weight gain. It's not just the growing bump that makes sleep tricky; hormone changes can affect how well you breathe too. For example, increased levels of estrogen boost blood flow to the mucous membranes, which can lead to nasal swelling and congestion. This condition, known as "pregnancy rhinitis," can make it harder to breathe through your nose and disrupt your sleep.

Hormonal changes contribute to higher rates of both insomnia and sleep apnea during pregnancy. In fact, research shows that 15–20% of obese pregnant women develop OSA.[25] Since sleep apnea can lower oxygen levels for both the mother and baby, early medical evaluation is essential if symptoms such as loud snoring, gasping for air during sleep, or excessive daytime fatigue arise.

> "I think years of broken sleep [from caring for a child with sleep issues] has created my insomnia. That and **the joys of menopause, waking in the night as your body temperature rises, and inability to go back to sleep, which is a HUGE silent epidemic for us mid- age women.**
>
> I find **breathing helps to calm me and slow my thoughts.** Especially if I count my breath, it gives my brain a task and stops the constant negative mental assault that only comes in the wee small hours!"

Menopause: Why Sleep Becomes Harder During Midlife

Menopause is the natural end of a woman's reproductive years, occurring when menstrual periods stop permanently, typically between ages 45 and 55. But for many women, it doesn't just mark the end of periods; it also marks the beginning of sleep problems. Sleep disturbances become more common, affecting 40–60% of menopausal women.[26] Many struggle with difficulty falling asleep, frequent nighttime awakenings, and waking up too early.

The decline in estrogen and progesterone during menopause plays a major role in sleep disruption. Lower estrogen can lead to hot flashes and night sweats that jolt you awake just as you were finally drifting off. At the same time, progesterone—an important respiratory stimulant—drops significantly, weakening the body's ability to keep the upper airway open. This helps explain why the risk of OSA increases by nearly 200% in menopausal women compared with those who are premenopausal.[27]

Add to that the stress of midlife; aging parents, busy work schedules, maybe even teenagers under your roof and it's no wonder cortisol levels creep up. Higher cortisol, the body's main stress hormone, can interfere with both sleep quality and quantity. Menopause has also been linked to a higher risk of restless legs syndrome, which causes uncomfortable sensations in the legs and a strong urge to move them especially at night, making rest even harder to come by.

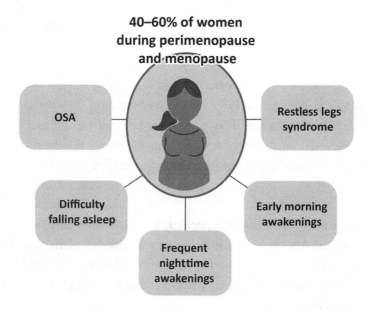

Sleep in Older Age: Why It Changes and How It Affects Health

Sleep problems become more common with age, affecting a large portion of the population. Research reports of the prevalence of sleep disturbances among older adults vary widely, ranging from 6 to 65%.[28] This is a significant concern because getting enough quality sleep is essential for maintaining cognitive function and protecting against chronic disease, while sleep deprivation has been linked to cognitive decline, depression, and even dementia.[29]

Several factors make sleep more challenging as we get older, including changes in sleep quality, nighttime awakenings, and shifts in our natural sleep-wake cycle.

1. **Sleep quality and quantity declines with age.** As we age, the amount of deep, restorative sleep we get decreases due to natural changes in the brain. By the time we reach our mid-to-late forties, we only get about 60–70% of the deep sleep we had as teenagers. By age 70, that number drops even further—many older adults have lost 80–90% of their deep sleep.[30]

   > "As I've got older, deep sleep has declined. Taping increases deep sleep and improves my HRV [heart rate variability]. If I wake up in [the] night, then I use the light breathing technique to get back to sleep, and it works very effectively. Light breathing with the relaxation audio works very well in relieving daytime fatigue."
   >
   > *Isabel, 58, England*

2. **Sleep becomes more fragmented, and nighttime bathroom trips increase.** Another common change with age is fragmented sleep, meaning more frequent awakenings throughout the night and reduced sleep efficiency—the percentage of time spent in bed actually sleeping.

   If you've ever wondered why you wake up more often now than you did years ago, or why you're up at 3 a.m. making your way to the bathroom, you're not alone. As we get older, sleep tends to become lighter and more broken. For older adults, less efficient sleep has real consequences, including:[31]

   • Higher risk of mortality
   • Worse physical health
   • Increased forgetfulness
   • Lower energy levels
   • Higher rates of depression

   One major cause of disrupted sleep in older age is nocturia, the need to wake up and use the bathroom during the night. This is particularly common in older adults with insomnia or sleep-disordered breathing conditions like OSA.[32–34]

Interestingly, breathing through the nose instead of the mouth has been shown to reduce sleep fragmentation and lessen the need to urinate at night.

"Until recently, I would wake up frequently during the night needing the loo, and sometimes I couldn't get back to sleep. I always felt that I wasn't getting any deep sleep at all, and this added to feeling tired during the day, so I would have cat naps to get me through.

Since starting the breathing and mouth taping, I feel a lot more centered and energized, and clearer in my head than I was before, and, although I still wake to pee in the night, it's just once, and I feel I am sleeping much deeper and spend less time awake in the night."

3. **Melatonin production declines, shifting sleep-wake cycles.** Melatonin, often called the "sleep hormone," plays a crucial role in regulating sleep patterns. By middle age (around 40–45), melatonin levels begin to drop.[35] By age 70, the nocturnal peak of melatonin can be significantly reduced or even absent in some people.[36] This decline contributes to the sleep difficulties commonly seen in older adults, such as the reductions in sleep quality, quantity, and efficiency already noted, meaning older people tend to have a reduced total sleep time and lighter, more fragmented sleep.

   To make things trickier, aging doesn't just reduce melatonin levels; it also affects the body's internal clock, or circadian rhythm. As we get older, the timing of melatonin release shifts. This means:

   • Melatonin levels start dropping earlier in the morning, leading to earlier wake-up times.
   • Melatonin production peaks earlier in the evening, making older adults feel sleepy earlier.

This shift helps explain why many older adults find themselves going to bed early, waking up before sunrise, and sometimes nodding off during the evening news. But here's the catch: those evening naps, while tempting, can make it harder to fall asleep or stay asleep later that night. And once you're up too early the next morning, the cycle continues. It becomes a frustrating loop: tired but unable to sleep deeply, waking too soon, and not feeling fully rested.

"Before nasal breathing, I would wake up a couple of times during the night and not sleep past 2 AM-ish. And I went to bed between 9–10.

Now I go to bed between 8:30–9:30 and get a good 7 hours of sleep. . . . I have better-balanced energy throughout the day now."

RandyLynn, 75, USA

Safety Tip: For older adults who wake up frequently at night, especially to use the bathroom, it's important to have motion-activated nightlights or easily accessible dim lighting in hallways and bathrooms to reduce the risk of trips and falls.

LOOKING AHEAD: MANAGING SLEEP

Although hormonal changes and aging impact our sleep, that doesn't mean we are sentenced to an endless cycle of restless nights and daytime fatigue.

In the chapters ahead, we'll take a closer look at some of the most common sleep challenges and more importantly, what you can do about them.

CHAPTER 10

AN OVERVIEW OF ADULT SLEEP DISORDERS

In Chapter 1, I focused on giving you the essential tools—the breathing exercises and step-by-step guidance to start transforming your sleep. This chapter, however, is here to deepen your understanding. It's about not just the "how" but also the "why." Here, we'll dive into the science behind breathing and sleep, exploring the intricate mechanics of what's really going on when you're lying awake at night or struggling with sleep-disordered breathing.

By the time you've finished this chapter, you'll have a greater appreciation for just how complex we humans are and how addressing sleep disorders requires more than just a one-size-fits-all solution. Human physiology, emotions, and habits all intertwine in ways that can either support or sabotage your sleep.

I'll give a brief overview of various approaches to improving sleep, with a particular focus on the Buteyko breathing technique. Think of this as an adjunct to the tools you've already learned, an additional layer to complement the arsenal of approaches you may already have at your disposal. This isn't about replacing what works for you; it's about enhancing it with techniques that target the root of many sleep struggles—your breathing.

The market is filled with supplements and "sleep remedies" that promise better health and deeper sleep. Some health influencers even promote "supplement stacking," the practice of combining multiple supplements, which could work out to be a costly avenue to pursue. Stacking supplements in the pursuit of optimal health seems to have reached new extremes. Take Bryan Johnson, for example, a man who's determined to hack his way to eternal youth.[1] If you haven't seen it yet, his story is featured in a Netflix documentary. His daily routine reportedly involves taking up to 100 supplements a day. While cost is certainly a barrier for most, I can't help but marvel at how anyone has the time or energy to devote themselves so fully to improving their health.

What's particularly interesting about Bryan, though, is his unwavering dedication to sleep. In his relentless pursuit of longevity, sleep is one of the cornerstones of his regimen—something that doesn't require a fortune and is entirely within reach for the rest of us. As he puts it:

> "Take sleep as seriously as you do your job. You show up on time, you respect it, you're very rigorous about it, you're disciplined, you take pride in it."

For all the cutting-edge science, expensive supplements, and life-hacking gadgets Bryan uses, this one piece of advice remains universally applicable. Sleep is one of the most powerful, restorative, and accessible tools we have for our health—and it doesn't cost a penny.

Rather than reaching for supplements as a first solution, sleep experts advise that focusing systematically (every night) on regulating your sleep-wake cycle, adhering to sleep hygiene recommendations, and regulating stress will be more helpful in helping you achieve better sleep.[2]

Breathing is perhaps the most overlooked aspect of sleep, despite being the function most affected by sleep disturbances—it's even in the name: "sleep-disordered breathing." Yet breathing re-education isn't just for those with diagnosed sleep disorders. It's a powerful tool for anyone struggling with a restless body or a mind stuck in overdrive due to heightened stress responses.

This isn't just for those with obstructive sleep apnea or upper airway resistance syndrome (UARS); it's for anyone who wants to settle their body and calm their nervous system before bed whether you're dealing with stress, poor sleep quality, or just want to feel more rested in the morning. When you include breathing techniques in your nighttime routine, you're not just doing another sleep hack; you're tuning into something essential. You're addressing a core part of the sleep process that's often ignored but quietly shapes how well you rest and recover.

COMMON SLEEP DISORDERS

As we have learned, sleep disorders are surprisingly common and can have a major impact on your daily life, especially when they lead to excessive daytime sleepiness and difficulty functioning. These conditions are grouped into categories, including insomnia, sleep-related breathing issues (like sleep apnea), and disorders that affect your body's internal clock or cause unusual behaviors during sleep.

Each type of sleep disorder comes with its own challenges, but understanding them is the first step toward better rest. Table 10.1 outlines the most common sleep disorders, their key features, and how often they occur. Whether you're curious about your own sleep or want to help someone else, this guide can be helpful—you may even recognize some symptoms you have experienced yourself.

Table 10.1   *Common Sleep Issues and Disorders*

Sleep Disorder and Example	Brief Description	How Common?[3]
Insomnia Disorders		
Chronic Insomnia Disorder	Those with insomnia may experience challenges in falling asleep, maintaining sleep, and/or early-morning wakefulness.	Globally, approximately 8–10% of the adult population suffers from chronic insomnia.[4]
Sleep-Related Breathing Disorders		
Snoring	While not considered a sleep disorder, snoring is a common symptom of sleep-disordered breathing, which ranges from upper airway resistance to OSA. Snoring can impact your (and your partner's) sleep and cause daytime sleepiness.	In the US, among adults aged 30 to 60, 44% of men snore regularly compared with 28% of women.[5]
Upper Airway Resistance Syndrome (UARS)	In those with UARS, the airway partially collapses or narrows during sleep, creating resistance in breathing and increased breathing effort. This increased effort can disrupt sleep, causing frequent awakenings and daytime sleepiness.[6]	Approximately 6–11% of the general population.[7]

Table 10.1 *Common Sleep Issues and Disorders (continued)*

Sleep Disorder and Example	Brief Description	How Common?[3]
Obstructive Sleep Apnea (OSA)	OSA involves repeated breathing interruptions during sleep, associated with snoring, pauses in breathing, snorting and gasping. This interrupted sleep causes daytime sleepiness and fatigue and is associated with many negative health consequences (please refer to Chapter 10D).	In a 1993 study in the United States, moderate-to-severe OSA was prevalent in 11% of men and 4% of women.[8] According to a 2013 follow-up study, the number increased to 14% of men and 5% of women.[9] In 20 years, the prevalence of OSA in US adults aged 30 to 70 increased by 27% in men and 25% in women.[10] In the UK and Ireland, the prevalence is 24·5%.[11]
Central Disorders of Hypersomnolence		
Narcolepsy	A chronic disorder that causes periods of extreme daytime sleepiness (hypersomnolence), including sudden brief episodes of deep sleep.	Approximately 0.02–0.05% of the US adult general population.
Circadian Rhythm Sleep-Wake Disorders		
Delayed Sleep Phase Disorder Advanced Sleep Phase Disorder	Conditions where an individual's internal body clock, or circadian rhythm, is out of sync with the natural environment. Delayed sleep phase disorder or delayed onset of sleep and waking, is commonly observed in teenagers. Advanced sleep phase disorder, or early onset of sleep and waking, is commonly found in elderly people.	Approximately 7–16%[12]

(continued on next page)

Table 10.1   *Common Sleep Issues and Disorders (continued)*

Sleep Disorder and Example	Brief Description	How Common?[3]
Sleep-Related Movement Disorders		
Restless Legs Syndrome (RLS)	A neurological disorder that causes uncomfortable sensations in your legs and an irresistible urge to move them. Symptoms are often most intense at night and can severely disrupt sleep.	RLS affects approximately 3% of the US population, but if you count mild or occasional symptoms, the real number might be closer to 7–10%. It is more common in females. Symptoms typically become more frequent and last longer with age.
Sleep-Related Bruxism (SB)	Characterized by involuntary grinding, clenching, or gnashing of the teeth during sleep. Can lead to damaged teeth, jaw pain, TMJ disorder, headaches, and disrupted sleep. Stress and anxiety increase the likelihood of bruxism. Jaw clenching or grinding may be a response to the need to maintain an open airway.	The global prevalence of SB in pediatric and adult populations is estimated at 21%.[13] In those with OSA, the prevalence of SB reaches 37.1%, correlating with increased muscle tone during sleep and suggesting that SB in OSA patients is related to overall sleep-disordered breathing.[14]

In the chapters that follow, we will take a closer look at some of the most common sleep disorders—insomnia, snoring, UARS, and OSA—and discuss strategies for restoring functional nasal breathing to improve their management.

DAVINA'S STORY: FROM SLEEPLESS NIGHTS TO LIFE-CHANGING RESULTS

Davina, age 46, a primary school teacher from Northern Ireland, had battled late-onset asthma, chronic insomnia, and fatigue since her early twenties. No matter how many inhalers or medications she tried, her health only seemed to decline. But everything changed when she stumbled upon an article about the Buteyko Method. Skeptical but desperate for a solution, she booked a class with Patrick McKeown.

That decision changed her life.

"My asthma became very severe very quickly. I had a lot of chest infections, I had pneumonia, I was in and out of hospital, and it was becoming progressively worse. It was a very difficult time. Things were just spiraling out of control. My asthma was uncontrolled. I was on more and more inhalers and steroids. My sleep was terrible.

"I found out that Patrick had face-to-face classes, and I got booked in as soon as I could. I thought—I'll try this out and see what it's like—and do you know what? It just completely changed my life for the better! The Buteyko Method made complete scientific sense, and it was so simple. I think whenever I went to the first class, my CP [Control Pause] was about 8, you know I was able to just do about 12 steps. I was very ill."

By learning to breathe through her nose, retraining her breathing patterns, and using mouth tape at night, Davina began to notice small but powerful shifts.

At first, her asthma symptoms gradually eased. She found herself using her inhalers less frequently. Her sleep improved dramatically—no more suffering through restless nights. However, about six months into her breathing practice, she began experiencing frequent throat infections and tonsillitis.

A visit to an ENT specialist confirmed she needed her tonsils removed. After undergoing surgery, she continued her Buteyko breathing practice and kept using mouth tape at night to ensure she maintained nasal breathing.

The results? Life-changing!

"It improved my life, improved my sleep, improved everything. The mouth tape was invaluable, as well as the breathing exercises and the surgery. They transformed my life!"

Paying It Forward

Inspired by her recovery, Davina went on to train as one of the first Buteyko Clinic Instructors, eager to share the techniques that had turned her health around.

And the benefits didn't stop with her—her son, Henry, faced similar health struggles, and through the same breathing techniques, he too experienced a dramatic improvement (his story is told in Chapter 12).

Davina's story illustrates how breathing better can be a game-changer—not just for asthma but for insomnia, energy levels, and overall health. By learning to breathe through your nose, taping your mouth at night, and retraining your breathing habits, you, too, can experience the profound effects of better sleep and easier breathing.

If you're struggling with poor sleep, why not give it a try? It just might change your life.

CHAPTER 10A

INSOMNIA—HIDDEN DRIVERS AND EFFECTIVE SOLUTIONS

Insomnia is one of the most common sleep challenges. It's when you have trouble falling asleep, staying asleep, or getting good-quality rest. For some, it's short term (acute insomnia) and resolves on its own, but for others, it can drag on for months or even years (chronic insomnia). While it may seem like insomnia just comes out of nowhere, it's often linked to something deeper, like stress, anxiety, or even how we think about sleep itself.

For many people, the real culprit is hyperarousal—when the nervous system is stuck in overdrive. It's like your body is constantly on high alert, not just at night but all day long. By the time you lie down, it's impossible to unwind. Your body feels jazzed up, and the mind won't turn off. It's not just the racing thoughts; it's your whole system refusing to settle.

Once poor sleep becomes a pattern—lasting more than three months—it often creates a vicious cycle. You start to believe it's just who you are. People start labeling themselves as "bad sleepers." You might think, "I've always been this way," or "My mother was a bad sleeper, so I must have inherited her bad sleeping genes." The mind clings to this identity, replaying the bad nights over and over while forgetting the good ones. Each difficult night becomes proof that you're simply not capable of sleeping well. Before long, sleep isn't something you look forward to; it becomes something you brace yourself for. Instead of feeling like a time to recharge, it starts to feel like something to dread.

> "I used to take an hour to get to sleep, but since learning **Buteyko I now get to sleep in 5 to 10 minutes.** It has been a lifetime of struggling to get to sleep so this has made a huge difference to my life. I feel like I need less sleep now as well."
>
> *Sandy, 53, South Africa*

But here's the thing: the more we repeat that story, the more we reinforce it; until it feels like fact. And over time, it can become a self-fulfilling prophecy. If you believe you're a bad sleeper, you begin to expect poor sleep, worry about it before bed, and approach the night with tension instead of ease.

The truth is, you have more control over your sleep quality than you might think. It's not about blaming yourself. It's about gently challenging old beliefs and calming the systems that may be keeping you stuck.

This is where Chapter 8 also comes in. It's all about observing your thoughts and asking yourself: "Is this way of thinking helpful? Is it productive? Is it even true?" By shifting your mindset and retraining your nervous system, you can move toward better, more restful sleep. With Buteyko breathing, you can let go of the "bad sleeper" label and help ease the stress response, giving the mind and body a chance to truly relax and reset.

How Common Is Insomnia?

Acute Insomnia

Around one-third of adults—between 30 and 36%—report experiencing at least one symptom of insomnia.[1] These can include difficulty falling asleep, trouble staying asleep, or waking up feeling unrefreshed (what's often called "nonrestorative sleep"). Judging by these numbers, it's clear that having the occasional bad night of sleep is actually quite normal.

This might come as a relief, especially if you use a sleep-monitoring device. It's a helpful reminder that a poor night's sleep now and then isn't the end of the world. Your body is resilient, and one restless night doesn't mean your overall sleep health is doomed. So, if your device shows a less-than-stellar sleep score, take it in stride—it's okay to have an off night every once in a while.

Chronic Insomnia

Chronic insomnia isn't just a few nights of bad sleep—it's a long-term struggle that spills over into your days, draining your energy, focus, and sense of well-being. And that's the real issue—it's not just about the tossing and turning at night, but how it impacts you when you're awake.

Here's something to think about the next time you find yourself lying in bed with the mind racing, hopping from one thought to the next. The clock is ticking, your brain won't settle, and you feel like you're running out of time to fall asleep. The frustration builds, the pressure to fall asleep kicks in, and you feel stuck. But instead of getting caught up in the mental battle, what if you flipped the script? What if you used this time as an opportunity to rest, even if sleep doesn't come right away? Think about it: the room is quiet and dark, and your bed is likely warm and cozy. It's the perfect setup to give yourself some attention. Shift your focus away from the mind and onto your breathing. If your mind won't settle, give it a gentle focus like following the inhale and the exhale, or tuning in to a guided audio.

If you'd like, you can listen to the guided audio I've created. It walks you through relaxing your body and quieting the mind, step by step. Simply scan the QR code to download the audio file for sleep.

There's nothing to force. Nothing to fix. Just a chance to rest your body and let your nervous system settle down. And if sleep follows, that's a bonus. Now what about those mornings when you wake up groggy, already dreading the day ahead? Instead of pushing through and piling on the pressure, take 20 minutes to rest and reset. I do this myself. In fact, I listened to the same audio this morning while working on the final proofs of this book. It didn't knock me out like deep sleep might, but it gave me the clarity and focus I needed to get back into the day. Just enough to lift the mental fog. Simply scan the QR code, download, and give it a go. They're free and easy to use whenever you need a break.

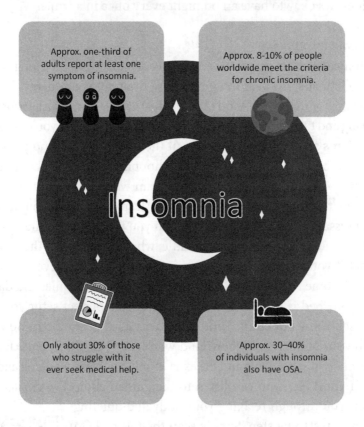

Approx. one-third of adults report at least one symptom of insomnia.

Approx. 8-10% of people worldwide meet the criteria for chronic insomnia.

Insomnia

Only about 30% of those who struggle with it ever seek medical help.

Approx. 30–40% of individuals with insomnia also have OSA.

To meet the clinical definition of chronic insomnia, it has to happen at least three times a week, last for three months or more, and interfere with your daytime functioning or overall well-being.

There are two main types of chronic insomnia. The first is *sleep-onset insomnia*, which is when falling asleep feels like the biggest hurdle. The second is *sleep-maintenance insomnia*, which means staying asleep is the problem—whether that's waking up in the middle of the night or far too early in the morning. And yes, many people deal with both at the same time.

While insomnia can feel overwhelming, small changes in how you approach your nights—and even your days—can start to make a difference. Whether it's shifting your mindset about those sleepless moments, resting and resetting during the day, or practicing breathing exercises to calm the mind, these tools can help you start reclaiming your sleep and your energy.

Approximately 8–10% of people worldwide meet the criteria for chronic insomnia, which translates to about 42 million adults globally.[2,3] However, it's worth noting that insomnia is vastly underreported. Studies suggest that only about 30% of those who struggle with it ever seek medical help.[4] This means the actual numbers are likely much higher.

Understanding the Causes of Insomnia: Risk and Contributing Factors

As you might expect, people with irregular sleep schedules, poor sleep habits, and high stress levels are more likely to experience insomnia. Additionally, insomnia is more prevalent in certain groups and conditions, including:[5]

- **Gender.** Insomnia occurs more frequently in females than in males, potentially due to hormonal changes and life-stage events such as pregnancy or menopause.
- **Age.** Older adults experience a higher prevalence of insomnia, often due to changes in sleep patterns and increased likelihood of chronic health conditions.

- **Shift work.** Insomnia is more common in those who work irregular or rotating shifts, as their schedules disrupt the natural sleep-wake cycle and reduce overall sleep quality.
- **Sleep disorders.** Many people with insomnia also have other sleep disorders. For instance, 30–40% of individuals with insomnia may have OSA, and 30–50% of those with OSA report insomnia symptoms.[6]
- **Mental health conditions.** Insomnia is significantly more common in people with mental health challenges. Up to 70% of individuals with major depressive disorder experience insomnia, and those with insomnia face at least twice the risk of developing depression and anxiety.[7]
- **Physical health conditions.** Insomnia is also more common in people with comorbid or co-occurring conditions such as chronic obstructive pulmonary disease, heart failure, and chronic pain.

Being aware of these potential contributing factors can help manage insomnia better in these vulnerable groups.

I'd like to turn your attention now to exploring a key mechanism underlying insomnia: hyperarousal.

Hyperarousal: The Hidden Driver of Insomnia

Insomnia often has an unexpected culprit: an overactive autonomic nervous system. At the heart of it lies a state called "hyperarousal," where your body feels stuck in overdrive, unable to properly relax. The sympathetic nervous system—commonly known as the "fight, flight, or freeze" response—takes control, while the parasympathetic system—which governs "rest, digest, and repair"—is pushed to the side. This imbalance doesn't just affect your ability to fall or stay asleep; it keeps your body on high alert when it should be winding down, disrupting the delicate transitions between wakefulness and rest.[8]

Now, let's talk about the word "sympathetic." Normally, it brings to mind kindness or compassion, but in this context, it comes from the original meaning of "acting together." The sympathetic nervous system is like your body's emergency response team—it rallies all your resources to face a threat. It mobilizes energy, speeds up your heart rate, and sharpens your focus, all to help you react quickly to danger. In those moments when you need to escape a threat or handle an urgent situation, it's incredibly useful, even life-saving.

When the sympathetic nervous system is constantly activated, like it often is in people with insomnia, it becomes a different story. Instead of protecting you, it prevents you from truly relaxing. Your body stays on high alert, unable to shift into a state of calm, and sleep becomes a challenge rather than the restorative process it's meant to be. While the sympathetic system is designed to help you in moments of need, being stuck in overdrive keeps the mind and body in a perpetual state of "ready for action."

On the other side is the parasympathetic nervous system, which acts as a counterbalance. Picture the two systems like a seesaw: when one side goes up, the other naturally goes down. When the sympathetic system is in charge, your body is on edge, ready to respond to threats. But when the parasympathetic system takes over, the seesaw tilts the other way, and your body can finally relax. Your heart rate slows, your digestion works efficiently, and the mind finds peace—this state of calm is essential for good sleep.

For people with insomnia, though, the seesaw gets stuck. The sympathetic system dominates, leaving little room for the parasympathetic system to step in. Instead of winding down at night, the body remains revved up, making it difficult to fall asleep or stay asleep once you do. This imbalance keeps the cycle of poor sleep and heightened alertness going, preventing the restful recovery your body and mind desperately need.

So, how do you know if you're stuck in this hyperaroused state? It often feels like being "wired but tired." The mind races, jumping from one thought to the next, and your body feels restless, almost as if it's buzzing with unused energy. Even small things—a creak in the floorboards, a slight shift in thought—can jolt you awake. It's as if your body is constantly bracing for impact, even when there's no real threat. Some people describe it as feeling like "the bear is always there," as if a predator is lurking in the background.

This hypervigilance doesn't just disrupt your nights; it spills into your days. You wake up feeling drained, emotionally fragile, and unable to focus. The stress of poor sleep triggers even more sympathetic activity, further fueling hyperarousal and setting the stage for another restless night. Over time, this creates a vicious cycle of fragmented, shallow, and unsatisfying sleep, leaving you stuck in a loop of exhaustion and frustration.

The good news? You can tip the balance back. You can help the body shift out of "emergency mode" and back into a state of calm. One of the easiest ways to do this is through your breath. Breathing is a direct line to your nervous system—when you slow and soften your breath, you send a signal to your brain that it's safe to relax.

ADDRESSING INSOMNIA

When it comes to treating insomnia, the focus is often on tackling the hyperarousal that keeps you wired but tired. The most common approaches include Cognitive Behavioral Therapy for Insomnia (CBT-I), sleep medications, or a combination of the two.

Cognitive Behavioral Therapy for Insomnia

CBT-I is like therapy for your sleep—it helps you untangle the messy web of negative thoughts and habits that feed sleepless nights. It might involve questions like, "What's the worst that could actually happen if you don't sleep tonight?" or even, "Have you had good days after poor sleep before?" These questions might sound a bit surprising, but they're meant to challenge the catastrophizing thoughts that often come with sleeplessness.

CBT-I also works on practical habits, like cutting out late-night caffeine, setting a consistent bedtime, and avoiding the endless doom scroll on your phone in bed. The idea is to rebuild a healthy relationship with sleep, so you stop dreading the moment your head hits the pillow.

So, how does Buteyko breathing compare? This approach offers something unique—it goes straight to the source of the problem: your autonomic nervous system. While CBT-I helps reframe your thoughts and behaviors around sleep, it doesn't touch your breathing or address your respiratory physiology. Breathing, on the other hand, is like a secret lever you can pull to tell your body, "Hey, we're safe. It's okay to relax."

With Buteyko breathing, you focus on slowing down your breath, breathing lightly, and using your nose. This helps shift your body out of "fight or flight" mode and into "rest and digest" mode, where relaxation and sleep come more naturally. Many people with insomnia unknowingly over-breathe or breathe irregularly, which can make their hyperarousal worse. Buteyko retrains your breath, calming the mind and body in a way that CBT-I can't.

Now, imagine combining the two approaches. A therapist might help you challenge your racing thoughts with questions like, "What evidence do you have that you won't fall asleep tonight?" while you use your breathing to physically calm down and tell your nervous system, "It's okay to switch off now." Together, these tools can tackle insomnia from both mental and physical angles, giving you a much better chance of breaking the cycle of sleepless nights.

Sleep Medications

Sleep medications can feel like a quick fix, offering relief by helping you fall asleep faster or stay asleep longer. But they come with baggage. Many are habit-forming and only meant for short-term use under strict medical guidance. They can leave you feeling groggy or foggy the next day, and for older adults, they increase the risk of falls and confusion. And while they may temporarily help you sleep, they don't address the underlying reasons why sleep isn't coming naturally.

Here's the irony with sleep medications: while they might help you fall asleep or stay asleep longer, they can quietly rob you of the very thing your body needs most—deep, restorative sleep. Many of these pills reduce slow-wave sleep, the stage of sleep that's crucial for physical recovery, immune function, and memory consolidation.[9] It's the phase that truly refreshes you, leaving you ready to face the day.

So, while the meds might seem like a helpful ally at first, giving you more hours in bed, they're also taking something away on the other end. It's a bit like using a credit card to pay for something essential. You get what you need right away, but there's a cost down the line. Over time, this reduction in slow-wave sleep can leave you feeling less refreshed, even if you're clocking more hours of sleep.

To complicate matters further, recent studies have linked the use of some sleep medications to cognitive decline later in life. As Dr. Chris Winter highlights in *The Sleep Solution,* "Reports linking these drugs to cognitive decline in life have emerged, but the old guard docs still use them like crazy."[10]

A memorable example of the pitfalls of sleep medication was highlighted in *The Mary Tyler Moore Show* episode, "Mary's Insomnia," which aired in 1976.[11] In this episode, Mary Richards, played by Mary Tyler Moore, turns to sleeping pills after struggling with insomnia, only to realize she's becoming dependent on them. Her boss, Lou Grant, intervenes, challenging her to skip the pills and explore a more natural approach. The humor-laden episode culminates with Lou encouraging Mary to breathe deeply, wrapping her in an afghan, and singing her to sleep. Against all odds, the simple act of focused breathing helps Mary relax and finally drift off.

Set in the 1970s, *The Mary Tyler Moore Show* used humor and relatable scenarios to address real-life issues, including sleep struggles. This lighthearted yet impactful story underscores a critical point: while medications can be effective in the short term, they are not a sustainable solution for chronic insomnia.

Supplements

Some people turn to supplements such as melatonin, the so-called "sleep hormone," to combat insomnia. Melatonin levels are generally lower in those with insomnia, especially in cases of long-term insomnia, indicating that the severity of the disorder may increase over time.[12]

Melatonin often gets a lot of attention as a natural sleep aid, and while it can be helpful in specific situations—like recovering from jet lag or supporting older adults whose melatonin levels naturally decline—it's not the perfect solution. For chronic insomnia, the evidence is mixed. Some studies suggest it can help, while others find little-to-no benefit. And it's not entirely free of drawbacks. At higher doses or with long-term use, side effects like daytime grogginess, dizziness, and headaches can occur, making it less appealing for everyday use.

One common question is whether melatonin can be addictive. The good news is that melatonin is not physically addictive, meaning you won't experience withdrawal symptoms if you stop taking it. However, people can become psychologically dependent on it—essentially convincing themselves that they can't sleep without it. This reliance can create its own challenges, especially when the real root cause of sleep problems isn't being addressed.

Interestingly, melatonin's availability varies around the world. In the United States, you can pick it up over the counter at almost any pharmacy or grocery store. But in countries like Ireland and the UK, melatonin is classified as a prescription-only medication. Why? These stricter regulations aim to ensure that melatonin is used appropriately and only when it's genuinely needed. It's also a way to prevent misuse or overuse, as taking melatonin unnecessarily or in high doses can disrupt your body's natural production of the hormone. Over-the-counter availability in some countries has led to people self-dosing without guidance, sometimes taking far more than needed, which increases the risk of side effects.

So, while melatonin can have its place in short-term sleep management, it's important to approach it thoughtfully. It might help you get over a rough patch, but it won't fix what's really keeping you up.

A Different Approach: Light, Slow, and Deep Nasal Breathing

Beyond therapy, pills, and supplements lies a powerful, side-effect-free approach to tackling insomnia. Since disrupted sleep is closely tied to increased activity in the sympathetic nervous system—the "fight, flight, or freeze" response—changing how you breathe can be a game-changer for people dealing with insomnia.

> "Before I used these techniques I would wake up feeling like I had not slept at all and this also had an impact on my energy.
>
> Now I wake up feeling amazing and always start my day in the garden doing my breathing techniques which will set me up for the whole day."
>
> *Mark, 47, UK*

Dr. Ravinder Jerath and his team shared an interesting perspective on insomnia in a 2019 article published in *Frontiers in Psychiatry*.[13] They proposed that slow, deep breathing, combined with relaxation techniques and good sleep hygiene, could be a game-changer for people struggling with insomnia—potentially even more effective than relying on sleep medications.

Jerath describes insomnia as a "mismatch disease," where the body's "fight or flight" system—the overactive sympathetic nervous system—takes charge at the very time it should be winding down for rest. By practicing light, slow breathing, the goal is to reset this imbalance, tipping the seesaw in favor of the parasympathetic "rest and digest" system. This calms the nervous system and helps ease the overwhelming pressure to fall asleep—a pressure that often backfires and makes sleep even more elusive.

What's surprising is that, while relaxation techniques and sleep hygiene are well-documented tools for addressing insomnia, very little research has focused on the power of light, slow breathing. Jerath hopes this fresh perspective will inspire further studies and ignite discussions about its potential as a natural, effective way to combat insomnia.

Light, Slow, and Deep Breathing to Promote Relaxation and Sleep

When it comes to breathing, the three key dimensions are breathing light, slow, and deep. Each of these techniques plays a role in calming the mind and restoring balance to the autonomic nervous system. Studies show that slow breathing enhances vagal tone and increases heart rate variability—key indicators of parasympathetic activity— helping the body relax and paving the way for higher-quality sleep.[14,15]

Vagal tone reflects how well your vagus nerve, the powerhouse behind your parasympathetic "rest, digest, and repair" system, is balancing the sympathetic "fight, flight, or freeze" side.

Even more fascinating, slow, deep breathing has been linked to increased melatonin production, further enhancing parasympathetic tone, calming sympathetic activity, and helping induce sleep.[16] Slow, deep breathing also lowers levels of the stress hormones norepinephrine and epinephrine. Along with cortisol, these hormones are often elevated in insomniacs and contribute to alertness, body movement, and arousal.[17] But through the simple act of slowing your breath, you can counter this unwelcome hormonal state and set the stage for deeper, more restorative sleep. The best part? It's free, natural, and accessible to anyone, anytime.

A small study on the efficacy of slow, paced breathing for insomnia demonstrated that slow breathing performed before or at bedtime can improve sleep as measured by polysomnography. The study included 14 insomniacs and 14 controls and found that sleep onset latency, number of awakenings, and awakening time during sleep were decreased and sleep efficiency was increased when insomniac participants practiced slow, paced breathing exercises for 20 minutes before going to sleep.[18] In simple terms, the study revealed that practicing these exercises allowed participants to fall asleep more quickly, wake up less often during the night, and enjoy longer periods of restful sleep, ultimately enhancing their overall sleep efficiency.

Over the years, my personal favorite has been the *Breathe Light Exercise*. There's something uniquely powerful about it. It not only calms the nervous system but also quiets overactive brain cell activity, all while anchoring your attention to the breath.

The *Breathe Light Exercise* is a simple yet powerful way to calm the body, enhance vagal tone, and promote parasympathetic dominance. It involves light, soft, and reduced breathing, creating a gentle sensation of air hunger. This subtle reduction in breathing volume quiets the nervous system and redirects your focus away from racing thoughts, helping to ground you in the present moment. When practiced before bed or during those frustrating middle-of-the-night wake-ups, *Breathe Light* can be an effective tool to prepare your body and mind for deep, restorative sleep.

Exercises and Recommendations for Addressing Insomnia Using the Breath

Practicing the following exercises and recommendations, along with good sleep hygiene, may just be the key to relieving your struggle with insomnia.

1. **Difficulty falling asleep.** To help quiet the mind and ease into sleep, it's important to slow and lighten your breathing, letting the brain know it's safe to relax. Here are a few ways to achieve this:

- **Breathe through your nose as much as possible.** Practice breathing through your nose consistently throughout the day, during rest, exercise, and sleep. Nasal breathing naturally encourages a calm, steady breath that carries into the night. If you often wake with a dry mouth, consider using MyoTape or a similar nasal breathing support to promote nose breathing.

- **Work toward a CP score of 20+ seconds.** A CP score of over 20 seconds is a reliable sign that your breathing is stable and functional, which is a key factor in promoting quality sleep.

- **Practice *Breathe Light* for 10 minutes before bed.** This exercise helps to calm both the mind and body by slowing down your breathing rate, preparing you for sleep. For ease, you might try listening to my guided audio for insomnia, which includes the *Breathe Light Exercise*. You can access it using the QR code to download it to your phone.

2. **Waking in the middle of the night.** Earlier, I mentioned using soft, slow breathing to calm the mind and activate your body's natural relaxation response. And yes, this can work wonders. But if you're lying awake in the middle of the night with the mind racing and thoughts spiraling out of control, you already know— it's not always that simple. Sometimes, no matter how hard you try to focus on your breathing, those intrusive thoughts just keep barging in, making it nearly impossible to relax.

   That's when it helps to hand over the reins to something else—something that takes the pressure of "trying" completely off your shoulders. Instead of battling with the mind or working to consciously slow your breath, try putting on a set of headphones, playing a guided audio session, and letting yourself relax into the process. No effort, no overthinking—just listen and let go.

Even if your thoughts are loud or sleep doesn't come right away, that's okay. Play the track again if needed. You're still giving your body a chance to rest deeply, and here's the thing—even rest alone can make a world of difference. You might not wake up feeling like you've had the perfect night's sleep, but you'll almost certainly feel better than if you'd spent those hours tossing, turning, and stressing. Sleep doesn't have to be perfect. The real goal is to give yourself enough rest to recharge and face the day ahead without feeling completely drained.

Guided audio sessions are an excellent way to shift your focus and ease your body and mind into relaxation. Listening to a calming voice gives your busy mind something soothing to focus on, naturally redirecting your attention and quieting your thoughts. (Yes, my calming voice—what can I say; even I enjoy the sound of it!) Before you know it, you're drifting off. And even if you don't fall asleep right away, the deep rest you're getting is still incredibly valuable. Your body and mind will thank you for it the next day. For a practical way to explore this, try the guided audio. You can access it using the QR code to download it to your phone, making it easy to use whenever you need a little extra help winding down.

By incorporating these practices into your routine, you'll build a strong foundation for deep, restorative sleep. As your breathing stabilizes and your CP score improves, you'll experience fewer nighttime disruptions, better sleep quality, and more energy to greet each morning.

In the following pages, I share the story of a Ukrainian woman named Alina, who successfully used these techniques when her sleep and well-being were shattered by the relentless stress of war.

ALINA'S STORY: FROM SURVIVING WAR AND HYPERAROUSAL TO HEALING THROUGH THE POWER OF BREATH

Alina, a 35-year-old marketer from Ukraine, was forced to flee her home city and endure the chaos of war. She faced immense physical and emotional challenges. As a result of her living in a state of constant hyperarousal and hypervigilance, her body and mind were unable to switch off. Yet through intentionally working with her breath, she recalibrated her nervous system, reclaimed peace, overcame anxiety, and restored her sleep. She hopes her journey will inspire others navigating high-stress situations.

The Impact of War on the Nervous System

When war erupted in 2022, Alina's life was upended overnight. She had to leave Kyiv, abandoning her career and security. The stress was relentless—an unending cycle of fear, adrenaline, hyperarousal, and survival mode. The impact was devastating—disrupted sleep, panic attacks, memory loss, and severe hormonal imbalances.

"I was in Ukraine when the war started. I had to move from my hometown to another city. That meant leaving everything—my home, my job, my family. It was terrifying. Every day, I feared for my life. The stress was overwhelming. I noticed physical changes—weight gain, lost periods, no energy. Low memory. I couldn't even focus enough to read a book. So many women around me experienced the same thing—missing periods, cognitive fog, chronic exhaustion."

Her nights were no better. Air raid sirens shattered any sense of rest, forcing her into shelters at all hours. Sleep became shallow, restless, and filled with disturbing dreams.

"Sleep was completely out of my control. I would wake up, hear the alarms, and run to the bathroom for shelter. Even when I wasn't running, I tossed and turned, drenched in sweat, having nightmares."

Rebuilding a Life Amid Uncertainty

Despite the ongoing war, Alina sought to regain some control. She immersed herself in healthy habits—swimming, running, functional movement, and sleep hygiene. But the stress was relentless.

"You can eat well, you can exercise, but when you are constantly in fear, it's never enough. No matter how hard I tried, the reality was that I could die at any moment."

In early 2023, a medical checkup revealed another blow: her ovarian reserve had plummeted due to extreme stress. Doctors warned that without intervention, she might lose the chance to have children.

"It was another level of stress—knowing that war had not only stolen my present but was threatening my future."

Alina eventually relocated elsewhere in Europe in 2024, but stress still clung to her body. Despite her being physically safe, her nervous system remained in a state of hyperarousal. That's when she discovered the power of breathwork.

Discovering Breath as a Tool to Regulate the Nervous System

Inspired by James Nestor's *Breath* and guided by the Oxygen Advantage®, Alina began practicing nasal breathing, light, slow and deep (LSD) breathing, and mouth taping. These simple yet powerful techniques rewired her nervous system, helping her shift from survival mode to a state of calm.

"When I moved, I finally felt safe. But safety alone wasn't enough. My nervous system was still stuck in a trauma response. That's when I started breathwork. At first, it was just nose breathing and mouth taping at night, which helped. But when I added LSD breathing, everything changed."

She noticed a profound shift. Her anxiety diminished, her sleep deepened, and her panic attacks disappeared. Significantly, her dreams also changed—no longer filled with war and fear, but regular, peaceful dreams she hadn't experienced in years.

"I use nasal breathing during the day and while exercising, except when swimming. I practice LSD breathing in the morning and evening, and that's where I felt the biggest transformation. It signaled to my body: *we are safe now*. It activated my parasympathetic nervous system, moving me out of fear and into a state of relaxation. I hadn't realized how much I needed that."

Breathing Re-education: A Lifeline for Sleep and Nervous System Regulation

Alina's healing experience was so profound that she trained as a breathing coach. Now, she is dedicated to teaching others—especially those in war-torn or high-stress environments—how to harness the power of their breath to regain control over their nervous system.

"I want people to know that even in the worst circumstances, there is something you can do. You may not control war, alarms, or explosions, but you *can* control your breath. Breath is free, it's always with you, and it's the fastest way to calm your nervous system."

Her mission is to teach breathwork as an emergency tool—helping people find calm in the chaos, resilience in the face of uncertainty, and rest even when the world around them is unstable.

"I've been in moments where I had nothing. No medicine, no comfort, nothing but fear. And in those moments, breath was the one thing I could count on. It helped me regain control. That's what I want to share with others—how to breathe their way back to safety, even in the darkest times."

Today, Alina sleeps deeply, free from panic and fear. Her energy has returned, her mood has lifted, and she's no longer trapped in survival mode.

"Breathwork reprogrammed my nervous system. It switched me from *surviving* to *living* and *thriving*. And I want others to know that no matter how bad things seem, there is hope. There is always a way to come back to yourself."

Alina's story is truly a testament to the profound effect that using simple, accessible techniques such as light, slow, and deep nasal breathing can have. I'm incredibly grateful to Alina for her generosity in sharing her story as a source of hope and inspiration to others who are facing stressful situations.

CHAPTER 10B

SLEEP-DISORDERED BREATHING AND SNORING

Let's turn our attention now to sleep-disordered breathing. Even though it's often treated as separate from insomnia, the two frequently go hand in hand. These disorders, ranging from snoring to the silent interruptions of sleep apnea, fragment rest and deprive the body of the deep sleep it needs to repair, restore, and thrive. Left unchecked, they can permeate into nearly every aspect of health. In the following chapters, we'll explore the most common types of sleep-disordered breathing and, more importantly, what you can do to restore optimal breathing and optimal sleep. But let's begin by exploring the topic of breathing resistance, as this underlies sleep-disordered breathing.

AIRWAY RESISTANCE

When we breathe, air should flow effortlessly through our airways—smoothly, silently, and unrestricted. For adults, breathing during sleep should not be audible; for children, it should *definitely* not be heard. But when the nasal passages are narrow or the throat tightens, airflow gets disrupted. That added resistance makes it harder to breathe smoothly and can easily disturb your sleep.

Snoring is like the first alarm bell when it comes to breathing resistance during sleep. It's the audible warning sign that something isn't quite right. And let's be honest—snoring comes in all shapes and sizes, from the occasional mild snore to the kind of racket that shakes the walls. To give you an idea of just how loud snoring can get, the Guinness World Record goes to Kåre Walkert from Sweden, whose snoring hit a staggering 93 dBA while he was being monitored at Örebro Regional Hospital in 1993.[1] To put that into perspective, 93 dBA is about as loud as a jackhammer or a motorcycle revving up. Imagine trying to sleep through that!

But snoring isn't just a noise problem—it's often the first step on a slippery slope. If left unchecked, it can escalate to hypopneas. These are episodes where airflow is so restricted that your blood oxygen levels drop by at least 3% for 10 seconds or more, putting additional strain on your body and disrupting sleep even further.

The Cycle of Airway Resistance and Collapse in Sleep-Disordered Breathing

Sleep-disordered breathing often follows a self-reinforcing loop. As breathing becomes harder and more labored, the body responds by trying to pull in more air. But this increased effort can actually make things worse by sucking soft tissue inward and narrowing the airway even more. If the airway is already compromised—whether due to weak muscle tone, excess tissue, or a naturally narrow airway—this negative pressure can cause hypopneas or apneas, where airflow is significantly reduced or completely stops. The brain detects oxygen desaturation or rising CO_2 levels, triggering an arousal response to restore muscle tone, reopen the airway, and resume breathing. However, this repeated cycle of arousals leads to sleep fragmentation, increased respiratory effort, and ongoing airway instability, ultimately worsening sleep-disordered breathing over time.

You might not remember these wake-ups, but they fragment your sleep, leaving you exhausted in the morning without knowing why.

Stages of Airway Resistance and Collapse

1. **Increased resistance.** Airflow is restricted due to nasal congestion, mouth breathing, faster and harder breathing patterns, or a naturally narrow airway, making breathing more effortful.
2. **Negative pressure effect.** The increased inspiratory effort generates negative pressure inside the airway, pulling soft tissues inward.
3. **Partial collapse.** If the airway is already predisposed to narrowing—whether due to anatomical factors, weak muscle tone, or excess tissue—the negative pressure can further restrict airflow or cause partial obstruction, resulting in hypopneas (30–50% airflow reduction).
4. **Complete collapse and arousal.** With further resistance, the airway can fully collapse, leading to apneas (cessation of airflow for 10 seconds or more). In response, the brain detects oxygen drops or rising CO_2 levels and triggers an arousal, restoring airway function—but at the expense of sleep continuity.

As shown in Table 10B.1, the level of airway resistance directly affects the sound and quality of breathing during sleep, progressing from *no resistance*, where breathing remains silent and effortless, to *very severe resistance*, where the airway becomes completely obstructed. Identifying where an individual falls along this spectrum is crucial for early intervention before symptoms progress to more severe sleep-disordered breathing. By addressing breathing resistance and airway instability, interventions can help improve airflow, reduce respiratory effort, and promote deeper, more restorative sleep.

Table 10B.1 *A Scale of Breathing Resistance*

0	1	2	3	4
No Resistance	**Mild Resistance**	**Moderate Resistance**	**Severe Resistance**	**Very Severe Resistance**
Breathing is silent and effortless, occurring in and out through the nose, driven by the diaphragm with minimal effort.	Audible breathing without snoring. Airflow remains nasal or oral, still primarily diaphragm-driven but with slight turbulence.	Turbulent airflow in the airway leads to mild snoring as resistance increases. UARS where breathing effort is increased, sleep is disrupted by frequent arousals, but full airway collapse does not occur.	More pronounced snoring or hypopnea, where airflow is reduced by 30–50% due to partial airway collapse, lasting 10 seconds or more, and associated with oxygen desaturation or sleep fragmentation.	Complete airway collapse leads to apneas and more severe hypopneas, where breathing pauses entirely for 10 seconds or more. Snoring is interspersed with breath stops, indicating repeated airway obstruction.

Resistance

No ⟶ Mild ⟶ Moderate → Severe ⟶ Very Severe →

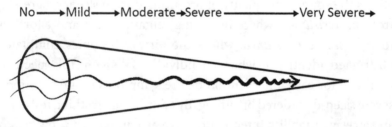

Breathing

Silent → Audible → Snoring ⟶ Hypopnea ⟶ Apnea ⟶

SNORING—A WARNING SIGN

When your airway is obstructed, even slightly, resistance builds. This can create turbulence, the kind that manifests as snoring—a telltale sign of air struggling to squeeze through a narrowed passage. In the rest of this chapter, I'll break down the different kinds of snoring, what's behind them, and, most importantly, how to quiet things down. With simple, effective solutions, you (and anyone within earshot) will be well on your way to silent, more restful nights.

Mouth Snoring

Snoring often happens when a large amount of air is forced through a flexible airway, causing the soft palate to vibrate. This type of snoring is known as *palatal* snoring, and it's the most common form. The soft palate is the muscular part of the roof of your mouth near the back of the throat, and when airflow becomes turbulent, usually because of mouth breathing, nasal congestion, or poor muscle tone, it starts to flap and rattle, creating that familiar snoring sound.

Palatal snoring is most often associated with mouth breathing during sleep. When the mouth is open, the airway changes shape and becomes more collapsible. The tongue falls back, the jaw drops, and airflow has a direct path to hit the soft palate, causing it to vibrate. In contrast, nasal breathing helps keep the airway more stable and reduces the chances of these vibrations.

Here's the surprising part—palatal snoring often stops when the mouth is closed during sleep. So, if you wake up with a dry mouth, it's a clear sign that you've been breathing through your mouth all night.

Some people might argue that it doesn't matter if you breathe through your nose or mouth during sleep, but waking up with a dry mouth is actually a warning sign. It's not just an annoyance; it's a potential marker for sleep issues. A study involving Greek male soldiers revealed that those waking with a dry mouth ("morning hyposalivation") experienced poorer sleep quality compared with others.[2] This groundbreaking research is one of the first to objectively link dry mouth with sleep disturbances—and the results are striking. Dry mouth was associated with poor sleep quality, excessive daytime sleepiness, a higher risk of obstructive sleep apnea, and even sleep bruxism (teeth grinding).

The researchers emphasized the need for larger studies to confirm these findings, but the message is already clear: dry mouth isn't just a dry mouth—it's a red flag. Dentists, in particular, are uniquely positioned to spot signs of xerostomia (dry mouth) early and play an important role in addressing sleep-related concerns. This highlights yet another reason why dentists should be involved in their patients' sleep health discussions.

So, what can you do? A simple but effective solution is using mouth tape to promote nasal breathing during sleep. Keeping your mouth closed helps prevent mouth snoring, improves nasal airflow, reduces soft palate vibration, and may significantly enhance sleep quality.

It might feel a bit odd at first, like putting a seatbelt on your lips, but many people report that once they get used to it, they wake up feeling more refreshed and less groggy.

If you're curious about trying this, I've included tips on mouth taping at the end of this chapter to help you get started. Small changes like this can make a big difference in how well you sleep—and how you feel the next day.

Nose Snoring

Think of your nasal passages like a series of alleyways, carefully designed for air to flow freely and efficiently. These alleyways have an important job: they slow down the air you breathe, giving it time to be warmed, moistened, and humidified before it reaches your lungs. They also act as messengers, passing crucial information from the air to your brain—like detecting allergens, irritants, or even threats in your environment.

But what happens if these alleyways get blocked? Imagine a clear road suddenly cluttered with traffic—air can't move as freely, and the smooth flow becomes turbulent. This disruption can lead to nasal snoring, which often happens where the nasal passage meets the throat. Instead of a smooth ride, the air bumps around, creating vibrations that cause that familiar snoring sound.

Several factors can create this "traffic jam" in your nose. Nasal congestion, for instance, is like roadwork in your airways, narrowing the space and making it harder for air to pass through. A deviated septum—where the wall dividing your nasal passages isn't straight— can also reduce airflow and increase resistance. Even having naturally smaller nasal structures can contribute, making it harder for air to move quietly and efficiently.

When air has to squeeze through a smaller or obstructed space, it moves faster and more erratically, causing turbulence. This turbulence not only leads to snoring but also disrupts the natural processes that your nasal passages are meant to handle—warming, humidifying, and filtering the air. Essentially, blocked nasal alleyways turn your nose into a noisy, inefficient air tunnel instead of the smooth, quiet system it's designed to be.

So, if you're dealing with nasal snoring, it's worth investigating what's causing the blockages. Addressing these issues—whether through clearing nasal congestion, considering treatments for a deviated septum, or practicing nasal breathing exercises—can help restore the balance and quiet the turbulence, leading to better, quieter sleep for everyone.

Not Just the Airways: The Role of Breathing in Snoring

Snoring isn't just about narrow or collapsed airways—it's also about *how* you breathe. Fast, forceful breathing can take what might be a minor airflow issue and turn it into a symphony of turbulence. And here's the fascinating part: snoring sounds differ depending on whether they're coming from your mouth or nose. If you've ever had the dubious pleasure of hearing snoring up close, you'll know what I mean.

Picture this: a husband adamantly denies snoring, brushing off his wife's complaints as exaggerations—until one morning she plays him a recording of his nighttime racket. The proof is undeniable, and he's left sheepishly admitting, "Okay, maybe I do snore." What he doesn't realize is that snoring sounds can reveal more than just embarrassment—they can pinpoint the source of the issue. Nasal snoring has a distinct, higher-pitched, nasally quality, while mouth snoring tends to be deeper, throatier, and often louder. This difference helps identify whether the turbulence is in the nasal passages or further back in the throat.

To understand how breathing affects snoring, try this quick experiment. First, imitate mouth snoring: open your mouth, tighten your throat slightly, and draw air in quickly. Feel that vibration at the back of your mouth? That's the turbulence caused by fast airflow meeting a partially collapsed airway. Now, close your mouth and try to snore through your mouth. Notice how mouth snoring disappears when you breathe only through your nose.

Next, let's re-create nasal snoring. Breathe quickly and forcefully through your nose, and you'll hear the distinctive high-pitched vibration of nasal snoring. To reduce this, slow your breathing. Take a gentle inhale through your nose, followed by a slow, relaxed exhale. Try snoring as you breathe this way—it's much harder, isn't it? That's because slower, softer breathing reduces turbulence and vibrations, making nasal snoring less likely.

Snoring is fundamentally about turbulence, and the speed and force of your breathing play a major role. When you breathe rapidly or forcefully, chaotic airflow causes tissues in your nose or throat to vibrate. Slowing your breath smooths the airflow, cutting down on vibrations and making snoring less likely. This means something as simple as focusing on slower nasal breathing can help reduce snoring.

"My wife complained about my loud snoring, and I felt 'hungover' (without drinking) every morning. Since I started using sleep tape my snoring is almost non-existent. . . .

The difference I feel, not only in the morning, but throughout the day, is extraordinary. . . .

At night as soon as I apply the tape my body goes 'we feel the tape, it must be time for bed' and I'm asleep in minutes. It literally changed my life."

THE WILD WEST AND SNORING: A CAUTIONARY TALE

Few stories highlight the frustrations of snoring quite like one from the Wild West. In 1871, infamous outlaw John Wesley Hardin was staying at a hotel in Abilene, Kansas, when he became so irritated by the snoring of Charles Couger, a man in the adjacent room, that he reportedly fired his gun through the wall, killing him.[3] According to some accounts, Hardin even leapt out of a second-story window to avoid arrest. The local sheriff, Wild Bill Hickok, chose not to pursue him—perhaps out of fear, or maybe just out of respect. It's hard to say. This tale became one of the many legends that cemented Hardin's reputation as one of the Wild West's most dangerous gunslingers.

The Wild West, characterized by lawlessness and frontier justice, was a time when disputes—no matter how trivial—often escalated quickly. Hardin's extreme reaction might sound absurd today, but anyone who's lost night after night of sleep due to a partner's snoring can probably relate to the feeling of desperation. Thankfully, we've come a long way since the days of settling snoring disputes with gunfire.

How Common Is Snoring?

Many snorers are blissfully unaware that they snore. Indeed, it is often the weary partner who brings the issue to the snorer's attention. This makes it more difficult to determine how many people snore. Oftentimes, although not always, the snorer is male. In adults between 30 and 60 years old, it is estimated that 44% of men and 28% of women snore regularly.[4] Over the age of 60, the numbers increase, and around half of all people snore regularly.[5]

Understanding the Causes of Snoring: Risk and Contributing Factors

Snoring may be caused by a combination of breathing patterns, structural factors, and lifestyle choices that narrow the airway and create turbulence as air moves through. In other words, snoring usually isn't caused by just one thing; it's the result of a few culprits working together. Some of the most common contributors include:

Breathing and Anatomical Factors

- **Dysfunctional breathing patterns.** A low Control Pause (CP) score, faster breathing, and increased breathing volume can contribute to turbulence in the upper airway.
- **Mouth breathing.** Breathing through the mouth instead of the nose increases nasal congestion and the likelihood of snoring.
- **Chronic nasal congestion.** Blocked nasal passages force breathing through the mouth, worsening snoring.
- **Enlarged tonsils, tongue, or soft palate.** Extra tissue can partially block the airway during sleep.
- **Poor tongue posture.** When the tongue falls back instead of resting against the roof of the mouth, it can obstruct airflow.

- **Deviated septum or nasal polyps.** Structural nasal issues make it harder to breathe properly through the nose.
- **Small or recessed jaw.** A smaller airway space increases the likelihood of snoring.

Lifestyle and Other Contributing Factors

- **Obesity.** Excess weight, especially around the neck, can put pressure on the airway.
- **Alcohol consumption.** Drinking alcohol relaxes throat muscles, making airway collapse more likely.
- **Smoking.** Smoking irritates and inflames the airway, contributing to congestion and obstruction.
- **Sedative medications.** Sedatives further relax throat muscles, increasing airway restriction.
- **Pregnancy.** Hormonal changes and weight gain can lead to increased airway resistance.
- **Sleeping on your back.** This position allows the tongue and soft tissues to collapse backward, partially blocking the airway.

By understanding these risk factors, you can begin taking steps to optimize your breathing and reduce snoring, leading to *better sleep quality and overall health* (for both you and anyone who shares your bed!).

ADDRESSING SNORING

There are plenty of ways to quiet snoring, but most solutions only focus on keeping the airway open—they miss a big piece of the puzzle: how you breathe. The way you breathe throughout the day and night plays a huge role in whether or not you snore. That's why I recommend tackling any unhealthy breathing habits first, along with other simple, effective strategies to help you enjoy quieter, more restful sleep.

To Reduce Mouth Snoring

Use a Gentle Nasal Breathing Support Tape, Such as MyoTape
MyoTape is a simple yet effective tool designed to encourage nasal breathing during sleep by gently keeping the mouth closed. Since snoring through the mouth can only occur when the mouth is open, using MyoTape can significantly reduce or even eliminate mouth snoring, promoting quieter, more restorative sleep.

Made from elasticated cotton, MyoTape is both gentle on the skin and comfortable to wear. To use it, gently stretch the tape about 30% before applying it. Place the tape around the lips, ensuring it surrounds the mouth without adhering directly to the lips. This unique design provides comfort and safety while supporting nasal breathing throughout the night.

Unlike traditional "mouth tapes" that completely cover the mouth, MyoTape doesn't seal the mouth shut. Instead, it works as a nasal breathing support, allowing for natural airflow and providing a safer, more effective way to encourage healthy breathing patterns during sleep.

Some quotes from our community who used the Buteyko Method to address snoring:

"I've snored most of, if not all, my life. I found that as I got into my 30s, that I was finding it **very difficult to wake up in the morning due to grogginess, as well as my increasing daytime fatigue.**

Within a few days of trying mouth tape I started to find I was **no longer waking during the night and that I was able to wake up in the morning much more easily.**

I can easily say that **it has changed my life.** If I go even one night without it I feel a massive difference in how I feel the next day."

"In the past I used to snore and it seemed as if I was a mouth breather during sleep. On awakening I'd often find it very it challenging to get up and would feel tired after sleep or a little worn out.

"When I started using tape, my experience was that the sleep was better quality and I'd wake up feeling more rested or I could sleep a shorter duration and still wake up feeling refreshed. I also noticed feeling less thirsty. . . ."

Ciarán, 47, USA

"I've been using tape at night and nose breathing per Patrick's book, *Shut Your Mouth*, for 6 years. It has improved my quality of sleep, calmed my emotions, and trained me to nose breathing during the day. It has increased my athletic ability and endurance.

My partner refuses to try taping, so we have to sleep in separate rooms because of his snoring. His loss!"

"I have **snored** for years. **Really disruptive to my husband.**

I tried taping my mouth and have not snored since. **I was thrilled but it didn't end there.** In follow-up visits to my dentist I was asked WHAT was I doing as my **gum health had dramatically improved. I'm converted!"**

Phyllis, 69, Canada

"I started mouth taping 2 years ago. **I wake up so grumpy and tired if I don't mouth tape. I don't snore anymore. My teeth are better with less cavities, my asthma is non-existent, I'm less anxious [. . .] I'm more alert and my memory is better.**

I don't pee at night. I finally sleep through the night. I wake up refreshed instead of yawning and I don't take as long to get out of bed because I'm actually refreshed.

I re-trained my breathing and stopped mouth breathing for everything, even exercise. By doing this I have **NO asthma** anymore and I don't need steroids for chest infections at least twice per year. **I'm a changed woman.**"

Rowena, 35, Australia

To Reduce Nasal Snoring

The list below might feel a little overwhelming at first glance, but don't worry—you don't have to tackle everything at once. Many of these suggestions naturally support each other, making them easier to implement than they might seem. The good news? Most of these strategies can be seamlessly incorporated into your daily routine, creating lasting habits that support better sleep and breathing.

- **Clear the nose with a nose unblocking exercise.** This simple exercise can help temporarily decongest the nose, making it easier to breathe. Remember, the nose works better the more it's used. Kind of like a muscle; the more you train it, the better it performs. Regularly practicing nose breathing and improving your CP score can enhance nasal function over time.

- **Establish consistent nasal breathing.** Commit to nasal breathing during the day—whether at rest or during physical activity. Yes, even while out for a brisk walk, focus on breathing through your nose. If the sensation of breathlessness becomes too intense, simply slow your pace. The more you reinforce this habit during the day, the easier it will be to maintain at night. Remember: the nose is for breathing!

- **Reduce breathing volume with the *Breathe Light Exercise*.** Practicing the *Breathe Light Exercise* for 10 minutes, four times a day, can help reduce the speed and volume of airflow. This not only makes nasal breathing more effective but also lessens the intensity of nasal snoring. Think of it like turning down the volume on your breathing; less turbulence, more silence.

- **Improve your Control Pause score.** Aim for a CP score of 20 seconds or more. This milestone is crucial for easier nasal breathing and a less congested nose. A higher CP score reflects improved breathing efficiency, and when your breathing is more efficient, your sleep tends to follow.

- **Use nasal dilators or snore strips.** These tools can help open nasal airways by flaring the nostrils, reducing resistance to airflow, and making nasal breathing easier. They're a practical option for minimizing snoring caused by restricted nasal airflow.

- **Sleep on your side.** Sleeping on your back can worsen snoring by allowing the tongue to fall backward, partially blocking the airway. Side sleeping encourages the tongue to rest on the roof of the mouth and keeps the lower jaw forward, helping to keep the airway more open. Even a small increase in airway diameter can make a big difference.

- **Make lifestyle adjustments (if applicable).** Factors like excess weight, smoking, and alcohol consumption can all contribute to snoring. Weight loss and sleep are interconnected, so addressing one often helps the other. Quitting smoking and reducing alcohol intake, especially before bed, can also make a noticeable difference. (We'll delve deeper into these topics later.)

Each of these steps plays a role in reducing nasal snoring. Together, they can help you achieve better sleep, quieter nights, and healthier breathing habits.

MARINKA'S STORY: FROM SNORING AND FATIGUE TO RESTFUL SLEEP AND RESILIENCE

For years, Marinka, a 37-year-old Oxygen Advantage® Instructor from the Netherlands, accepted her restless nights, morning fatigue, and occasional snoring as just part of life. She'd wake up exhausted, despite getting a full night's sleep, and during stressful periods, she found herself waking in the middle of the night, unable to drift back into rest. Her husband faced similar struggles—chronic snoring and morning grogginess were a daily reality.

At first, Marinka's interest in breathwork was purely practical—she wanted to improve her ability to handle altitude sickness on high-altitude hikes. But what she discovered along the way completely transformed not just her physical endurance, but her sleep quality, stress levels, and daily energy.

The Game-Changer: Nasal Breathing and Mouth Taping

During her Oxygen Advantage® Instructor training, Marinka learned something that stopped her in her tracks: the way she was breathing was affecting her sleep, energy, and overall health.

Determined to test what she had learned, she started using breathing exercises and mouth taping to keep her airway open and promote nasal breathing while she slept. She chose MyoTape, a tape that surrounds the lips rather than sealing them shut. At first, she was hesitant.

"That first night, I wasn't sure I liked it—I kept thinking, 'There's something around my mouth!' But by the second night, it was no problem at all. And the difference? Unbelievable. I slept WAY better. I woke up with no dry mouth, feeling refreshed and completely rested."

Although initially skeptical, after seeing Marinka's results, her husband—who had been a chronic snorer for 13 years—decided to give mouth taping a try as well.

The results were immediate.

His snoring completely disappeared. He started waking up energized, needing less sleep, and feeling more refreshed than he had in years. He quickly became a firm believer in the power of nasal breathing and now tapes his mouth every night.

Marinka used breathing techniques to improve her ability to handle stress and fall back asleep if she woke during the night.

"When I'd wake up in the middle of the night with my mind racing, I'd do the *Many Small Breath Holds Exercise*. It helped me focus, calm my nervous system, and before I knew it, I'd drift back to sleep."

By using slow, controlled breathing, she was able to signal safety to her body, shifting away from stress and back into deep rest.

A Boost in Endurance and Energy

By switching to nasal breathing and practicing daily breathwork exercises, Marinka's BOLT score (a measure of breathing efficiency, equivalent to the Control Pause) jumped from 15 to 35—a huge improvement that directly boosted her physical endurance, fitness, and energy levels.

"I originally wanted to improve my endurance, but what I didn't expect was how much better my sleep and overall health would become," she says.

Marinka's story is a reminder that something as simple as how we breathe can make all the difference. By switching to nasal breathing, mouth taping, and breathwork exercises, she and her husband transformed their sleep, eliminated snoring, and built greater resilience to stress and fatigue.

For anyone struggling with poor sleep, snoring, or low energy, her message is clear: start with your breath—it might just change everything.

CHAPTER 10C

UPPER AIRWAY RESISTANCE SYNDROME— THE OVERLOOKED SLEEP STRUGGLE

Upper airway resistance syndrome (UARS) is a sleep-related breathing disorder that can be easily overlooked. It doesn't come with the telltale sounds of snoring or the dramatic pauses in breathing and oxygen level drops seen in obstructive sleep apnea (OSA). Instead, UARS operates in a much subtler way, quietly wreaking havoc on your sleep and overall health. Yet its impact can be just as debilitating, leaving people exhausted and struggling to function during the day.

You could think of UARS as bridging the gap between normal sleep and OSA—a gap that's anything but small. Sleep doctors were likely baffled by patients who felt persistently tired, even after spending plenty of time in bed and having sleep studies that showed no apneas, hypopneas, or major oxygen desaturations. It was this puzzling pattern that led pioneering sleep researcher Dr. Christian Guilleminault to first identify UARS in children in 1983.[1] A decade later, in 1993, he expanded the term to include adults. That 11-year gap underscores the complexity of defining UARS as its own distinct condition.

At its core, UARS occurs when the airway is just slightly too narrow, creating increased resistance to airflow. This narrowing usually happens at the back of the mouth where it meets the throat or in the throat itself. While it doesn't lead to the significant oxygen drops seen in OSA, it does make breathing more effortful. Your body senses this increased effort almost like it's suffocating, triggering repeated micro-arousals—those brief wake-ups you may not even notice. These arousals fragment your sleep, preventing you from reaching the deep, restorative stages your body and mind need to feel truly rested.

Diagnosing UARS requires looking beyond the typical markers of sleep disorders like OSA. For example, people with UARS often have an apnea-hypopnea index (AHI) of less than five events per hour, meaning they don't experience frequent full or partial pauses in breathing.[2] Their oxygen saturation levels typically stay at or above 92%, indicating their blood oxygen remains normal throughout the night. The real clue comes from the respiratory effort-related arousal (RERA) index. A RERA index of 5 or more shows frequent arousals caused by the extra effort needed to breathe through a slightly narrowed airway. This combination—few or no apneas, normal oxygen levels, but frequent arousals—makes UARS a unique and elusive condition.

Dr. Christian Guilleminault's groundbreaking research on UARS offered a compelling argument that it is a distinct sleep disorder, separate from OSA.[3] His study of 400 UARS cases revealed that the average age of patients was 38 years, with 56% being women and 32% of East Asian origin. These findings stand in stark contrast to the typical profile of OSA, which is more commonly associated with older, overweight men. This demographic difference, coupled with the unique symptoms of UARS, emphasized that it wasn't merely a milder form of OSA but a condition with its own defining characteristics.

Despite Guilleminault's detailed research, UARS remains a topic of debate among sleep experts. Some argue that it is a stand-alone disorder, while others suggest it exists on a spectrum ranging from mild snoring to full-blown OSA. Guilleminault, however, was unwavering in his belief that UARS was its own syndrome. In his 2000 study, he stated, "There is a false assumption that UARS forms a continuum between primary snoring and OSAs. In our series of 400 cases of UARS, 93 have 'pure' UARS. These patients frequently complain of insomnia, sleep fragmentation, and fatigue."[4] For Guilleminault, this wasn't simply a less severe version of sleep apnea—it was a unique condition with distinct challenges that required specific attention.

This ongoing debate among sleep professionals underscores just how elusive UARS can be. Because it falls outside the conventional diagnostic markers of sleep apnea, many patients are left undiagnosed or misdiagnosed, their struggles dismissed or misunderstood. But for those living with UARS, it's far more than just subtle airway resistance. It's a nightly disruption that fragments sleep, leaving them drained and struggling to get through the day.

The result? Broken sleep and an unrelenting sense of exhaustion, even if you believe you're spending enough hours in bed. You wake up feeling anything but refreshed, and that tiredness sticks with you throughout the day, making it hard to focus, stay alert, or even function. Many people mistake UARS for simple insomnia, never realizing that the true culprit is hidden airway resistance during sleep. Recognizing and addressing UARS as a distinct and impactful sleep disorder is essential to breaking this cycle of sleepless frustration.

Adding to the challenge, UARS often comes with heightened anxiety.[5] This constant state of alertness makes it even harder for the body to relax and recover during sleep, setting off a vicious cycle: the effort to breathe at night leads to fragmented sleep, which fuels daytime fatigue and anxiety, leaving the body stuck in overdrive. Over time, this loop can spiral into symptoms that look a lot like other conditions, such as fibromyalgia or chronic fatigue syndrome. The result is an overwhelming sense of exhaustion and frustration, despite spending what feels like "enough" time in bed.

If you're waking up feeling exhausted despite spending plenty of time in bed, and no one has ever mentioned that you snore—or perhaps you've even had a sleep study where the doctor assured you that your sleep quality is fine—UARS could be the missing piece of the puzzle. It's a reminder that sleep disorders aren't always dramatic or obvious. Sometimes, it's the quiet, subtle disruptions, like those caused by UARS, that silently wreak havoc on your health and leave you wondering why rest feels so elusive.

How Common Is UARS?

Pinning down how common UARS is can be tricky, but it's no surprise that it's often underdiagnosed. Traditional sleep studies focus on the big, obvious markers like apneas or oxygen level drops, while the more subtle signs of UARS—like respiratory effort-related arousals—tend to slip through the cracks. And let's be honest: how often does your doctor ask about your sleep? Your blood pressure gets measured routinely, but sleep? That's rarely part of the conversation.

Studies estimate that UARS affects around 6–11% of the general population.[6] But even that figure might be conservative, given how often it flies under the radar. After all, if you're a young, fit, and slender individual, is your doctor really going to assume you have a sleep disorder? Likely not. Yet, UARS often affects exactly this group, making it one of the most overlooked sleep conditions.

Understanding the Causes of UARS: Risk and Contributing Factors

UARS is often nicknamed "fit female syndrome" because it tends to affect younger, healthy, slender women, although men, children, and other women can also experience it. Sleep issues like snoring or OSA are often associated with older, overweight men. This stereotype means that when someone who looks healthy and fit struggles with sleep, their condition is more likely to be overlooked or dismissed.

Many people with UARS share certain anatomical traits, like a high and narrow palate. This often develops when the upper jaw doesn't fully grow during childhood, leading to a narrower roof of the mouth and a more restricted airway.

There's often a history of orthodontic work in people with UARS including early tooth extractions not limited to wisdom teeth. Unfortunately, some orthodontic treatments, while intended to straighten teeth, can unintentionally narrow the airway. It's surprising, but true; a well-meaning orthodontist might be focused on aesthetics without considering how the treatment affects long-term breathing and sleep. And shockingly, this practice still continues today.

The position of the teeth and jaws directly impacts the airway, which is why airway health should absolutely be a part of modern dentistry. Thankfully, there are dentists and orthodontists who understand the critical connection between the airway and dental structures. However, not all do. If your dentist is recommending extractions, it's worth getting a second opinion—ideally from a dentist who specializes in airway health. Making sure the treatment plan considers your airway can make a big difference in your long-term sleep and overall well-being.

Dr. Michael Gelb, a renowned airway specialist, has observed a consistent pattern among his UARS patients: many of them report having their wisdom teeth removed early on. Research supports this observation. Studies show that 88% of UARS cases have a history of early wisdom tooth extraction or congenital absence, suggesting a link between these dental interventions and narrowed airways.[7]

Writer Rachael Combe shared her personal experience with UARS in *Elle* magazine, describing how her sleep issues began in her early thirties. She would wake up gasping for air, and her Fitbit revealed she was only getting about four hours of sleep per night. What started as occasional insomnia snowballed into severe exhaustion—she struggled to stay awake during the day for more than 15 minutes at a time.

During a consultation with Dr. Gelb in New York, she finally got some answers. Gelb asked about her anxiety, her history of wisdom tooth removal, and whether she'd been told she needed a palate expander as a child. When he diagnosed her with UARS, he jokingly said, "You have UARS. It's the young, thin, beautiful women's sleep disorder. You should write about it!"

What's striking is how much UARS—and its more dramatic counterpart, OSA—impacts quality of life. Research shows that individuals with these conditions experience a quality of life that's five to six times worse than that of the general population.[8] What does this mean in real terms? It means constantly waking up exhausted, struggling with focus, feeling emotionally drained, and battling persistent fatigue—all of which make everyday activities feel harder. It's not just about missing a good night's sleep; it's about how that sleep deprivation spills over into every aspect of life, affecting relationships, work, and overall well-being.

This highlights a crucial point: sleep health isn't just a luxury or something to think about when you feel tired. It's foundational to your quality of life, and conditions like UARS deserve far more attention than they currently get. If you're constantly feeling drained despite spending enough time in bed, it's worth considering that the issue might be something more subtle, like UARS.

"I have upper airway resistance syndrome. I became so interested in the connection with breath/vagus nerve and sleep patterns. I completed the Oxygen Advantage® Functional Breath Instructor course. I learned to breathe functionally 24/7.

No medical specialist ever checks breathing patterns. I have seen over 15 doctors/specialists. I used to be awake for hours, but I sleep through the night now and only get up once for the toilet.

At 61 years of age, I feel the best I've felt in a long time. Thank you, Patrick, I'm very grateful."

Zarn, 61, Australia

ADDRESSING UARS

While treatments like continuous positive airway pressure (CPAP) and mandibular advancement devices (MADs) are commonly used to keep the airway open and reduce resistance, their effectiveness can be amplified when paired with breathing-focused techniques like those offered by the Buteyko Method. Since UARS is fundamentally a breathing issue—caused by increased effort due to narrow airways—addressing breathing patterns alongside traditional treatments can make a significant difference in sleep quality and overall well-being.

In Chapter 10A, we explored the role of hyperarousal in insomnia and how it disrupts sleep. Interestingly, hyperarousal is also a key feature of UARS, as both conditions involve heightened activity of the sympathetic nervous system—the body's "fight, flight, or freeze" mode. That's why the tools that help calm the system for insomnia also work well for UARS. The aim is to calm the nervous system, stabilize breathing, and promote relaxation. When you do that, you're giving yourself the best possible shot at consistent, deep sleep.

CPAP and MADs: The Traditional Options

CPAP delivers a steady flow of air pressure to prevent airway collapse during sleep. It's particularly effective at maintaining an open airway, but many people find it challenging to use consistently due to discomfort or difficulty adapting to the equipment. On the other hand, MADs gently hold the lower jaw forward, reducing airway collapses by providing structural support. These devices work well for many individuals and can complement approaches that focus on improving breathing patterns and nasal airflow.

The Role of Breathing in Managing UARS

UARS isn't just about mechanical airway resistance—it's also about how your body reacts to it. People with UARS often have a low arousal threshold, meaning they wake up easily in response to even minor increases in breathing effort. This sensitivity is linked to heightened sympathetic nervous system activity, which keeps the body hyper-reactive and on edge, even during sleep. This creates a cycle of fragmented sleep, daytime fatigue, and increased stress, which is similar to what we discussed earlier in the context of insomnia.

The Buteyko Method offers practical tools to address these underlying issues, helping to stabilize breathing patterns and balance the autonomic nervous system.

Supporting Nasal Breathing and Airway Function

- **Decongest your nose and practice nasal breathing.** Nasal congestion can worsen airway resistance, but nose unblocking exercises can help clear nasal passages and promote consistent nasal breathing. Pairing this with proper tongue posture—resting the tongue on the roof of your mouth during sleep—helps keep the airway open and reduces resistance.
- **Consider nasal dilators or snore strips.** For individuals with significant nasal resistance, these tools physically open the nasal passages, easing airflow and reducing breathing effort during sleep.

Normalizing Breathing Volume and Patterns

- **Raise your CP score.** The CP score is a simple way to assess your breathing patterns and how well they are regulated. A CP of 20 seconds or more indicates stabilized breathing, reducing airway resistance and lowering the risk of waking up unnecessarily.
- **Practice light, slow, and deep breathing.** These three elements support stable breathing and help quiet the nervous system. Lighter breathing reduces turbulence. Slower breathing reduces overall

effort. Deeper breathing engages the diaphragm, which helps to stabilize the upper airways and supports consistent airflow.

Each five-second improvement in your CP score is a sign that your breathing is getting more functional—and your sleep will follow suit.

Balancing the Autonomic Nervous System

The heightened sympathetic drive seen in UARS and insomnia often leaves the body in a constant state of hyperarousal. This makes it difficult to relax, unwind, and stay asleep. The Buteyko Method helps shift the autonomic seesaw toward the parasympathetic "rest and digest" state by slowing the breath, reducing heart rate, and signaling safety to the brain. This balance improves sleep quality and reduces sensitivity to minor breathing disturbances. It's a subtle reset button, but one that can make a powerful difference when practiced consistently.

LISA'S STORY: FROM UARS AND DISRUPTED SLEEP TO LIFE-CHANGING REST AND A NEW DENTAL SPECIALTY

I previously highlighted the critical link between airway health, dentistry, and sleep—a connection that many dentists are unaware of. Lisa, a 48-year-old dentist from Colorado, experienced this firsthand. What started as a personal, lifelong struggle with UARS, nocturia (waking up at night to urinate), and insomnia not only changed her life but also reshaped her entire approach to dentistry.

For Lisa, everything changed five years ago when she stumbled upon my book, *The Oxygen Advantage*®. The idea that nasal breathing could dramatically improve sleep intrigued her, so she decided to try mouth taping at night.

The results? Nothing short of life-changing!

"The first time I wore mouth tape, it was like my whole life changed overnight! For as long as I can remember, I would wake up in the middle of the night to pee . . . and then I couldn't go back to sleep for two hours. I even wet the bed until I was about nine or ten. Doctors told my mom I was just a deep sleeper. But in hindsight, it was all connected to my breathing."

That very first night of keeping her mouth closed with tape, Lisa slept through the night for the first time in years. No dry throat. No restless tossing and turning. No waking up exhausted.

"The first night I ever wore mouth tape I just remember waking up and feeling immediately better. Like I got a well-rested sleep. I slept through the night. My throat didn't feel dry; I felt so much better. So, I've been addicted to MyoTape. If I ever fall asleep without wearing it, I can tell in the morning. It makes a huge difference in how I feel."

Thereafter, Lisa's fascination with breathing and airway health grew, influencing her professional path. She is now training in functional airway dentistry and is passionate about educating her patients and friends about breathing and airway health.

Lisa trained in performing tongue-tie releases and was shocked to discover she had a tongue tie herself—something that had impacted her swallowing, speech, and even her posture her entire life.

"I was at a lunch with other dentists, and as they were describing tongue-tie symptoms, I realized—I was literally chopping my food into tiny pieces, struggling to swallow without water, and the last to finish eating."

A simple tongue-tie release relieved years of neck pain and headaches, problems she never realized were connected.

MyoTape: A Small Tool with a Big Impact

Lisa is now a fierce advocate for nasal breathing and MyoTape—so much so that she carries tape in her pocket and hands it out to patients, friends, and even people she meets while hiking!

"I have friends whose lives changed after just one night of using mouth tape. They wake up feeling like they slept well for the first time in years. I've got a few friends that are really passionate about MyoTape now."

She wears MyoTape every single night, along with a nasal dilator to support her breathing. And she's on a mission to educate others—especially in the dental world—about the critical connection between airway health and overall well-being.

"Doctors never diagnosed me. I had to figure it out myself. In America, it's often up to airway-focused dentists to recognize these issues because most traditional dentists still don't see the connection. They would still be skeptical and make fun of this kind of stuff."

Lisa's story is a testament to the importance of nasal breathing and airway health. What started as a personal experiment turned into a lifelong passion—one that's already changing the lives of her patients and children.

CHAPTER 10D

UNDERSTANDING AND MANAGING SLEEP APNEA

Sleep is meant to be a time of rest and recovery, allowing your body and brain to recharge for the day ahead. If you've ever woken up gasping for air, felt exhausted despite a full night's rest, or been told you snore loudly or stop breathing in your sleep, you may be dealing with sleep apnea.

Sleep apnea is one of the most common and serious sleep-related breathing disorders. It causes repeated pauses in breathing throughout the night, disrupting oxygen flow to the brain and body. And here's the thing: left untreated, sleep apnea can lead to serious health consequences.

In this chapter, we'll break down the different types of sleep apnea, the risks and factors that contribute to it, and the challenges in getting a proper diagnosis. Most importantly, we'll explore effective solutions, with a particular focus on the critical role of functional breathing in managing and improving sleep apnea.

There are two primary types of sleep apnea, each with its own unique characteristics:

1. **Central sleep apnea (CSA).** This less common form of sleep apnea happens when the brain fails to send the proper signals to the muscles responsible for breathing. In other words, the brain "forgets" to tell your body to breathe, causing temporary

pauses in breathing. It's not about a blocked airway but rather a communication breakdown between the brain and the breathing muscles.

2. **Obstructive sleep apnea (OSA).** By far the more common type, OSA occurs when the upper airway becomes partially or fully blocked during sleep. Here's what's happening: while you're awake, your airway stays open thanks to the dilator muscles, which keep the throat supported and unobstructed. But during sleep, those muscles naturally relax. For people with OSA, this relaxation goes too far, causing the airway to collapse and restrict airflow.[1]

The thing about OSA is that the brain is still sending the signal to breathe—it's not like central sleep apnea, where the signal is missing altogether. If you've ever shared a bed with someone who has OSA, you may have noticed that they're actively trying to breathe during an episode. Watch closely, and you might see their diaphragm and chest muscles contracting as they work hard to pull air into their lungs. The problem? Their throat is collapsed, so despite all that effort, air simply can't pass through.

This struggle leads to the classic symptoms of OSA: loud snoring, complete silence, followed by gasping for air during sleep. These episodes usually end when the brain senses a drop in oxygen levels and sends a "wake-up call" to the body, triggering a brief arousal just long enough to dilate the airway and restore breathing. While the sleeper may not consciously remember these wake-ups, these micro-arousals prevent them from entering the deep, restorative stages of sleep that are so critical for physical and mental health.

To understand why these oxygen drops matter so much, let's talk about the brain. Although the brain only accounts for about 2% of the body's weight, it demands 15% of the blood flow from the heart and consumes 20% of the body's oxygen supply.[2,3] Pound for pound, the brain uses roughly 10 times more oxygen than most other parts of the body. Oxygen is the brain's lifeline, fueling everything from regulating your heartbeat to forming memories. When oxygen levels drop even slightly, the brain kicks into high gear to restore balance. It's a survival mechanism, but it comes at the cost of restful sleep.

OSA isn't just about loud snoring or momentary disruptions; it's about the significant strain it places on the body and brain. Every time the airway collapses, the brain and muscles are forced to work overtime to compensate for the lack of airflow. This constant struggle leaves the person feeling drained and exhausted, regardless of how many hours they spend in bed.

The bottom line? Both types of sleep apnea disrupt the brain's essential oxygen supply, and when it comes to sleep, oxygen isn't negotiable. Sleep apnea, whether central or obstructive, isn't just a nighttime problem—it's a 24/7 issue that can ripple through every aspect of your health.

HOW COMMON IS OSA?

Obstructive sleep apnea is one of the most widespread and disruptive health conditions affecting modern civilization. To put it into perspective, the global population today stands at over 8 billion people. Within that, a staggering 1 billion adults aged 30–69 years are estimated to have OSA, according to a 2019 review published in *Lancet Respiratory Medicine*.[4] This figure is based on an apnea-hypopnea index (AHI) of five or more events per hour, which measures how often breathing is disrupted during sleep. An AHI of five or more events per hour means that, at least five times every hour, a person either stops breathing completely for ten seconds or more (an apnea) or their breathing becomes so shallow that it significantly drops their oxygen levels (a hypopnea).

The number with moderate-to-severe obstructive sleep apnea—for which treatment is generally recommended—was estimated to be almost 425 million. According to data from the study, in some countries, more than 50% of the population was thought to have

OSA, but prevalence was lower in the United States (33.2%) and in the UK and Ireland (24.5%).

OSA is more prevalent among certain demographics:

- Older adults
- Males (though female prevalence increases postmenopause)
- Specific ethnic groups (including African Americans, Native Americans, and Hispanics)

Despite the potentially serious health implications of sleep apnea, the condition often goes undiagnosed. Shockingly, nearly 93% of women and 82% of men with at least moderate sleep apnea have no idea they have it.[5] This raises the question: how has sleep apnea become so common, yet so often left undiagnosed, that it has quietly turned into one of the biggest hidden health problems of our time?

Understanding the Causes of OSA: Risk and Contributing Factors

Several factors can increase the risk of OSA by contributing to airway obstruction, reduced muscle tone, or inflammation. These can range from physical traits and lifestyle factors to medical conditions and of course breathing patterns. Some of the key risk and contributory factors include:[6–8]

- Obesity or being overweight—particularly if you have a large neck circumference—since it is common for overweight people to have excess tissue at the back of their throat, which can result in a blocked airway during sleep
- Large neck circumference, even in young, fit individuals like rugby players or American footballers, can narrow the airway and increase the risk of obstruction
- Male gender
- Being older (risk increases with age)
- Family history

- Menopause
- Certain genetic or endocrine disorders
- Poor facial development and smaller airways
- Nasal congestion, asthma, and COPD (inflammation)
- Mouth breathing and faster and harder breathing
- Waking up with a dry mouth
- Taking sedatives

Can Alcohol Worsen Sleep Apnea?

A glass of wine in the evening might feel like a reward after a long day, but if you have sleep apnea, alcohol could be quietly making things worse, especially for your breathing. I know several people who've decided to cut back on alcohol, not because they were drinking heavily, but simply based on what their wearable devices were telling them. Even one or two drinks led to noticeably poorer sleep and a spike in heart rate, sometimes ten percent higher the next day. Studies have shown that alcohol increases the number and severity of breathing disruptions in people with OSA.[9] It lowers oxygen levels, makes airway collapse more likely, and can turn mild cases of sleep apnea into something far more serious.

The problem is that when most people go for a sleep study, they typically haven't been drinking alcohol beforehand. (If you have, well . . . I think you might have a different issue!) So, if you're someone who regularly drinks in the evening, can you fully trust the results of your sleep study? If alcohol significantly worsens your breathing, but you were sober during the test, the study may not reflect how bad your sleep apnea truly is on a typical night.

Why Does Alcohol Make Sleep Apnea Worse?

Alcohol affects sleep and breathing in several ways:[10]

- **It relaxes the airway muscles.** The muscles in the throat and tongue are supposed to stay slightly active to keep the airway open during sleep. Alcohol causes them to relax more than usual, making it easier for the airway to collapse and block airflow.

- **It makes it harder to wake up.** Normally if breathing is restricted, the brain wakes you up just enough to get things moving again. But alcohol raises your "arousal threshold," so the body stays asleep longer even when oxygen levels dip. This leads to longer and more severe apnea episodes.

- **It can cause nasal congestion.** Alcohol affects blood vessels in the nose, leading to congestion that makes it harder to breathe through the nose. Since nasal breathing plays a huge role in keeping the airway stable, blocked nasal passages can make sleep apnea worse.

- **Timing and amount matter.** Drinking right before bed means alcohol is still in your system while you sleep, having its maximum impact on breathing. The more you drink, the stronger the effect—especially for older adults, who tend to be more sensitive to alcohol's impact on muscle tone and sleep quality.

The Bigger Picture

It's not just about snoring or sleep quality. Alcohol makes sleep apnea more dangerous. People with untreated OSA already have a higher risk of drowsy driving, and adding alcohol to the mix only makes things worse. Impaired alertness and slowed reaction times can make accidents more likely.

If you have sleep apnea and regularly drink in the evening, it may be worth experimenting with reducing alcohol or cutting it out for a few weeks to see how your sleep improves. And if you've had a sleep study but suspect that alcohol might be making your apnea worse than the results suggest, it's something worth discussing with your doctor.

At the very least, if you do drink, try to give your body a few alcohol-free hours before bed. Your sleep and your brain will thank you for it.

The Hidden Dangers of Sleep Apnea

A person with sleep apnea may experience hundreds of breathing interruptions in a single night, severely disrupting sleep quality and overall health. The drop in oxygen caused by the breathing interruptions due to OSA places strain on the heart. Over time, this continuing strain takes a serious toll on health, potentially leading to:

- Hypertension, cardiovascular morbidities, and stroke[11-13]
- Type 2 diabetes[14,15]
- Cognitive impairment[16]
- Depression or mood changes[17]
- Reduced quality of life[18]
- Increased risk of premature death[19,20]

Given these serious health risks, early diagnosis and treatment of OSA are crucial. Catching it early can prevent long-term complications and dramatically improve sleep, energy, and overall well-being.

DIAGNOSIS

The Realities of a Sleep Study: How Reflective Is It of Your Breathing?

To diagnose OSA, doctors use a clinical sleep study. For many people, the idea of doing a sleep study sounds like the ultimate way to get answers about their sleep quality. But here's the thing: how well does it actually reflect how you sleep on a typical night?

With the latest Apple Watch and other wearable devices beginning to track breathing disturbances during sleep, tens of thousands of people are going to start seeing data that suggests something might be off. If your watch shows frequent breathing disruptions, it's a sign worth paying attention to. It might not mean you have sleep apnea for sure, only a formal sleep study can confirm that, but it could be the nudge that gets you to look deeper and take action to protect your sleep and health.

A sleep study, or polysomnography, is a diagnostic test that tracks brain waves, breathing patterns, oxygen levels, heart rate, muscle activity, and eye movements to assess for sleep disorders. It's commonly used to diagnose sleep apnea, insomnia, restless legs syndrome, and narcolepsy. Sounds straightforward, right?

Now here's where things get real: is a sleep study really capturing how you sleep on a typical night?

Imagine this: instead of your cozy bed at home, you're lying in a strange room, on a strange bed, in a hospital or sleep clinic. There are sensors taped to your chest and forehead, wires snaking around your body, and a technician monitoring you from another room. Bright hallway lights leak in through the door, and the air carries that sterile "hospital smell." Then you're told: "Okay, go to sleep now."

Let's be honest; it's not the most restful setup. Other factors can also skew the results of a sleep study, such as alcohol consumption and nightly variation in sleep apnea severity. The reality is that a sleep study is a snapshot—a single night in an environment that's very different from home. While the results provide valuable insights, they may not fully capture your typical sleep patterns. In some cases, this could lead to false or misleading conclusions, either overestimating or underestimating the severity of sleep apnea.

Recent research shows that OSA severity can vary markedly from night to night, which has big implications for diagnosis and treatment. A study by Lechat and colleagues analyzed sleep data from 67,278 people using multinight, in-home sleep monitoring, rather than traditional sleep lab testing.[21] The findings were eye-opening: up to 1 in 5 people diagnosed with OSA based on just one night of testing may have been misclassified. And for those with mild to moderate OSA, the chance of misdiagnosis jumped to 1 in 2.

Why such a big difference? Because sleep varies. Some nights we sleep deeply, other nights we're restless. Breathing may be more disrupted by things like alcohol, stress, allergies, or sleeping position. So if you only test once; on a night that doesn't reflect your typical sleep, you might get a diagnosis that overstates or understates your condition.

This study is significant not only because of its massive sample size, but also because it used multinight at home data, which may more accurately reflect how we actually sleep in our everyday lives. It calls into question the reliability of single night sleep studies, which are still considered the gold standard in diagnosing OSA. For many people, especially those with fluctuating symptoms it might not tell the full story.

That said, sleep studies remain the gold standard for diagnosing sleep apnea. The key is not just identifying that sleep apnea is present, but understanding what to do next. Because whether someone accepts CPAP (continuous positive airway pressure) treatment, tries a mandibular advancement device, or explores breathing re-education, the goal isn't just about a diagnosis—it's about getting better sleep in the real world.

What Is Assessed During a Sleep Study?

In terms of sleep-related breathing disorders, a sleep study gathers critical data on how often a person experiences partial or complete airway collapses during sleep:

- Hypopnea is when the airway partially collapses for at least 10 seconds, and it causes your blood oxygen levels to drop by 3% or more. Breathing doesn't stop completely, but there is a reduction in airflow.
- Apnea is a full collapse of the airway that lasts at least 10 seconds. During this time, breathing completely stops.

These events are key indicators used to evaluate breathing disturbances and assess the severity of sleep-related breathing disorders. The total number of hypopneas and apneas is calculated per hour of sleep measured by the apnea-hypopnea index (AHI).

Here's how it's classified in adults:

- Mild sleep apnea. AHI of 5 to 15 events per hour.
- Moderate sleep apnea. AHI of 15 to 30 events per hour.
- Severe sleep apnea. AHI of more than 30 events per hour.

If someone's AHI score is over 20, they're usually recommended for CPAP therapy. The AHI, the most widely used measurement for diagnosing OSA, was developed by Dr. Christian Guilleminault, one of the pioneers of sleep research. While it's considered the gold standard for assessing OSA severity, it's not without its flaws.

One of the biggest issues is that AHI treats apneas (complete breathing pauses) and hypopneas (partial restrictions) as equally significant, even though apneas often have more severe physiological consequences. A complete airway collapse can cause a bigger drop in oxygen levels and put more stress on the heart and brain than a partial blockage—yet AHI counts them the same.

Another limitation is that AHI doesn't consider important details that can make a big difference in how sleep apnea actually affects someone. For example:

- The duration of each event matters. A long apnea event can cause much deeper oxygen desaturation than a short one; yet AHI doesn't weigh this factor.
- Not all sleep stages are equal. Breathing disruptions during deep sleep (slow-wave sleep) or REM sleep can have a bigger impact on restorative sleep quality and cardiovascular health than those occurring in lighter sleep stages; yet AHI treats them all the same.

While AHI is still the standard for diagnosing OSA, it's clear that it doesn't tell the whole story. Understanding sleep apnea isn't just about counting breathing events—it's about looking at how they affect the body and overall sleep quality.[22] That's why some researchers have started calling for a new index; one that paints a fuller picture of OSA's true impact.

> "I had a lot of stress when I was initially diagnosed with apnea. Several years later I lost 80 pounds which seemed to help. The initial diagnosis was severe sleep apnea.
>
> I used a CPAP for several years. Once I lost the weight I started using an oral device my dentist made. That helped but it messed up my teeth alignment.
>
> It was about that time I discovered Patrick [McKeown] and started practicing some of the breathing techniques.
>
> When he started advocating using the MyoTape, I began using that. Most nights I sleep quite well, and if I do wake up at night I get back to sleep quickly.
>
> Now I use the Oxygen Advantage® app to guide me more easily with the breathing exercises."

Understanding the Phenotypes of Sleep Apnea

When most people think of OSA, they picture a blocked or narrow airway. And while airway anatomy plays a big role, research since 2013, led by Dr. Danny Eckert and others, has shown that sleep apnea isn't just about airway size.[23,24] It's more like a puzzle with several pieces; some of which are hidden beneath the surface. It involves how the brain controls breathing, how easily a person wakes up during sleep, and how the body reacts to small changes in oxygen and carbon dioxide levels.

In fact, about 70% of people with sleep apnea have one or more non-anatomical traits that contribute to their condition. This explains why some people continue to struggle with symptoms even when using CPAP or other treatments. If sleep apnea were purely a structural issue, these treatments would work for everyone—but that's not always the case.

Dr. Eckert, a world-renowned sleep scientist and director of the Adelaide Institute for Sleep Health at Flinders University, has classified sleep apnea into four key contributing factors, known as the PALM classification.[25] These represent different "phenotypes" of sleep apnea, meaning that people can have different underlying causes.

- **P (Pcrit).** Airway collapsibility (how easily the airway closes during sleep)
- **A (arousal threshold).** How easily a person wakes up in response to breathing disturbances
- **L (loop gain).** Stability of breathing control (whether the body overcorrects for breathing changes)
- **M (muscle recruitment).** How well the muscles of the throat and airway work to keep the airway open

A phenotype is like a personal blueprint—it's a combination of traits shaped by both genetics and environment. When it comes to sleep apnea, your phenotype can help explain whether your breathing stops due to a floppy airway, a highly sensitive brain, or an overreactive response to the smallest shifts in gases like CO_2.

For example, some people have a naturally narrow or collapsible airway, making it easier for their throat to close during sleep. Others have weak muscle tone in the throat and tongue, which means their airway doesn't stay open as it should. Some experience unstable breathing control, where breathing repeatedly stops and restarts because of an overactive response to small changes in oxygen and carbon dioxide levels. Others wake up too easily in response to minor breathing disruptions, preventing deep, restorative sleep.

Understanding your phenotype is key to finding the right treatment. If unstable breathing control is the main issue, a CPAP machine may not fully fix the problem. If frequent awakenings are driving sleep apnea, treatments focused only on airway size won't be enough. The more we understand the "why" behind the apnea, the better we can choose tools that work.[26]

In the next section, we'll explore the different phenotypes of sleep apnea, explaining how they affect breathing and what can be done to improve them. This is where breathing and airway training techniques, like the Buteyko Method and myofunctional therapy, can be valuable. The Buteyko Method focuses on nasal breathing, light and slow breathing patterns, and CO_2 regulation, helping to reduce erratic breathing and airway instability. Myofunctional therapy strengthens the tongue, throat, and facial muscles, improving airway function and reducing airway collapse.

Alongside traditional treatments, these techniques can help stabilize breathing, support airway function, and address some of the underlying causes of sleep apnea—not just the symptoms.

P (Pcrit): Airway Collapsibility—How Easily the Airway Closes During Sleep

"Pcrit" (critical closing pressure) refers to how easily your upper airway collapses during sleep. If your airway closes partially or fully with even the slightest suction pressure, this indicates a high Pcrit, meaning your airway is highly collapsible and more prone to obstruction. Ideally, the airway should be able to withstand a good amount of suction pressure without collapsing.

Several factors contribute to high Pcrit, including obesity, which increases fat deposits around the tongue, throat, and abdomen, making the airway more vulnerable to collapse.[27] However, up to half of all people diagnosed with OSA are not obese,[28] meaning that airway collapsibility is not solely linked to weight. Structural factors such as a narrow airway, a retruded jaw, or poor muscle tone can also play a major role in airway obstruction.

CPAPs and MADs are commonly used to help keep the airway open by mechanically preventing collapse, but for many people, especially those with mild to moderate sleep apnea, addressing breathing patterns and airway muscle function is just as important.

With the mouth closed and the tongue resting on the roof of the mouth, the airway is naturally wider, reducing resistance to airflow.

Your everyday breathing pattern directly influences how you breathe during sleep. If you habitually breathe through your mouth, take big breaths, or breathe fast and heavily, you create greater negative pressure in the airway, making it more likely to collapse. Buteyko breathing teaches light, slow nasal breathing, which reduces the force of air moving through the airway, helping to keep it stable.

Another important factor is diaphragmatic breathing. When you breathe deeply and engage your diaphragm properly, it provides physical support to the throat muscles, thanks to a fascinating mechanical link between the diaphragm and upper airway.[29] This means that training yourself to breathe through your nose, lightly, and with good diaphragm recruitment during the day can help lower Pcrit and improve airway stability at night.

A (Arousal Threshold)—How Easily a Person Wakes Up in Response to Breathing Disturbances

Some people with sleep apnea don't necessarily have a blocked airway as their main issue—instead, they wake up too easily in response to minor disruptions. This is known as having a "low arousal threshold" (low AT), and it affects about 30 to 50% of individuals with OSA.[30] Research has shown that these individuals wake from sleep in response to very small increases in breathing effort, as measured by negative esophageal or epiglottic pressure swings. In other words, even a slight increase in resistance to breathing can trigger an awakening, leading to fragmented sleep.

When someone with low AT experiences a brief pause in breathing, a small drop in oxygen levels, or even an external disturbance like a minor noise, their brain overreacts and wakes them up instead of allowing the body to naturally adjust. This leads to fragmented sleep, where the person repeatedly wakes up throughout the night, often without even realizing it. Even if their breathing isn't severely obstructed, they still feel exhausted in the morning because they never get into deep, restorative sleep.

A common misconception is that a low arousal threshold is the same as insomnia. While both conditions involve waking up easily, insomnia is more about struggling to fall asleep or stay asleep due to psychological or behavioral factors, whereas low AT is a physiological response to minor airway instability. However, the two often overlap. Studies have shown that the presence of insomnia among OSA patients reduces CPAP adherence, suggesting that when insomnia is present, it should be treated alongside OSA.[31]

Many standard sleep apnea treatments don't address low AT. For example, MADs, which hold the jaw forward to prevent airway collapse, do not help with low AT.[32] A patient with this phenotype may still wake up frequently and feel exhausted, even if their airway remains physically open throughout the night.

Some researchers have explored the use of sedative/hypnotic agents to increase arousal threshold, allowing the body to tolerate minor breathing disturbances without waking up.[33] These medications help accumulate respiratory stimuli during stable sleep, which then activate the pharyngeal dilator muscles, stabilizing the upper airway. While some improvements in the AHI have been observed, they have generally been modest and mostly documented in single-night studies.

However, sedative/hypnotic agents also carry risks. In some cases, they could prolong apneas and lead to more severe oxygen desaturation (hypoxemia) before the brain triggers an arousal.[34] This means that while they may be beneficial for some people, they could be harmful for others, particularly those prone to longer apneas.

Instead of relying on sedatives, the Buteyko Method offers a natural way to help reduce unnecessary awakenings by stabilizing breathing patterns. When breathing is heavy, fast, or erratic, the brain is more likely to detect it as a problem and trigger an arousal. By practicing lighter, slower, and more rhythmic nasal breathing, Buteyko helps keep breathing stable and reduces the likelihood of unnecessary wake-ups.

Since the brain is constantly monitoring breathing during sleep, nasal breathing plays a crucial role in ensuring deeper sleep and less time spent in light sleep. When the mouth is closed and the tongue is resting on the roof of the mouth, the airway remains more stable. This reduces resistance and helps prevent the small disturbances that often trigger awakenings, especially in individuals with a low arousal threshold (low AT).

There's also the nervous system piece. People with low AT often experience hyperarousal, meaning their nervous system remains on high alert even during sleep. Buteyko breathing techniques activate the parasympathetic nervous system, shifting the body into a state of relaxation and promoting deeper, more restorative sleep.

How Can You Tell if You Have a Low Arousal Threshold?

Researchers have developed a way to predict a low arousal threshold from a standard diagnostic sleep study.[35] A clinical scoring system by Edwards et al. assigns 1 point for each of the following criteria:

- **Nadir SpO$_2$ (lowest oxygen saturation) > 82.5%.** This means that even at your lowest oxygen level during sleep, your blood oxygen saturation stays above 82.5%. People with severe airway blockages often have much lower oxygen levels, but if your levels remain above 82.5%, it may suggest that frequent arousals rather than major oxygen drops are disturbing your sleep.
- **Fraction of hypopneas > 58.3%.** Hypopneas are partial blockages of the airway, where airflow is reduced but not completely stopped. If more than 58.3% of your breathing disturbances are hypopneas (rather than full apneas), it indicates that your airway is not fully collapsing but still causing frequent arousals. This pattern is often seen in people with low AT, as their brain wakes them up before a complete airway collapse occurs.
- **Apnea-hypopnea index < 30 events per hour.** AHI measures the number of apneas (complete blockages) and hypopneas (partial blockages) per hour of sleep. People with a low arousal threshold often have an AHI below 30, meaning their breathing disturbances may not appear severe on paper but they still

experience frequent awakenings due to heightened sensitivity to minor changes in airflow or breathing effort.

If someone scores 2 or more on this system, it strongly suggests a low arousal threshold. This means that their sleep disturbances are not just due to airway obstruction, but also because their brain wakes them up too easily in response to minor breathing changes.

L (Loop Gain)—Stability of Breathing Control

"Loop gain" is a term borrowed from engineering that helps us understand how stable or unstable a person's breathing is during sleep. It's a way of measuring how the body responds to small changes in breathing—specifically, how sensitive the brain is to fluctuations in CO_2 levels.[36] Since breathing during sleep is regulated by CO_2 levels, a person's loop gain helps explain whether their breathing is well balanced or prone to overcorrections that can make sleep apnea worse.

At its core, loop gain is the ratio of the response to the disturbance that caused it. In other words, if something slightly disrupts breathing—like a partial airway blockage—the brain is supposed to react in a controlled, measured way, restoring breathing without overdoing it. But in people with high loop gain, the body overreacts, triggering a response that is far too strong. This exaggerated reaction drops CO_2 levels too much, which then suppresses the brain's drive to breathe.[37]

To understand why this happens, it's important to remember that carbon dioxide is the primary driver of breathing. When CO_2 builds up in the blood, the brain detects this rise and signals the body to take a breath. But in people with high loop gain, this system is too sensitive. When the airway collapses and breathing stops, CO_2 levels rise because it's not being exhaled. When breathing resumes, it does so with exaggerated, gasping breaths that rapidly blow off too much CO_2, causing levels to drop too low. And when CO_2 drops too low, the brain doesn't send the signal to breathe. This is what's known as "central apnea"—a pause in breathing that occurs because the brain simply isn't triggering a breath.

For the worrying partner lying awake, this cycle is easy to spot. It often starts with loud snoring, as the person struggles to keep their airway open. Then suddenly—silence. They've stopped breathing altogether. The pause can last several seconds before their brain finally forces them to take a breath. But when they do, it's not a gentle recovery—it's a loud, gasping inhale, often followed by fast, hard breathing through an open mouth as they desperately try to catch up. This exaggerated breathing flushes out too much carbon dioxide, and once their CO_2 levels drop too low, the brain no longer sends a strong enough signal to keep breathing steadily. Another pause follows, and the cycle repeats throughout the night.

This pattern of unstable breathing control doesn't just cause central apneas—it also ties into obstructive sleep apnea. When the brain doesn't send a signal to breathe, it also reduces the signal to the upper airway dilator muscles—the muscles that keep the airway open. If these muscles don't receive strong enough activation, they fail to do their job properly, making it even easier for the airway to collapse. This is why high loop gain can make obstructive sleep apnea worse, even when there isn't an obvious anatomical issue.

For at least 30% of people with OSA, high loop gain is a major part of the problem. It's why some people struggle with sleep apnea even when their airway obstruction is only partial or brief—because the issue isn't just obstruction, but unstable breathing control. This also explains why certain treatments, like MADs or upper airway surgery, often fail for these individuals.[38] These treatments focus on keeping the airway open but don't address the unstable breathing rhythm that keeps driving the problem.

Scientists have found a way to estimate a person's loop gain without needing a full sleep study. Dr. Ludovico Messineo, a research fellow at Harvard Medical School's Division of Sleep and Circadian Disorders, has made significant contributions to sleep medicine, particularly in understanding respiratory control mechanisms in OSA. In his 2018 study titled "Breath-Holding as a Means to Estimate the Loop Gain Contribution to Obstructive Sleep Apnea," published in the *Journal of Physiology*, Dr. Messineo explored the relationship between breath-hold duration and loop gain.[39] The researchers found that individuals with higher loop gain had shorter maximal breath-hold durations during wakefulness. In other words, the less time someone could hold their breath, the more unstable their breathing regulation tended to be during sleep. Another measurement, the second breath response, looked at how hard a person breathed immediately after a 20-second breath-hold; if they took deep, gasping breaths afterward, it suggested high loop gain and unstable breathing control.

While this test is not exactly the same as the CP used in the Buteyko Method, both provide insight into chemosensitivity to CO_2 or how reactive the brain is to increases in carbon dioxide levels. The CP is a simple way to check if your breathing patterns need improvement. If you have sleep apnea and measure your CP at 20 seconds or less, it's a strong sign that your breathing is dysregulated.

By improving CO_2 tolerance and reducing excessive breathing effort, Buteyko helps break the cycle of overreaction and instability that defines high loop gain.

If high loop gain is driving your sleep apnea, improving breathing control isn't just helpful—it's essential. If breathing instability is the real problem, targeting how you breathe may be just as important as treating where you breathe.

M (Muscle Recruitment)—How Well the Muscles of the Throat and Airway Work to Keep the Airway Open

One of the key factors in sleep apnea is how well the muscles in the throat respond to airway narrowing during sleep. Ideally, when the airway starts to collapse, the brain should activate the muscles around the throat, tongue, and soft palate to keep it open.[40] But for some people, this muscle response is too slow or too weak, allowing the airway to fully close before the muscles kick in. This is known as "poor pharyngeal muscle responsiveness," and it's a major contributor to sleep apnea in about 30% of people with OSA.[41]

The upper airway is made up of both rigid structures such as the jaw (mandible), upper jaw (maxilla), and hyoid bone, and soft tissues, including the tongue, throat muscles, and fat pads around the airway. While structural factors like a narrow jaw or retruded maxilla can make the airway more vulnerable to collapse, the real problem for many people is poor muscle function. This is especially true in the velopharyngeal area, the space just behind the soft palate, which is a common site of collapse for most people with OSA.

Even during sleep, the body has built-in mechanisms to keep the airway open. When breathing resistance increases—due to negative pressure in the throat or shifts in oxygen and carbon dioxide levels— the brain should send signals to activate the upper airway muscles, keeping them engaged enough to maintain airflow. But in some people, the signal arrives late. Their dilator muscles don't kick in until after breathing has stopped for a while, allowing the airway to collapse again and again throughout the night.

Some treatments attempt to correct this by stimulating the hypoglossal nerve, which controls tongue movement and helps keep the airway open. In select cases, hypoglossal nerve stimulation has been shown to reduce the AHI by up to 70%, significantly improving sleep apnea symptoms.[42] But this approach isn't suitable for everyone, and up to one-third of patients don't respond to it. Instead of relying on machines or implants, another approach is to train the muscles themselves so they naturally respond better. That's where orofacial myofunctional therapy (OMT) comes in.

OMT was first described in 1918 by Dr. Alfred Roger, who recognized the importance of tongue posture and proper oral function for airway health.[43] OMT consists of exercises that strengthen and coordinate the tongue, throat, and facial muscles, improving their ability to keep the airway open during sleep. It targets key areas like the lips, tongue, soft palate, and facial muscles, and also incorporates breathing, swallowing, speech, and chewing exercises. A systematic review found that OMT can reduce AHI by nearly 50%, improve oxygen levels, and reduce daytime sleepiness.[44]

Despite these promising results, effectiveness varies from person to person. Scientists are still working to understand exactly how muscle training improves airway function so that treatment can be better tailored to each individual. Research by O'Connor-Reina and colleagues found that when patients used a smartphone app to follow myofunctional exercises, adherence to therapy was significantly higher—90% in the app group compared with 50% in the group without the app.[45] The increased adherence may be due to direct feedback from the app, as well as easier access to health professionals for guidance.

Another study by Diafëria et al. showed that CPAP adherence nearly doubled when it was combined with myofunctional therapy. In their study, adherence to CPAP alone was only 30%, while adherence in the CPAP + OMT group was 65%.[46] This suggests that training the airway muscles makes CPAP more tolerable, possibly by reducing the pressure required to keep the airway open.

As awareness of OMT and its role in sleep health grows, organizations like the AOMT (Academy of Orofacial Myofunctional Therapy) are leading efforts to expand education and training in myofunctional therapy for both healthcare professionals and the general public. The AOMT was founded in 2013, building on decades of pioneering work by Joy Moeller in the field of myofunctional therapy. Joy's dedication to advancing OMT laid the foundation for its integration into modern healthcare, and her son Marc, along with Samantha Weaver, established the AOMT to expand education, training, and awareness of myofunctional therapy. Their work has been instrumental in bringing OMT to the forefront of sleep medicine, emphasizing its vital role in improving airway health and breathing function for both children and adults.

Many children with sleep-disordered breathing have oral myofunctional issues, such as low tongue posture, mouth breathing, or weak airway muscles, which, if left unaddressed, can lead to lifelong breathing problems. Catching these early and correcting them through OMT can support healthy facial development, promote nasal breathing, and lower the risk of developing OSA later in life.

For adults with sleep apnea, OMT provides a non-invasive way to improve muscle responsiveness, reducing reliance on CPAP or other mechanical interventions. Combining OMT with the Buteyko Method can be particularly powerful. While OMT strengthens and tones the airway muscles, Buteyko breathing helps stabilize breathing patterns by promoting diaphragmatic breathing, which has a direct mechanical connection to the upper airway dilator muscles. Nasal breathing and correct tongue posture are also essential—when the tongue rests properly against the roof of the mouth and breathing is through the nose, the airway is naturally supported, reducing the risk of collapse.

For those with poor pharyngeal muscle responsiveness, improving muscle tone and breathing control is key to managing sleep apnea effectively.

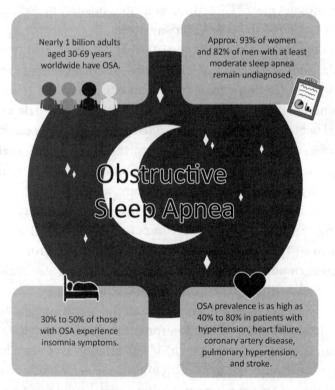

Why Understanding Phenotypes Matters

Dr. Eckert's research revealed that approximately 70% of people with OSA have one or more non-anatomical factors contributing to their condition.[47] This means that for many individuals, particularly those with mild-to-moderate sleep apnea, addressing breathing pattern disorders and incorporating OMT can play a meaningful role in treatment. Even for those using CPAP or MADs, practices like nasal breathing, Buteyko training, and OMT can help improve both effectiveness and long-term compliance.

In the next section, we'll look at the most common treatments for sleep apnea. CPAP is still considered the gold standard and works well for many people. But what about the millions who never get diagnosed or those who try CPAP and find it doesn't suit them? The second mainstay of treatment, MADs, also helps many people by holding the airway open, but as we've seen, they are not effective for those with low arousal threshold or high loop gain.

ADDRESSING SLEEP APNEA

Treatment for OSA varies based on its severity of the condition and underlying phenotype. CPAP therapy is commonly recommended for moderate-to-severe cases and remains one of the most effective treatments available.

Continuous Positive Airway Pressure

Let's talk about CPAP, the gold standard for treating OSA. Since its invention in 1981 by Australian doctor Colin Sullivan, CPAP machines have been helping people breathe better during sleep by delivering a steady stream of pressurized air. Think of it like a reverse vacuum cleaner. Instead of sucking air out, it pushes air through the airway to hold it open. It's simple yet effective, but the journey of CPAP from its inception to today is as fascinating as it is challenging. Back in the late 1970s, Dr. Sullivan, a respiratory physician and researcher at the University of Sydney, was studying how upper airways collapse during sleep. His subjects were bulldogs and other short-nosed dogs that are prone to breathing issues. Why bulldogs? Their tight jaws, thick necks, and crowded airways might look adorable, but they mirror many of the same structural challenges humans face when it comes to breathing during sleep.

There's even a story, passed around in sleep medicine circles, that Sullivan was inspired after watching his own bulldog, reportedly named Samantha, struggle to breathe at night. She would snort, gasp, and occasionally pause her breathing, just like a person with sleep apnea. Whether this happened exactly as the story goes is unclear, there's no hard evidence, but it's a charming story nonetheless.

Inspired, Sullivan began experimenting. Using surgical tubing, a makeshift nasal mask, and the motor from a reverse vacuum cleaner, he built the first prototype of what would later become the CPAP machine. First, he tested it on dogs. Then on humans. And it worked. People who had spent years waking up choking and gasping for air were finally sleeping through the night. For many, it was the first time in years they woke up feeling like themselves again.

The first CPAP devices were revolutionary but far from perfect. Imagine a machine so loud that it had to be placed in the room next door, with a long hose fed through the wall so the user could sleep in relative silence. That's how the earliest CPAP machines operated— transforming bedrooms into something out of a sci-fi movie. But their use also highlights just how desperate some people were, and still are, to find relief from the exhausting toll of sleep apnea. Thankfully, today's CPAP machines are quieter and more compact, but the principle remains the same: delivering pressurized air to prevent airway collapses during sleep.

So why are we humans struggling with airways that resemble those of bulldogs in the first place? A lot of it comes down to how modern life has reshaped us. Processed diets, soft foods, poor oral habits, and a general shift away from nose breathing have led to narrower faces, smaller jaws, and less room in the mouth for the tongue. That means smaller airways and a greater risk of those airways collapsing during sleep.

When you step back and look at it, this doesn't seem like progress. Our airways have narrowed instead of widened. Breathing has become harder, not easier. It raises a bigger question: if this is what modern living is doing to us, where is it all heading? Instead of moving forward, we seem to be going backwards.

Fast forward to today, and CPAP is a global cornerstone in the treatment of sleep apnea. Companies like ResMed, which Sullivan helped co-found, Philips Respironics, and Fisher & Paykel now dominate the CPAP market. It's a multi-billion dollar industry, valued at over 5.5 billion dollars and projected to top 7 billion in the coming years.

CPAP is undeniably effective at reducing OSA severity. By continuously delivering air, it prevents the throat from collapsing, ensures steady air flow, and helps eliminate the constant micro-arousals that disrupt deep sleep. But here's the catch: after more than 50 years of research into sleep apnea, CPAP is still the mainstay treatment. It's like Henry Ford's famous quote about the Model T: "You can have any color you want, as long as it's black." With sleep apnea, it feels like doctors are saying, "You can have any treatment you want, as long as it's CPAP."

Interestingly, CPAP's inventor, Dr. Colin Sullivan, never intended for it to become a lifelong solution. In a 2023 interview with *Salon*, he said:

> "CPAP was always intended as a temporary physical therapy measure, not a permanent solution. I don't think the significance of sleep apnea is still fully grasped often by the medical profession."[48]

Sullivan also highlighted how sleep apnea remains under-diagnosed, even in patients with other health conditions:

> "I am still astounded when I see patients who have various cardiac conditions, and no one's even asked them about what happens to them at nighttime in terms of sleep."

He emphasized the role of snoring as a warning sign, stating:

> "Snoring is a forerunner for so many people, probably the major-ity. A very large number of patients I've seen started snoring at 30 or 35, and then it kept going, and after 10 years or so, they developed apnea."

But here's something that rarely comes up in the CPAP conversation: the way you breathe while using the machine can make or break how well it works.

Most of the focus tends to be on pressure settings and finding the right mask. But underneath all that is a much more basic question: Are you breathing through your nose or your mouth?

That one detail can shape your entire CPAP experience.

Let's start with nasal breathing. Breathing through the nose, especially during sleep, naturally helps keep the lower jaw slightly forward and encourages the tongue to rest against the roof of the mouth. That tongue position plays a big role in keeping the airway open. When CPAP is added, the pressurized air works with your anatomy rather than against it. The result is smoother airflow, fewer interruptions, and better sleep.

Now compare that to mouth breathing. When the mouth is open during sleep, the tongue tends to fall back, the jaw drops, and the airway narrows. That same CPAP pressure now has to work overtime to keep things open. Often this means higher pressure settings, more air leaks, dry mouth, bloating, and general discomfort. In a way, mouth breathing can end up canceling out the very benefit CPAP is trying to provide. It is like trying to heat a room with the windows wide open.

So why aren't more doctors encouraging nasal breathing with CPAP, especially when it is clearly more effective?

Here's the thing. Most sleep doctors are not trained in breathing education. Their role is to diagnose and manage sleep apnea, often with devices and equipment. If a patient comes in breathing through their mouth, the solution is usually to prescribe a full-face mask to accommodate it. There is rarely a conversation about whether that mouth breathing could be changed.

In fairness, doctors may assume the person cannot breathe through their nose due to congestion or habit. But that is where the right tools and training come in.

Mouth breathing is not a fixed condition. It is a habit, and like many habits, it can be changed. Even a chronically stuffy nose can often be improved with simple exercises. The Buteyko Method teaches people how to unblock the nose, breathe more quietly and lightly, and transition gently to nasal breathing. This does not just make CPAP more tolerable. It helps it work the way it is supposed to.

A full-face mask might seem like the easiest option, especially if you have always breathed through your mouth at night. And yes, it allows for airflow through both the nose and mouth. But the downsides add up: more pressure, more discomfort, and more chance of giving up on therapy altogether.

On the other hand, using a nasal mask with nasal breathing can be a game-changer. It usually allows for lower pressure settings, fewer leaks, and better comfort. Sure, there may be an adjustment period, especially if the nose is blocked or the habit of mouth breathing is strong, but most people can overcome these challenges with the right guidance.

If nasal breathing still feels out of reach, that is where MyoTape can help. It gently supports the lips to stay closed, making it easier to breathe through the nose without feeling forced or restricted. Combined with the Buteyko Method, it is a simple way to create lasting change.

So if CPAP has not been going the way you hoped, if you are waking with a dry mouth, struggling with high pressure, or just not feeling rested, it might not be the machine. It might be your breathing.

When your breathing and your CPAP are aligned, it stops feeling like a battle. It becomes a partnership.

While CPAP works well for many, it's not without its challenges:

- **Low compliance rates.** Roughly 50% of patients stop using CPAP within a year, often due to discomfort or difficulty adapting to the mask and equipment.[49]
- **Claustrophobia and discomfort.** Around 34.6% of non-compliant users report feeling claustrophobic wearing the mask.[50]
- **Health risks from poor maintenance.** CPAP devices require regular cleaning to prevent the buildup of spores and fungi, which can affect users' respiratory health.[51]
- **Side effects.** Issues like dry mouth, nasal congestion, and air leaks can discourage consistent use.
- **"Smashed face syndrome."** Long-term use of CPAP masks can sometimes cause facial structure changes due to prolonged pressure.[52]
- **Device recalls.** Recent recalls due to foam degradation in some CPAP devices have raised health concerns and shaken user confidence.[53]

Out of all the individuals with OSA, 80 to 90% go undiagnosed, highlighting just how vastly underrecognized this condition is.[54] As noted earlier, for those who are diagnosed, the gold standard treatment is CPAP. However, the path to effective treatment is far from straightforward.

Of those advised to use CPAP, only 40% actually start the therapy.[55] And even among those who do, 46–83% eventually stop using it due to discomfort, inconvenience, or other challenges.[56-58] Despite advancements in behavioral interventions and patient coaching over the past 20 years, adherence rates have not significantly improved.

To break it down for context:

- Out of every 100 people with OSA, 80 to 90 remain undiagnosed.
- That leaves only 10 to 20 individuals who actually receive a diagnosis.
- Of those diagnosed, roughly 4 to 8 will start using CPAP.
- However, after a year, only 1 to 4 individuals will still be using CPAP consistently.

So what happens to the other 96–99%? Many continue to struggle with the serious consequences of untreated OSA, such as daytime fatigue, poor sleep quality, and increased risks of heart disease and stroke. This enormous gap between diagnosis, treatment, and sustained use shows us that a one-size-fits-all approach just doesn't work. We need more tools in the toolbox.

"About 13 years ago I was living with my girlfriend (now my wife), and she would frequently tell me that she'd hear me stop breathing at night, and then gasp for air in my sleep. It freaked her out. She had just finished med school, and knew I had sleep apnea. She'd always say, 'Don't die on me.'

At first, she gently started pointing it out to me when she noticed me mouth breathing. As I got older, and more responsible, I reduced my drinking, which ultimately helped my sleep, but it really wasn't until about 5 years ago, when I became aware of the Buteyko Method, that I fully committed to nasal breathing, and mouth taping at night.

Now I am certified in both Buteyko and Oxygen Advantage®. I have an evening routine that includes about 20 minutes of slow and reduced breathing; then I tape my mouth (or sometimes tape before reduced breathing), sleep on my left side, and my sleep quality is generally excellent.

Since I began mouth taping (which I took to quite easily), my wife has never commented that she hears me gasping for air in my sleep. In fact, I don't even snore anymore."

Ben, 42, USA

Mandibular Advancement Device

Over the years, I've heard so many positive reports from people using mandibular advancement devices (MADs). For some, they've made a real difference, especially for those who couldn't tolerate CPAP masks or simply never got used to them. When CPAP doesn't feel right, a MAD can offer a more comfortable, less intrusive alternative.

A MAD is a small, custom-made plastic device that fits in your mouth, kind of like a mouth guard or orthodontic retainer. Its job is simple: it pulls your lower jaw and tongue forward to help keep your airway open during sleep. But there's one important detail that often gets overlooked: MADs can sometimes lead to more mouth breathing at night. Since the device positions the jaw forward, it can make it harder to keep the lips sealed, leading to open-mouth breathing.[59] And as you probably know by now, mouth breathing is no small thing; it's linked to a less stable airway, drier airways, and poorer sleep quality overall.

In the next section, we'll take a closer look at mouth taping; how to do it safely, the different things to consider, and how it can actually enhance the effectiveness of a MAD by promoting nasal breathing through the night.

Mouth Taping: Helpful or Harmful?

Now, I want to talk about something that was a game-changer for me: breathing through the nose during sleep. I mentioned this earlier in the book, but it's worth taking a deeper look because this one change had a huge impact on my sleep and overall health.

To this day, I still wear a nasal breathing support—specifically, MyoTape, which, yes, happens to be my own product. You might be wondering, "If nasal breathing is so natural, why do you still use it?" The truth is, I don't need it anymore the way I did in the beginning. But now, it has become a habit, almost like a sleep cue. As soon as I put it on, my body recognizes it's time to wind down. It's strange, but it works. The simple act of applying the tape signals to my brain that it's time for deep, restful sleep.

But enough about me, let's talk about why nasal breathing matters so much during sleep. If you wake up with a dry mouth, there's a very high chance that you're breathing through your mouth while you sleep. And while this might not seem like a big deal, mouth breathing can worsen sleep apnea, increase snoring, and reduce sleep quality.

Mouth breathing during sleep is incredibly common, especially in people with OSA. Research by Zhang et al. found a strong link between dry mouth and sleep apnea, highlighting just how important this symptom is.[60] In a study of 912 participants, 54% of snorers reported waking up with dry mouth, compared with just 30.5% of non-snorers. In another group of 207 patients suspected of having OSA, those who were ultimately diagnosed with sleep apnea were far more likely to experience dry mouth. The researchers concluded that dry mouth is such a strong predictor of sleep apnea that they recommended adding it to *The STOP-Bang Questionnaire*, one of the most widely used screening tools for OSA.

So, if you're waking up parched and dehydrated, it's not just an inconvenience—it's a red flag that your breathing is disrupted during sleep.

If you've been scrolling through social media, you might have noticed that mouth taping is everywhere. People are raving about how it helps with snoring, energy levels, and even skin hydration. But does it really work? It's worth noting that the research done so far looked at mouth taping on its own, not paired with breathing retraining. So what they measured was the effect of simply sealing the lips, not necessarily improving how someone breathes.

One of the first studies to test this was a pilot study by Huang and Young. They studied 30 patients with mild sleep apnea (AHI between 5 and 15) who also had a habit of mouth breathing.[61] The patients' Epworth Sleepiness Scale (ESS) scores dropped from 8.1 to 5.2, showing they felt less exhausted during the day. Their snoring intensity dropped from 49.1 decibels to 41.1 decibels, and their snoring frequency fell from 146.7 events per hour to just 40 events per hour. Most importantly, their AHI dropped from 12 to 7.8, meaning they had fewer breathing disruptions during sleep.

Another study by Labarca et al. looked at how combining an adhesive mouth strip (AMT) with a MAD could improve sleep apnea treatment. The idea was that preventing mouth breathing while using a MAD could make the device even more effective. The study included 21 adults with moderate-to-severe OSA (AHI 10–50) and compared different treatment setups: MAD alone, AMT alone, and MAD + AMT combined.[62]

The results showed that adding mouth taping to a MAD made a big difference. The median AHI in the MAD-only group was 10.5, but in the MAD + AMT group, it dropped to just 5.6—a much greater improvement. 76% of participants using MAD + AMT achieved an AHI of less than 10, compared with just 43% with MAD alone. The conclusion? Using a mouth strip alongside a mandibular advancement device significantly improved treatment success by keeping the airway open and reducing mouth breathing.

Another recent study by Lee et al. tested mouth taping on patients with mild OSA who were mouth breathers. The results were consistent with earlier studies: 65% of participants saw their snoring cut by at least 50%, and their AHI dropped by 47%, from 8.3 to 4.7 events per hour.[63] Even for those who primarily struggled when sleeping on their back, their supine AHI dropped from 9.4 to 5.5.

Despite these promising results, mouth taping is still controversial, and many doctors hesitate to recommend it, mostly for two key reasons. Both of those concerns are valid, and they're exactly what this book is designed to help you overcome. When nasal breathing is restored using the Buteyko Method, and mouth taping is done safely using MyoTape which still allows for mouth puffing, those concerns are no longer barriers. The first concern is straightforward: can the person breathe comfortably through their nose? If nasal congestion is an issue, forcing the mouth closed can make things worse. This is where nasal unblocking and retraining the breath really matter. One way to test it is to try six rounds of the *Nose Unblocking Exercise*. Then sit and breathe quietly through your nose for three minutes. Easy? Great. Now try walking while still breathing through your nose. If that's uncomfortable, it may signal a need to improve nasal airflow, either with practice or by checking for structural issues like a deviated septum.

The second concern is mouth puffing. This happens when a person instinctively tries to expel air through their mouth during sleep, usually in response to airway restriction. Oral breathing is extremely common in people with OSA, often occurring right before and after apnea or hypopnea events. For some, mouth puffing is a natural mechanism to release excess air when nasal breathing alone isn't enough. If the mouth is completely sealed, it could create discomfort or even make breathing disturbances worse instead of improving them.

This issue gained attention after a clinical case study reported that a patient's sleep apnea worsened when their mouth was taped during sleep. After an otorhinolaryngological checkup, doctors observed that the patient was experiencing intermittent mouth puffing (IMP), an unconscious attempt to breathe through the mouth despite the tape preventing it. The researchers then conducted a study to further investigate the role of mouth puffing in OSA, as well as how mouth taping might impact sleep apnea severity.[64]

The study included 71 participants aged 35 to 60 years, each with varying degrees of OSA severity. They found that people with severe OSA had significantly higher intermittent mouth puffing percentages compared with those with mild or moderate OSA. The breakdown of participants was as follows:

- 33.78% had severe OSA.
- 22.38% had moderate OSA.
- 14.55% had mild OSA.

The study found that mouth taping helped some people but worsened symptoms in others. Specifically, 51.72% of participants had improved oxygen desaturation index scores when mouth taped, while 48.28% actually worsened.[65] This means that for nearly half of the participants, blocking the mouth created more breathing difficulties rather than solving them.

A key finding was that the percentage of mouth puffing was positively associated with OSA severity. In simple terms, the more someone engaged in oral or oronasal breathing, the worse their sleep apnea and oxygen saturation (SpO_2) levels were.

Body weight is another important factor. Research shows that a higher BMI is linked to more severe OSA and an increased likelihood of mouth puffing during sleep. This makes it especially important to identify risk groups. If you have a higher BMI and severe OSA, completely taping your mouth shut at night could worsen your sleep apnea and even be risky.

One morning, while exercising on an elliptical trainer in our office, I stuck to my usual habit of breathing through my nose. As I increased the intensity, I could feel my breathing becoming more labored. Then, without even thinking about it, my body forced my mouth open to release the excess air—my nose simply couldn't handle the volume quickly enough. In that moment, I got a real, firsthand understanding of what mouth puffing is. It's not a conscious action; it's a natural response when airflow needs to escape quickly and the nose alone isn't enough. This is likely what happens during sleep—if breathing becomes restricted and nasal airflow isn't sufficient, the body instinctively finds another route, and air exits through the mouth. This experience reinforced for me why covering the mouth completely during sleep can be problematic for some people; if the body needs to release air and can't, it could disrupt breathing rather than improve it.

I developed MyoTape specifically for my clients, many of whom had a real psychological fear of having their mouth completely taped shut at night—which I completely understood. The thought of being unable to breathe properly can be unsettling, especially for those with sleep apnea or nasal congestion. Fortunately, MyoTape allows for mouth puffing, making it a safer and more comfortable alternative.

Unlike traditional mouth tape, MyoTape doesn't seal the lips shut—instead, it gently surrounds them, bringing them together without blocking airflow. You can test this yourself: put on the tape, breathe in through your nose, and exhale through your mouth. You'll notice that the air can still escape freely, which is crucial for those who experience mouth puffing during sleep. This way, nasal breathing is encouraged, but not forced, ensuring a natural and adaptable breathing pattern throughout the night.

> "Taping my mouth during the night has removed sleep apnea completely and vastly reduced waking and periods of insomnia occurring during the night. I practice on average 1 session on breathing using the ButeykoClinic app per day but aim to schedule time for more."

If you've already had a sleep study, that's a great starting point—it provides a baseline of where you are right now. This means you have an opportunity to see real progress by applying the Buteyko Method and then doing a follow-up sleep study in a few weeks. How much will your apnea index improve? Will your breathing become more stable? The comparison could be fascinating—and it's a chance to see firsthand how small, consistent changes in your breathing can lead to measurable improvements in your sleep quality.

If you haven't had a sleep study yet, then the next few weeks are crucial. This is the time to fully commit to Buteyko breathing and myofunctional therapy, giving your body the best chance to improve before your test. Sleep studies are the gold standard for diagnosing sleep apnea, so following the instructions below will help you get the most accurate results—whether it's your first test or a follow-up after practicing these techniques.

How to Prepare for Your Sleep Study

1. **Open Your Airway to Prevent Collapse**
   - **Practice nasal breathing with proper tongue posture.** Rest three-quarters of your tongue against the roof of your mouth to support airway stability and prevent collapse.
   - **Engage the diaphragm.** Focus on breathing low into the diaphragm, as this naturally stabilizes the airway by improving muscle tone in the throat.
   - **Use MyoTape for nasal breathing.** If you already wear MyoTape at night, continue to do so during the sleep study.
2. **Normalize Your Breathing Volume**
   - **Raise your Control Pause score.** Aim to gradually increase your CP score to 20 seconds or more as an indicator of improved breathing control.
   - **Adopt light, slow, and deep breathing patterns.** By practicing gentle, controlled nasal breathing throughout the day, you help train your body to adopt this healthier pattern automatically, even at night. Aim to practice for five minutes, four to six times a day, and gradually work up to a full fifteen minutes before bed. You'll find full descriptions of each exercise in Chapter 1, but one key point to remember is this: light breathing is the foundation.

What Could Change Between Your Sleep Studies?

By consistently following these breathing and airway techniques for a few weeks, many people find that their sleep apnea severity decreases—sometimes by 50% or more. Here's what you might notice when you compare your before-and-after sleep study results:

- A lower AHI—fewer breathing interruptions per hour
- Improved oxygen saturation levels
- Fewer sleep disturbances and deeper, more restorative sleep
- Less snoring and reduced airway resistance
- A more stable breathing pattern throughout the night

By taking these steps before your sleep study, you're not just collecting data—you're actively improving your sleep health. The results will show you just how much control you have over your sleep apnea and how making these simple changes can lead to profound, measurable improvements in your well-being.

> "I used to use a CPAP machine. I couldn't stand the mask. Plus I never felt that it helped me. Once I discovered mouth taping, my sleep has improved greatly."

> "Since my husband and I started using MyoTape, we sleep like rocks and longer each night. I used to wake at 2 or 3 in the morning and not be able to go back to sleep. This doesn't happen anymore.
> My husband snores really bad and uses CPAP. MyoTape prevents him from snoring and we both sleep."
>
> *Karen, 64, USA*

SEAN'S STORY: FROM SNORING AND SLEEP APNEA TO RESTFUL NIGHTS

Sean, a 60-year-old computing security consultant from England, spent much of his life struggling with snoring, poor sleep, and breathing difficulties. These challenges not only affected his energy levels but also raised serious health concerns as he grew older. It wasn't until Sean discovered the power of nasal breathing and mouth taping that his life—and his sleep—began to transform.

A Lifelong Struggle with Breathing and Sleep

Sean's issues with breathing began in childhood. He often found himself short of breath, unable to run long distances, and plagued by chronic snoring. Over the years, the problem worsened, disrupting his sleep and leaving him feeling exhausted during the day. Despite trying nasal strips and other over-the-counter remedies, nothing seemed to work.

"I always thought there was something wrong with my breathing," Sean recalls. "But I never believed there was anything I could do about it."

The turning point came during a minor hospital procedure when an SpO_2 monitor revealed that Sean's oxygen levels were lower than normal, particularly at night. Encouraged by his wife—who had noticed he occasionally stopped breathing during sleep—Sean consulted a specialist. The diagnosis was mild-to-moderate OSA, and he was prescribed a CPAP machine.

Struggles with CPAP Therapy

Initially, Sean found some relief with the CPAP machine, but the discomfort quickly outweighed the benefits. The device, designed to keep his airway open, became a source of frustration, often waking him in the middle of the night.

"I got on okay with it for a while, but after maybe a total of 6 months it was starting to keep me awake. By this time I was working on getting myself to sleep by breathing techniques and such like. So, I'd put the CPAP machine on, but wake up at maybe 2 o'clock in the morning. I'd try to get back to sleep, but you can't do any breathing techniques with this thing on your face. So eventually I stopped using it. I felt it was keeping me awake more than it was letting me sleep."

Determined to find another solution, Sean began experimenting with propping up his bed and sleeping on his side. However, it wasn't until he stumbled upon a podcast by James Nestor that everything changed.

Discovering Nasal Breathing and Mouth Taping

Inspired by the podcast's emphasis on nasal breathing, Sean committed to retraining his breathing habits during the day and night. Shortly after, he discovered my program and began incorporating breathing exercises and mouth taping into his routine.

The results were transformative. Sean found he could fall asleep faster and stay asleep longer. He woke up feeling refreshed, free from the dry mouth, headaches, and sore throat that had plagued him for years.

"Now, if I want to go to sleep, I just breathe, relax, and breathe myself to sleep," Sean explains. "Before, I'd have to read for hours just to fall asleep. Now, I'm still on the same book I bought a year ago!"

Sean also started tracking his oxygen levels using a smartwatch. The improvement was undeniable—his nighttime oxygen saturation, which used to dip as low as 70%, now consistently ranged between 93 and 96%.

The Impact on Overall Health

Sean's journey didn't just improve his sleep; it had a ripple effect on his overall health. He was diagnosed with atrial fibrillation (AFib), a heart rhythm disorder, and initially prescribed beta blockers. However, after incorporating nasal breathing and improving his respiratory health, Sean stopped taking the medication and hasn't experienced any AFib episodes since.

"I just wish I'd started doing this 40 years ago," Sean reflects. "I spent years thinking I couldn't breathe properly and that there was nothing I could do about it. It turns out the solution was simple."

Sean now advocates for greater awareness of nasal breathing and mouth taping as first-line solutions for sleep apnea and snoring. He believes that many people could potentially avoid the discomfort of CPAP machines by addressing the root cause of their breathing issues.

"The only time I was told to keep my mouth shut was when I was using the CPAP machine," Sean says with a laugh. "But in hindsight, keeping my mouth closed might have been all I needed in the first place. My apnea wasn't particularly severe, and I think the CPAP was overkill for me. If these techniques can help someone avoid a CPAP machine, it's worth it. Breathing through your nose is so much easier, and it's better for everyone. I just want people to know there's another way."

Through his journey, Sean has found restful nights and better health, proving that simple solutions can be life-changing. Sometimes, the best answers are right under our noses—literally!

SECTION 3

CHILDREN'S AND ADOLESCENT'S SLEEP

CHAPTER 11

CAUSES AND CONSEQUENCES OF POOR SLEEP FOR CHILDREN AND ADOLESCENTS

Have you ever watched your child sleep and noticed their mouth hanging open? Maybe they snore a little or shift around restlessly through the night. It might seem harmless, even a little cute, but it could be a quiet signal that their sleep is not as restorative as it should be.

Sleep issues in children and adolescents are far more common than most parents realize, and their impact extends well beyond restless nights. We all know that healthy sleep is vital for every child's growth, health, and well-being. What's less well understood, even in dental and medical circles, is that the ability to benefit from restful sleep is deeply connected to another vital function: *breathing*.

In children and teens, the relationship between breathing and sleep is particularly crucial, because their bodies and brains are in a constant state of growth and development. That means that poor sleep affects how they develop, think, and feel, which has huge significance for their ability to thrive in all aspects of life.

With the pervasive presence of digital technology, life for today's children and teenagers is a far cry from the simpler times of my own childhood. It's no wonder we're seeing a surge in sleep issues among these age groups. Issues like mouth breathing, snoring, and restless sleep are not just harmless habits—they are red flags signaling disrupted breathing patterns that can lead to long-term health and developmental issues if left unaddressed.

This chapter explores the intricate link between sleep and breathing in children and teenagers. Understanding this can provide insight into many childhood challenges, including attention difficulties, academic performance, emotional regulation, and even physical growth. By learning to recognize the signs of disordered breathing and knowing the exercises and practices that support healthy breathing during sleep, parents, caregivers, and healthcare providers can ensure that children receive the rest they need to grow into their full potential with healthier bodies and sharper minds.

HOW MUCH SLEEP DO CHILDREN NEED?

Children need sleep like they need food, water, and air—it's the foundation of their physical and mental health. Yet, in today's fast-paced, always-connected world, many children are falling short of the rest they need.

Depending on their age, children and teenagers require anywhere from 8 to 17 hours of quality sleep every night to support their growth, learning, and emotional resilience (please refer to Table 11.1).

Table 11.1   *US Centers for Disease Control and Prevention*
Daily Recommended Hours of Sleep[1]

Age Group	Age	Daily Sleep Recommended
Newborn	0–3 months	14–17 hours
Infant	4–12 months	12–16 hours (including naps)
Toddler	1–2 years	11–14 hours (including naps)
Preschool	3–5 years	10–13 hours (including naps)
School-age	6–12 years	9–12 hours
Teen	13–17 years	8–10 hours

Of course, as already noted, many children get less than the recommended amount of sleep. For example:[2]

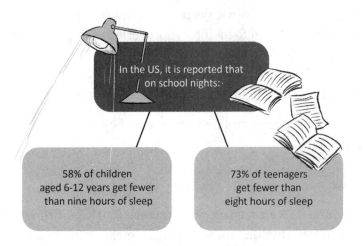

In the US, it is reported that on school nights:

58% of children aged 6-12 years get fewer than nine hours of sleep

73% of teenagers get fewer than eight hours of sleep

Considering these figures, no wonder it's difficult for children to pay attention and learn in class the next day!

How Do Sleep Habits Change as We Age?

Sleep requirements change significantly from infancy through to adolescence as the brain and body develop and mature. If you are a parent or caregiver, you may have wondered, "Why does my child wake so many times during the night?" or "Why can't I persuade my teenager to go to sleep at night yet can't persuade them to get out of bed in the morning?!"

To understand *how* and *why* sleep requirements and patterns evolve from birth through to age 18, let's revisit the concept of the circadian rhythm. You may recall from Chapter 6, that this internal clock regulates our cycles of sleep and wakefulness over 24 hours and generally shifts at three major stages of life: infancy, adolescence, and old age.

Infancy

- When babies are born, they haven't developed a circadian rhythm yet. A newborn baby's sleep cycle requires up to 17 hours of sleep, broken up into multiple short periods. Sleeping in multiple phases is also known as "polyphasic sleep."
- Babies develop a circadian rhythm around four to six months of age, at which point they tend to sleep in larger blocks of time.

Things change as children grow and they move towards their teenage years.

Adolescence

- Around 16% of teenagers experience a natural delay in their circadian rhythm, meaning their melatonin levels (which regulate the sleep-wake cycle) don't begin to rise until later in the evening.[3]
- This shift makes them feel more alert at night, often making it difficult to fall asleep before 11:00 p.m.
- With early school start times, many teens struggle to get the recommended 8 to 10 hours of sleep.
- This results in a sleep deficit, which can lead to problems with focus, mood, and overall health. Needless to say, this impacts their performance in school and daily life.

Sleep Quality, Quantity, and Consistency

When it comes to sleep, three things really matter: quality, quantity, and consistency. In other words, how well your child sleeps, how much sleep they get, and how regular their sleep schedule is. It's not enough for children and teenagers to just spend time in bed—they need deep, restorative sleep to truly reap the benefits.

Poor-quality sleep, whether it's due to insomnia, snoring, or a more severe sleep-related breathing disorder like OSA, can leave them feeling groggy, irritable, and unable to focus. Even when total sleep time seems adequate, short but fragmented sleep fails to meet the body's essential needs for recovery and growth. For young people, the combination of sufficient sleep time, a regular bedtime, and uninterrupted, high-quality rest is the key to supporting their physical health, emotional balance, and ability to learn and grow. If you would like to revisit the topics of sleep quality, quantity and consistency in more detail, please see Chapter 2.

What Causes Sleep Issues in Children?

Many factors can contribute to poor sleep in children, but they often share a common thread: *compromised breathing*. From nasal congestion and mouth breathing to enlarged adenoids and underdeveloped jaws, these seemingly minor issues can disrupt a child's ability to breathe easily during sleep, setting the stage for restless nights and long-term health challenges. Now, as you read on, you might notice that certain ideas come up more than once. And yes, you're right to spot it. That's not because I lost track or forgot I'd already mentioned something. It's because many of these issues are tightly woven together.

Take mouth breathing, for example. It can be caused by things like thumb sucking, bottle feeding, or a stuffy nose that never fully clears. But once it becomes a habit, it doesn't just stop there. It can affect how a child's face and airway develop, leading to a narrower airway, which in turn makes good-quality sleep even harder to achieve. That's why you may see some overlap in this chapter. Each section builds on the last, adding a new layer of understanding; from the habits that start it all, to the structural changes that follow, to the real-world impact on your child's sleep and wellbeing. These aren't isolated issues. They're part of a bigger story, and my aim is to help you connect the dots.

Here is a summary of the key factors that can impact sleep quality and quantity for children:

- **Breathing issues (e.g., sleep-disordered breathing).** Conditions such as habitual mouth breathing, snoring, and OSA, are significant contributors to poor sleep in children. These issues can result in interrupted sleep cycles, leading to daytime fatigue, irritability, and concentration difficulties. We will revisit these in more detail in the coming pages.
- **Allergies, asthma, and nasal congestion.** Conditions like asthma, chronic sinusitis, and allergies can cause nasal congestion and inflammation, impact the airways, and disrupt breathing, particularly at night. Chronic nasal congestion or a stuffy nose can lead to mouth breathing and poor sleep quality.
- **Anatomical factors.** Enlarged tonsils and adenoids are common in young children and contribute to blocked airways, leading to mouth breathing and interrupted sleep.

  High, narrow palates, missing teeth (due to extractions for orthodontic braces or congenitally missing teeth), poor jaw development, tongue tie, and small nasal passages restrict the size of the airway and hence airflow, predisposing children to mouth breathing and sleep-disordered breathing.

  Bottle-feeding during infancy can negatively impact craniofacial development, increasing the risk of structural issues like narrow palates and tongue mispositioning. Breastfeeding promotes nasal breathing and plays a crucial role in developing the oral and jaw structure in infants. The sucking action during breastfeeding develops facial muscles, widens the palate, and prevents malocclusions (crooked teeth), supporting long-term airway health. And of course, I'm very aware that societal pressures, high house prices, and large mortgages often require both parents to work, so it's never about placing blame on any mother who had to return to work early to help keep the household afloat.

- **Blue light exposure from screens.** Excessive screen time close to bedtime can interfere with melatonin production, making it harder for children and teens to fall asleep. Bright screens from devices like tablets, phones, and TVs are known to disrupt the natural sleep-wake cycle, or circadian rhythm.
- **Behavioral and psychological factors.** Anxiety and stress, which can arise from family issues, school pressures, or social media interactions, may interfere with a child's ability to relax before bed, resulting in insomnia or nightmares.

    Poor sleep hygiene, such as irregular bedtimes, or lack of a bedtime routine, also play a role. Bedtime resistance and difficulty winding down at night are common in younger children and can be exacerbated by inconsistent bedtime routines or overstimulation in the evening.
- **Medical interventions or treatments.** Some medications, including those for attention deficit hyperactivity disorder (ADHD) or asthma, may have stimulating effects or cause side effects that disrupt sleep.
- **Dietary factors.** Eating large meals or consuming sugary or caffeinated beverages close to bedtime can contribute to sleep disturbances. Sugary snacks or heavy meals can cause digestive discomfort. Caffeine in sodas (this can be a particular issue for teens, who can become fond of energy drinks), or chocolate can act as a stimulant, making it harder for children to wind down at bedtime.

Many of these issues can be counteracted by maintaining regular bedtimes and good sleep hygiene (see Chapter 6). However, if a child has breathing issues, their sleep problems are likely to continue until these are addressed.

The Importance of Nasal Breathing

Children are born natural nasal breathers, which is essential for the proper development of the face and airways. When children breathe through the nose, it helps regulate oxygen levels in the blood, supports efficient respiratory function, and promotes restful sleep— see Chapter 5 (Table 5.2) for a summary. Nasal breathing during sleep is essential to stimulate adequate ventilation and activate reflexes that help maintain the tonicity of the muscles that stabilize the upper airway.[4]

Mouth Breathing

Despite the wealth of benefits to be gained from nasal breathing, many children transition to mouth breathing. Estimates of the prevalence of mouth breathing in children vary broadly, ranging from 7 to 60%.[5-9] This dysfunctional habit can persist and is considered a hallmark of sleep-disordered breathing.

What Causes Mouth Breathing?
Mouth breathing in children can stem from various underlying causes, often related to issues that obstruct normal nasal breathing, though behavioral issues also play a role. Here are some common factors:

1.   Nasal Obstructions
     • Enlarged tonsils or adenoids. When enlarged, these may block airflow through the nasal passages, making mouth breathing

the easiest alternative. Adenoids, located at the back of the nasal cavity, are immune system glands that can swell in response to infection, often leading to mouth breathing in children between ages two and seven, until the adenoids typically shrink during adolescence.

- **Nasal polyps.** These small growths in the nasal lining can also obstruct airflow.
- **Deviated septum.** A misalignment of the nasal septum (the middle structure that supports the nasal cavity) can make it difficult for air to pass through one or both nostrils.

2. **Asthma, Allergies and Respiratory Infections**
- **Asthma, frequent colds, sinus infections, or upper respiratory infections.** These can cause temporary or chronic nasal congestion, leading to mouth breathing.
- **Allergic reactions.** Allergic reactions can cause swelling in the nasal passages, leading to congestion and mouth breathing.

3. **Anatomical Abnormalities**
- **Facial or jaw structure differences.** Some children have facial or jaw structure differences that can impact nasal airflow, such as a high-arched palate, a recessed chin, or a tongue or lip tie.

4. **Habitual Factors**
- **Thumb sucking.** Prolonged thumb sucking can alter the shape of the palate and the jaw, potentially leading to mouth breathing.
- **Pacifier or bottle use.** Extended use can impact the development of the mouth and palate, influencing the child's breathing habits.

Chronic allergies and enlarged tonsils or adenoids are the most common culprits behind mouth breathing. But here's the catch: even after these physical blockages are removed through surgery, many kids continue to breathe through their mouths simply out of habit.[10] This is where breathing re-education becomes essential.

"Both my children [teens] didn't have lots of energy in the morning and would wake up feeling tired.

  Since they have started adding nose breathing into as much of their day as possible they have started to feel better. Myself and my wife have seen a difference in their moods."

Mark, 47, UK

How Does Mouth Breathing Impact Children?

Children who mouth breathe often have disrupted sleep, wake up tired, and may appear inattentive in school due to chronic fatigue. Mouth breathing has been linked to developmental issues, cognitive impairments, and a range of health concerns:

- **Facial and dental development.** Chronic mouth breathing can alter facial and dental structures, often leading to a longer, narrower face, a high-arched palate, and dental malocclusions (misalignment of teeth). This happens because mouth breathing affects the positioning of the tongue, lips, and jaw. It's important that mouth breathing is addressed early in children, as maximal orofacial growth takes place during the first two years of life; by age six years, nearly 60% of the adult face has developed.[11]

- **Altered head, neck, and body posture.** Mouth breathing can lead to forward head posture, neck strain, and rounded shoulders as the body compensates to keep the airway open.[12] Poor breathing mechanics contribute to shallow chest breathing, tight chest muscles, and inefficient breathing patterns.

- **Increased risk of infections.** The nose acts as a filter for bacteria and allergens. Mouth breathing bypasses this filtration, increasing the risk of respiratory infections, throat infections, and allergies.

- **Dental health.** Mouth breathing dries out saliva, which is crucial for protecting teeth against bacteria. This increases the likelihood of tooth decay, gum disease, and bad breath.[13]

- **Sleep-disordered breathing.** Mouth breathing is associated with an increase in upper airway resistance and sleep-disordered breathing issues, like snoring and OSA.[14] Mouth breathing disrupts sleep quality by increasing the likelihood of snoring, sleep apnea, and oxygen desaturation during sleep.

- **Sleep fragmentation.** Children who breathe through their mouths often experience lighter sleep and wake up frequently throughout the night, which fragments their sleep cycles and prevents restorative deep sleep. This often leaves children feeling tired and lethargic during the day, impacting their ability to concentrate and stay alert, and can cause mood swings, irritability, and hyperactivity.

"My daughter [had a] bad sore throat in the morning and many bad dreams. With mouth taping (it's been a year), she has fewer nightmares she says, and she says she falls asleep faster with it on. Her morning sore throat is gone."

How Does Mouth Breathing Impact Facial Development?

When children breathe nasally, their lips remain gently closed, creating a sealed oral space. The tongue naturally rests against the roof of the mouth, supporting the upper jaw's growth and alignment. This balance between the tongue's internal pressure and the external muscles of the lips and cheeks is essential for the proper development of the upper dental arch. However, when a child mouth breathes, this balance is disrupted. The tongue drops from its ideal position, allowing the upper jaw to narrow and potentially leading to crowding of teeth, improper bite alignment, and even changes in facial structure over time. An improper bite or overcrowding of teeth can be a telltale sign that the jaw hasn't developed fully. And when jaw development is compromised, it can have downstream effects on the child's airway, increasing the risk of breathing difficulties, especially during sleep. These seemingly small shifts can have profound impacts.

A scientific paper titled "Mouth Breathing: Adverse Effects on Facial Growth, Health, Academics, and Behavior," by dentist Dr. Yosh Jefferson, outlines the negative consequences of mouth breathing and the need for better recognition from health professionals:

"The vast majority of health care professionals are unaware of the negative impact of upper airway obstruction (mouth breathing) on normal facial growth and physiologic health. Children whose mouth breathing is untreated may develop long, narrow faces, narrow mouths, high palatal vaults, dental malocclusion, gummy smiles, and many other unattractive facial features.

These children do not sleep well at night due to obstructed airways; this lack of sleep can adversely affect their growth and academic performance. Many of these children are misdiagnosed with attention deficit disorder (ADD) and hyperactivity.

It is important for the entire health care community (including general and pediatric dentists) to screen and diagnose for mouth breathing in adults and in children as young as 5 years of age. If mouth breathing is treated early, its negative effect on facial and dental development and the medical and social problems associated with it can be reduced or averted."[15]

Although these wide-ranging potential adverse impacts of mouth breathing were first reported over a century ago and have since been widely reported in the scientific literature,[16-18] mouth breathing in children sadly remains a prevalent but often overlooked issue within the medical and dental fields.

"I had been a lifelong mouth breather, as a child my bottom jaw always hung slightly open so that I could breathe. I suffered from dairy/casein intolerance, my nose was constantly blocked or running, my mouth was constantly dry.

I woke up each morning feeling tired although I slept for at least 10 hours. I had my tonsils and adenoids removed as a child. I stopped getting tonsillitis but it didn't change my breathing.

As an adult I consulted a renowned ENT . . . ; he corrected my deviated septum, and removed polyps from my nose but advised it was not possible for me to become a full time nose breather due to my small, narrow nasal passages. The septoplasty helped slightly, but I still could not breath through my nose freely. I was left with the understanding that my anatomy did not support nose breathing.

I heard Patrick [McKeown] being interviewed by John Douillard in 2020; this prompted me to book the one-on-one session with Ciaran [McKeown] that changed my life.

Additionally, I was diagnosed with ADHD and autism last year (at 42 years of age). I wonder if my breathing contributed to this."

Amy, 43, Australia

CONSEQUENCES OF POOR SLEEP FOR CHILDREN AND TEENS

Now that we are equipped with a better understanding of the relationship between breathing and sleep, let's explore the impact of poor sleep on children and teens.

When adults don't sleep well, we usually feel it in the form of fatigue, low energy, or trouble focusing. But kids often show it in completely different ways: irritability, hyperactivity, and poor school performance. It's not always obvious that sleep is the root cause, but more often than not, it's playing a major role behind the scenes.

And it's not just about how they act during the day. Because children and teens are still growing: physically, mentally, and emotionally, poor sleep can have a deeper, longer lasting impact. It's also worth pointing out that when a child doesn't sleep well, parents don't either. Especially in the early years, poor sleep tends to affect the whole household.

Overall, inadequate sleep can be linked to an array of negative effects on children and teens, impacting their physical and mental health, growth, immunity, physical and academic performance, and social functioning.

Physical Health and Growth

- **Growth impairment.** During deep sleep, the body releases growth hormone, which stimulates the growth of bones, muscles, and other tissues and is essential for physical development. Insufficient deep sleep may limit growth hormone production, potentially impacting the growth and development of children and teens.[19]
- **Increased risk of obesity.** Poor sleep can disrupt hormones such as leptin and ghrelin that regulate hunger and satiety (feeling full after eating), leading to increased appetite and a higher risk of unhealthy weight gain.[20]
- **Higher risk of type 2 diabetes.** Sleep deprivation can alter how the body processes glucose, increasing insulin resistance and raising the risk of developing type 2 diabetes over time.
- **Reduced physical performance and coordination.** Tired bodies don't move as well. Poor sleep affects balance, strength, and how fast muscles recover. It can make kids more accident prone during sports or even just playing outside.
- **Headaches and migraines.** Sleep deficiency is a known trigger for headaches and migraines, and children and teens who don't get enough sleep may experience these more frequently. Both lack of sleep and too much sleep (such as sleeping in on the weekend) are triggers for migraine.[21]
- **Weakened immune system.** Poor sleep can compromise the immune system, making children and teens more susceptible to colds and infections.
- **Poor skin health.** Sleep helps repair skin cells and reduces inflammation. Lack of sleep can lead to dull skin, dark circles, and a slower healing process for cuts and acne.[22]

Mental Health and Well-Being for Adolescents

A large body of research has found that adolescents with sleep issues have worse outcomes for physical, mental, social, and academic performance than their peers who obtain appropriate sleep.[23] Early school start times may compound these issues by disrupting adolescents' natural circadian rhythms, leading to shorter sleep durations and poorer mental and physical health outcomes. Adolescents with inadequate sleep face heightened risks of mood disorders, such as anxiety and depression, with sleep disturbances often exacerbating these conditions. Additionally, adolescents who struggle with sleep may engage in riskier behaviors, including substance use, to cope with increased stress or poor sleep quality.[24]

The cumulative effects of poor sleep can impact a teenager's energy levels, resilience, and physical and mental health over time, highlighting how important it is to recognize and address sleep issues.

Cognitive and Behavioral Impacts

Many research studies have investigated the impact of sleep-disordered breathing on children's cognitive and academic performance. Studies report that even mild forms of sleep-disordered breathing, such as habitual snoring, can significantly impair various cognitive and academic functions.[25,26] Children with sleep-disordered breathing exhibit notable deficits in areas such as attention, memory, and executive functions (a set of cognitive processes that enable us to plan, focus attention, remember instructions, and manage multiple tasks effectively).

Attention-Deficit Hyperactivity Disorder and Special Educational Needs

Research has identified a link between sleep-disordered breathing and neurodevelopmental disorders. ADHD is estimated to affect around 5–10% of children worldwide and is more likely to be diagnosed in boys than girls. In the United States, the ratio of boys to girls with ADHD is 3:1.[27] Symptoms include inattention (not being able to keep focus), hyperactivity (excess movement that is not fitting to the setting), and impulsivity (hasty acts that occur in the moment without thought).

Children with ADHD are significantly more likely to experience sleep problems including difficulty falling asleep, frequent nighttime awakenings, restless sleep, and even sleep-disordered breathing. In some cases, these issues stem from core features of ADHD itself, such as racing thoughts, impulsivity, or an inability to unwind at the end of the day. Even the medications commonly used to treat ADHD can sometimes interfere with sleep if not properly timed.

At the same time, poor sleep quality can worsen the very symptoms associated with ADHD like difficulty concentrating, emotional reactivity, hyperactivity, and forgetfulness. This creates a cycle that is often hard to break: the child sleeps poorly, which worsens their daytime behavior, which then makes it harder to settle the next night.

This raises a critical question: Is it the ADHD that causes the sleep problems, or are sleep problems contributing to ADHD like symptoms? It's a classic "chicken or egg" scenario, and in many cases, it's likely both. For some children, underlying sleep disturbances such as snoring, mouth breathing, or sleep apnea may be the primary issue, and when those are addressed, symptoms that resemble ADHD can improve dramatically. For others, the ADHD is genuine and sleep difficulties are part of the broader picture.

Understanding this two-way relationship is important because it highlights that improving sleep can be just as crucial to a child's well-being as managing attention or behavior directly.

Studies show that 19% of children who snore also exhibit ADHD symptoms.[28] A large-scale study conducted within the Shandong Adolescent Behavior and Health Cohort revealed that frequent snoring, insomnia, and restless legs syndrome were significant predictors of subsequent ADHD symptoms in adolescents.[29] Similarly, children who snored or had OSA symptoms were found to have a twofold increase in the odds of being diagnosed with ADHD or exhibiting ADHD symptoms.[30]

A study published in the journal *Pediatrics* looked at over 11,000 British children between the ages of 6 months and 57 months and found a striking connection between breathing and brain development. Children who showed signs of sleep-disordered breathing (including mouth breathing, snoring, or pauses in breathing during sleep) by the age of 5 had a 40% higher risk of having special educational needs by the age of 8 if the issue went untreated.[31] The special educational needs categories included in the study were speech, language, and communication needs; specific learning difficulties; and behavioral, emotional, and social difficulties. In many cases, these challenges are labeled as ADHD or "behavioral problems" but what if the root cause is simply how the child is breathing at night? This study suggests that when sleep-disordered breathing is left unaddressed in early childhood, it can play a direct role in later attention, learning, and emotional difficulties.

What Does This Mean?

What's particularly notable from the findings of these research studies is that the impairments in cognitive functions appear across the spectrum of sleep-disordered breathing severities, ranging from snoring through to OSA. In other words, it doesn't take full-blown sleep apnea for a child's thinking, focus, or school performance to be affected. A child with sleep-disordered breathing, even if it's just regular snoring, might already be struggling to keep up with classmates, concentrate in class, or manage their emotions.

And this isn't just theory for me. I've lived it. As a teenager in high school, I struggled academically. I had all the classic signs: constant nasal congestion, mouth breathing and snoring. But no one ever asked about my sleep. I remember sitting in class, wondering why I couldn't hold my focus, why it felt like everyone else could absorb information so easily while I was stuck. I began to question if I just wasn't as intelligent. Looking back, it's clear that my breathing habits were interfering with my sleep and, as a result, my ability to learn.

And I know I'm not alone. It's likely that many children in school today are struggling academically, and society too often tells them they're not intelligent.

These children may be bright, even exceptionally bright, but because of undiagnosed sleep-disordered breathing, they're unable to reach their full potential.

And that's a shame. These kids are not just statistics. They're tired. They're trying. And they deserve better.

In the next chapter, we will dive into some of the most common sleep disorders and introduce exercises designed to improve your child's breathing both during the day and while they sleep. These practical strategies aim to reduce snoring, encourage deeper, more restorative sleep, and promote better overall health and well-being.

CHAPTER 12

UNDERSTANDING AND MANAGING SLEEP DISORDERS IN CHILDREN AND ADOLESCENTS

Sleep disorders in children and adolescents are more than just restless nights—they can profoundly affect a young person's growth and development. In infancy and early childhood, difficulties settling at bedtime and frequent awakenings can strain both the child and the family. As children grow, these issues evolve, with poor sleep hygiene and disrupted circadian rhythms becoming more common in adolescence. Left unaddressed, sleep problems can cause health issues, fuel anxiety and depression, and even lead to risky behaviors like drug taking.[1] The consequences of chronic sleep disruption are far-reaching, impairing attention, learning, and memory while creating a ripple effect of emotional challenges.[2]

COMMON SLEEP DISORDERS

In the next section, we'll delve into two primary categories of pediatric sleep disorders: *insomnia disorders* and *sleep-disordered breathing* (including snoring, upper airway resistance syndrome, and obstructive sleep apnea).

Insomnia Disorders

Occasional insomnia, which may involve difficulty falling asleep or staying asleep from time to time, is common and often linked to temporary factors such as stress, changes in routine, or environmental disturbances. While occasional insomnia can be disruptive, it generally resolves once the triggering factors are addressed.

A diagnosis of chronic insomnia requires assessment by a physician and a comprehensive approach.

Chronic insomnia in children is defined as:

> "Repeated difficulty with sleep initiation, duration, consolidation, or quality that occurs despite age-appropriate time and opportunity for sleep, which results in daytime functional impairment for the child and/or family."[3]

How Common Is Insomnia?
Insomnia is relatively common among children and adolescents. Here are some statistics: [4-7]

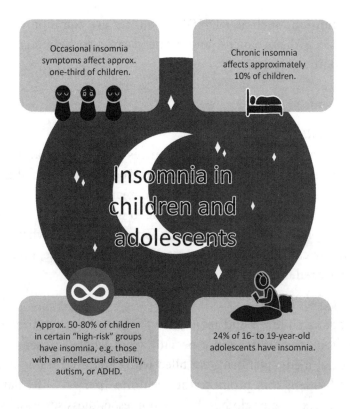

What Are the Risks/Contributory Factors for Insomnia in Children and Teens?

Several factors contribute to insomnia in children and teens, including biological, psychological, and social influences, and these can be age-specific.

School-Age Children

- For school-age children, sleep difficulties may stem from medical conditions like enlarged adenoids, which can lead to OSA, as well as non-allergic rhinitis and bedwetting.
- Too much screen time before bed, along with irregular sleep schedules, can disrupt the body's natural sleep wake rhythm and make it harder for children to fall asleep.

- Conditions such as ADHD and autism are commonly linked to sleep disturbances, and anxiety can also be a significant underlying factor.

Adolescents

Circadian Rhythm Changes

- During adolescence, natural changes in the circadian rhythm delay sleep onset, making it challenging for teens to fall asleep early, even when school schedules demand early wake times.
- This biological shift can contribute to what's known as "delayed sleep phase disorder," which is a form of insomnia where teens simply can't fall asleep at a socially acceptable time, no matter how tired they feel.

Psychological Factors

- Today's children and teens face pressure from all directions: school, social life, and especially from what they see online. Social media platforms are filled with carefully curated images and videos that promote the idea of a "perfect" life: flawless bodies, designer clothes, luxury homes, endless success. When children and teens see this over and over again, it begins to shape their expectations, not just of others, but of themselves. It subtly sends the message that unless they look or live a certain way, they are not good enough. This pressure can affect self-esteem, increase anxiety, and disturb sleep especially in girls, who are often more vulnerable to social comparison during adolescence. In fact, adolescent girls tend to report more insomnia symptoms than boys, which may be linked to a combination of hormonal changes, increased anxiety, and the emotional impact of unrealistic standards perpetuated on social media.[8] As a parent, this is not always an easy topic to bring up, but it's an important one. Helping your child or teen understand that what they're seeing is often staged, filtered, edited, and designed to get likes or attention can help take the pressure off. Remind them that their worth is not based on appearance or social media validation. Sometimes, simply opening that door to talk about it can take a bit of the pressure off and help them sleep a little easier.

- Growing evidence supports hyperarousal as the main causative factor in insomnia disorder in adolescents. Research suggests that abnormally elevated levels of cognitive activity (worry, rumination, intrusive thoughts) and abnormally elevated levels of physiological activity (e.g., inflammation, sympathetic nervous system activity) prevent individuals from falling asleep and having a restorative night's sleep.[9] For practical advice on how to support children who tend to overthink or get stuck in their heads (see Chapter 8 under the section "Helping Children and Teenagers Quiet the Mind").

WHAT IS HYPERAROUSAL?

The term "hyperarousal" refers to a state of heightened physiological and psychological alertness, where the body's stress response is activated even in the absence of immediate danger.

It is often characterized by an overactive sympathetic nervous system, which is responsible for the "fight, flight or freeze" response.

In hyperarousal, the body remains in a state of increased vigilance, with elevated levels of stress hormones like norepinephrine and cortisol, even during periods when relaxation or rest should occur, such as sleep.

Environmental Factors and Lifestyle Choices
- Excessive exposure to phones or other blue-light-emitting devices interferes with melatonin production, a hormone crucial for sleep, making it harder to fall asleep.

- High caffeine intake, for example, from energy drinks, similarly negatively affects sleep, by reducing sleep drive (the biological process that tells us when it's time to sleep).
- Early school start times are another significant factor. Studies show that adolescents with earlier school start times tend to get less sleep, which contributes to chronic sleep deprivation and associated mental and physical health issues.

Impacts of Insomnia

If left untreated, pediatric insomnia may be linked to a constellation of negative impacts in the affected child, including an increased risk of:[10]

- Health-related problems (e.g., obesity/overweight, pain, fatigue)
- Psychological issues (e.g., anxiety, depression)
- Interpersonal problems (e.g., poor family relationships, peer problems)
- Impaired daytime functioning (e.g., poor alertness, impaired school performance)
- Elevated levels of family stress
- Impaired parental mental health and quality of life

Please see Chapter 4 for a summary of the consequences of poor sleep. I'd like to focus here on several of these, relating to insomnia in children and teenagers:

Growth

- Sleep is essential for physical growth, particularly in children and adolescents who are undergoing rapid development. Growth hormone, which is critical for bone and muscle development, is released during deep sleep. Chronic insomnia, therefore, can deprive the child of sufficient deep sleep and lead to disruptions in physical development by reducing the production of growth hormone.[11] What this means is that the child may not grow in line with their age, potentially falling behind in height, muscle development, or overall physical maturity.

Cognitive Function and Decision-Making

- Cognitively, sleep (in particular deep sleep), is vital for memory consolidation, learning, and attention.[12] It follows that when children and adolescents experience insomnia, they may struggle to retain information, concentrate in class, or complete assignments effectively.

- Insufficient sleep in adolescents can lead to cognitive impairments, affecting critical thinking, decision-making, and problem-solving abilities, as well as increasing the risk of accidents due to drowsy driving and engaging in risky behaviors like taking drugs or fighting.[13] A large scale study conducted by Brigham and Women's Hospital in Boston examined data from over 67,000 high school students across the United States. The findings were concerning: students who slept fewer than six hours per night were much more likely to report behaviors such as using alcohol, tobacco, marijuana, or other drugs, as well as driving after drinking alcohol. According to sleep experts, adolescents need 8 to 10 hours of sleep each night for optimal health and development. Yet, more than 70% of high school students consistently fall short of this. Poor sleep doesn't just lead to daytime fatigue, it interferes with emotional regulation, increases impulsivity, and impairs the brain's ability to make sound decisions. These effects are especially problematic during adolescence, when the brain's prefrontal cortex, the part responsible for reasoning and self-control is still developing.[14]

As Dr. Elizabeth Klerman, senior author of the study, explains: "Insufficient sleep in youth raises multiple public health concerns, including mental health, substance abuse, and motor vehicle crashes." In other words, sleep loss in teens isn't just a personal issue; it has ripple effects that touch families, schools, and entire communities.

Mental Health and Behavioral Consequences

- Insomnia is strongly associated with mental health issues, including anxiety, depression, and behavioral problems in adolescents.[15] Persistent sleep disruptions can exacerbate symptoms of these conditions, creating a negative cycle where anxiety or depression worsens sleep, and poor sleep intensifies these mental health issues.

- Behavioral problems, such as impulsivity and aggression, heightened emotional reactivity, irritability, and a reduced ability to cope with stress are also more prevalent among sleep-deprived youth, which can strain relationships with peers, family, and teachers.[16,17]

Addressing Insomnia

Treatment for insomnia in younger children and adolescents includes lifestyle changes, such as establishing consistent sleep routines, limiting screen time before bed, and encouraging relaxation techniques. To revisit recommendations for sleep hygiene, please see Chapter 6.

Ensuring a dark bedroom is important, and blackout blinds may be a worthwhile investment to help achieve this. One large study carried out in China looked at the sleep habits of more than 200,000 children and teenagers living in fourteen cities. The researchers wanted to find out if artificial light from streetlamps and buildings, known as "outdoor light at night" was affecting children's sleep. Using satellite data, they measured how much nighttime light was shining into each child's neighborhood and then compared that to reports from parents about their children's sleep. What they found was quite striking: the more light exposure children had at night, the more likely they were to experience sleep disturbances. The results were strongest in younger children under the age of 12, who seemed particularly sensitive to nighttime lighting. This suggests that even something as simple as light coming in through a bedroom window can disrupt a child's ability to get deep, restful sleep. The researchers concluded that reducing light exposure at night, for example, by using blackout curtains could help improve sleep for children and teenagers.

Cognitive Behavioral Therapy for Insomnia (CBT-I) has proved effective in treating insomnia and may help young people develop healthier sleep habits. In adolescents, a combination of CBT-I and pharmacotherapy may be used.[18] Addressing insomnia early on is essential, as it can have substantial consequences across physical, cognitive, and emotional domains if not managed effectively.

Buteyko Method for Insomnia

Beyond medications, there's a simple and natural way to help children and teens who struggle with insomnia: a combination of CBT-I and better breathing. Sleep problems often stem from an overactive sympathetic nervous system, which keeps the body on high alert when it should be winding down. By addressing both unhelpful thought patterns and dysfunctional breathing habits, it is possible to calm the nervous system, making it easier to fall and stay asleep. While the focus of this book is on breathing, it's worth considering support from a psychologist or psychotherapist trained in CBT-I, as both approaches can complement each other and offer long-term tools for better sleep.

Insomnia in children and teens usually shows up in two ways. Some have trouble falling asleep at night. Others fall asleep fine but wake up in the middle of the night and find it hard to settle again. By improving breathing patterns, especially encouraging nasal breathing and practicing light, slow, and deep breathing, the body can shift into a relaxed state, paving the way for deep, restful sleep: no pills, no side effects; just gentler, more peaceful sleep.

For children and teenagers having trouble falling asleep, it's often because the mind is running on overdrive—whether from a stressful day, school pressures, anxiety, or even too much screen time before bed. But here's something most people don't realize: how you breathe plays a huge role in signaling to your brain that it's safe to sleep.

When a child's breathing is too fast or too hard, the brain can get the message that something is wrong, as if they need to stay on high alert. This keeps the body stuck in "fight, flight, or freeze" mode, making it harder to fully relax. And because sleep is a vulnerable state, the brain won't fully let go if it thinks it needs to stay watchful. The key to helping your child fall asleep more easily? Gentle, light, and slow breathing. This signals safety to the brain, allowing the body to shift into "rest mode" and settle into deep, peaceful sleep.

Helping Your Child Breathe for Better Sleep

Here are a few simple ways to support your child's breathing and help improve their sleep:

- **Encourage nasal breathing throughout the day.** Help your child get into the habit of breathing through their nose during rest, play, and gentle exercise. Nasal breathing helps create a calm, steady rhythm that naturally carries over into sleep.

  The main measurement of breathing in children and teenagers is the Steps Score. This is described in Chapter 1. It gives you a simple and practical way to track how well your child is breathing. For more information on supporting nasal breathing during sleep in children and teenagers, please see Chapter 1 under the section "Buteyko Exercises for Children and Adolescents."

  As your child's Steps Score improves, their breathing becomes more stable and efficient. Every 10-pace increase reflects progress in their breathing pattern. Reaching a Steps Score of 50 paces or more indicates reduced turbulence in the nasal passages and throat, making it easier for your child to breathe calmly at night. This often leads to deeper, more restful sleep with fewer nighttime awakenings.

- **Support nose breathing during sleep.** Breathing through the nose at night promotes lighter, slower breathing driven by the diaphragm. This can reduce snoring, improve sleep quality, and help your child wake up feeling more refreshed. If your child often wakes with a dry mouth, you might consider using MyoTape, a gentle support that encourages nose breathing without covering the mouth.

Important: Before using any nasal breathing support during sleep, it's essential to make sure your child can breathe comfortably through their nose.

- Practice *Breathe Light.* Children and teenagers who have trouble sleeping may find it helpful to listen to the guided audio for insomnia, which includes the *Breathe Light Exercise.* You can access it by scanning the QR code to download it to your phone.

Waking in the middle of the night can be just as disruptive and sometimes even more frustrating than having trouble falling asleep in the first place. Just like adults, children and teenagers can experience an overactive mind during the night, full of thoughts and mental noise. (For more on helping children quieten the "noise" in the mind, see Chapter 8.)

Even when they practice slow, steady breathing to shift attention from thoughts to the breath and to signal to the brain that the body is safe, restlessness can still linger, especially in the early hours. This is where the guided audio for insomnia can be a useful support. It gently helps redirect focus away from overthinking or the pressure to fall back asleep. As your child listens to the audio, their mind begins to settle and sleep often returns more easily.

By supporting your child to use these simple breathing practices, you're helping them build a strong foundation for deep, restful sleep. As their breathing pattern improves, you should notice fewer wake-ups during the night, better overall sleep quality, and a child who wakes up feeling more refreshed and ready for the day.

"My daughter is a very light sleeper; she wakes up easily, snores, and wakes up tired and in a bad mood. When she uses the mouth tape, she stops snoring and sleeps much better."

Sleep-Disordered Breathing

The term "sleep-disordered breathing" refers to a group of conditions that disrupt normal breathing during sleep, often leading to fragmented rest and poor oxygenation. These disorders, including snoring, upper airway resistance syndrome (UARS), and obstructive sleep apnea (OSA), can greatly impact a child's physical, emotional, and cognitive health.

Sleep-disordered breathing ranges from mild (audible breathing), to moderate (snoring), to severe (hypopnea) and very severe (apnea), as you can see in Table 12.1.

Table 12.1 *A Scale of Breathing Resistance*

No Resistance	Mild Resistance	Moderate Resistance	Severe Resistance	Very Severe Resistance
Breathing is silent and effortless, occurring in and out through the nose, driven by the diaphragm with minimal effort.	Audible breathing without snoring. Airflow remains nasal or oral, still primarily diaphragm-driven but with slight turbulence.	Turbulent airflow in the airway, leading to mild snoring as resistance increases. UARS where breathing effort is increased, sleep is disrupted by frequent arousals, but full airway collapse does not occur.	More pronounced snoring or hypopnea, where airflow is reduced by at least 30% due to partial airway collapse, lasting 2 breaths or more, and associated with oxygen desaturation or sleep frag-mentation.	Complete airway collapse, leading to apneas, where breathing stops for 2 breaths or more. Snoring is interspersed with breath stops, indicating repeated airway obstruction.

In terms of diagnosis, a key distinction between childhood and adult sleep disorders is that children with nocturnal breathing issues often do not have excessive daytime sleepiness. Rather, they may have nonspecific behavioral difficulties such as abnormal shyness, hyperactivity, developmental delay, or aggressive behavior, along with other symptoms such as poor appetite, speech issues, or difficulty swallowing.[19] Although sleep-disordered breathing is now recognized more than before, it remains a highly under diagnosed condition.

What follows is a guide to the different levels of resistance to breathing during sleep in children and teenagers, along with the sleep conditions commonly associated with each. Resistance, in this context, means anything that makes it harder for air to move in and out of the lungs during sleep. This could be caused by a blocked nose, a narrow airway, or poor breathing habits that require extra effort to breathe.

Resistance

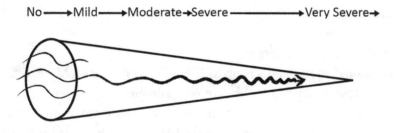

No ⟶ Mild ⟶ Moderate ⟶ Severe ⟶ Very Severe ⟶

Breathing

Silent ⟶ Audible ⟶ Snoring ⟶ Hypopnea ⟶ Apnea ⟶

Sleep apnea in children is often caused by physical and respiratory factors such as enlarged tonsils and adenoids, chronic nasal congestion, asthma, inflammation of the airways, narrow jaws, and habitual mouth breathing. These issues can restrict airflow during sleep and disrupt healthy breathing patterns.

For a closer look at what causes sleep-disordered breathing in children and teenagers, and how it can affect them, you'll find a full explanation in Chapter 11.

Now, let's delve into snoring, UARS, and OSA in more detail.

Snoring

Although often dismissed as harmless in children, snoring can be a key indicator of compromised airway health and poor-quality sleep. In children, breathing during sleep should generally be *silent*. When a child snores, it signals resistance in the airway that disrupts their natural breathing patterns and can lead to fragmented sleep.

Snoring is the sound that occurs when tissues in the throat, such as the pharyngeal walls, soft palate, tonsillar pillars, uvula, and tongue, vibrate as a child or teenager breathes during sleep. This vibration is usually caused by relaxed airway muscles, mouth breathing and a narrowing of the airway, which leads to turbulent airflow.

How Common Is Snoring?

Occasional snoring affects up to 25% of school-aged children, often due to temporary factors like colds or allergies.[20] However, habitual snoring—defined as snoring that occurs at least three nights per week—is reported in approximately 10% of preschool and primary school aged children.[21]

The impact of habitual snoring on children can be profound. Disrupted sleep interferes with cognitive development, potentially leading to difficulties with attention, memory, and academic performance. Some children may exhibit hyperactivity, fatigue, or behavioral issues that can resemble ADHD.

Habitual snoring in children has also been associated with a reduction in parasympathetic tone, indicating potential autonomic nervous system imbalance during sleep.[22] This means that children who habitually snore may have a dysregulated autonomic nervous system during sleep, meaning their parasympathetic nervous system, which promotes "rest, digest, and repair," is not functioning optimally, leading to less effective relaxation and recovery.

Upper Airway Resistance Syndrome in Children and Adolescents

UARS is a subtle form of sleep-disordered breathing first recognized in children by Dr. Guilleminault and colleagues in 1982. Guilleminault was a leading figure in research on breathing-related sleep disorders.

Unlike obstructive sleep apnea, which involves full or partial airway blockages, UARS is characterized by increased effort to breathe due to a narrowed airway. This resistance may not cause complete pauses in breathing but still disrupts sleep, causing frequent arousals and fragmentation, and places a strain on the body.[23]

Because UARS presents with more subtle symptoms, diagnosis is challenging and UARS often goes unnoticed—but it can still have a profound impact on health and development. Children and teens with UARS may appear restless during sleep, tossing and turning frequently. While they might not exhibit loud snoring or the classic signs of apnea, subtle symptoms like mouth breathing, teeth grinding, frequent waking, and daytime sleepiness or fatigue are common. When clinical symptoms indicate abnormal breathing during sleep but obstructive sleep apneas are not detected, physicians may mistakenly conclude that no sleep-related breathing disorder is present.[24]

How Common Is UARS?
UARS often flies under the radar because it lacks the classic pauses in breathing (apneas) or significantly reduced airflow (hypopneas) that doctors look for when diagnosing OSA. While the exact number of children and teens affected by UARS isn't well documented, research shows that the conditions that can increase the risk of developing sleep-disordered breathing apply to UARS.

For example, enlarged tonsils and adenoids (a condition called "adenotonsillar hypertrophy") are common causes of airway blockage in children, making it harder for them to breathe during sleep, sometimes leading to UARS or even full-blown OSA. Allergies (allergic rhinitis) can also be a culprit. When nasal passages get inflamed and swollen, airflow is restricted, which can disturb sleep and contribute to UARS.

Obesity is another major risk factor, as excess weight can put extra pressure on the airway, making breathing more difficult during sleep. Additionally, certain facial structures, like a small or recessed jaw, can create a narrower airway, increasing the likelihood of sleep breathing problems like UARS.

Addressing UARS

The first step in helping a child with UARS is to look closely at how they breathe each day. The way a child breathes has a direct effect on how easily air moves through their nose, throat, and lungs especially during sleep.

Simple habits like keeping the lips closed, breathing quietly through the nose, and helping the tongue rest in the correct position can make a big difference. Practicing the *Nose Unblocking Exercise* regularly can help ease nasal stuffiness, making nose breathing feel more natural and comfortable.

One of the most helpful practices is increasing your child's Steps Score, a simple breath-hold exercise sometimes known as *Dolphin Breathing*. When a child can comfortably reach a Steps Score of 50 paces or more, it leads to significantly reduced nasal congestion and a much better ability to maintain nose breathing throughout the day and night. (Please see Chapter 1 for a full description of these exercises.)

For some children, structural issues like enlarged tonsils or adenoids can make it harder to breathe freely during sleep. In cases like these, surgery, often an adenotonsillectomy may be recommended to help clear the airway and improve breathing. But surgery isn't always the only option.

The shape and development of a child's jaw and palate play a big role in how well they breathe. For example, a narrow upper jaw or high palate can limit space for the tongue and reduce airflow through the nose. In these cases, certain orthodontic treatments, like palatal expansion, can help widen the upper jaw and support better nasal breathing. You might hear this referred to as airway orthodontics, and it's a bit different from the traditional idea of simply straightening teeth.

What sets airway orthodontics apart is the bigger picture. The goal isn't just to align the teeth. It is also to develop the jaw in a way that supports proper tongue posture and healthy breathing.

Functional dentists or orthodontists who focus on airway development often work closely with practitioners trained in the Buteyko Method, and also incorporate myofunctional therapy which helps children improve their tongue posture, breathing habits, and swallowing patterns.

And that's important, because if a child continues to mouth breathe or has a poor swallowing pattern, the long-term results of their orthodontic work might not last. A lot of time, energy, and money can go into expanding the jaws and straightening the teeth, but if the underlying habits that contributed to small jaws or crowded teeth aren't addressed, the improvements may not hold.

Another thing worth mentioning is that dentists who understand airway development usually try to avoid removing teeth unless it's absolutely necessary. Their thinking is that if a child's teeth are overcrowded, it's often not because the teeth are too big, but because their jaw is too small. So rather than extracting teeth, the focus is on helping the jaw develop to the size it needs to be. That way, there's room for all the teeth and, just as importantly, the airway remains open and healthy.

This approach is quite different from some traditional orthodontists, where removing teeth is often part of the treatment plan. The concern with routinely taking out teeth is that it can reduce the overall size of the jaws. When the jaws become smaller, the airway can also become narrower and this may increase the risk of breathing problems like UARS, not just during childhood, but also later in life. So, when considering orthodontic treatment, it's worth looking beyond just how the teeth line up and thinking about how your child's jaw, tongue posture, and breathing patterns all work together. A healthy airway supports healthy sleep and it starts with how your child breathes, both day and night.

Addressing UARS early is key, not just for better sleep, but for your child's long-term health and well-being. The earlier it's recognized and treated, the better the outcomes, especially as growing children are more responsive to positive changes in breathing and airway development.

There's no single "gold standard" treatment for all children with UARS. For some, it may involve surgical intervention, such as removing enlarged tonsils or adenoids. In other cases, treatment might include orthodontic support to improve jaw development, or in rare situations, CPAP therapy may be considered.

For many children, a combination of the Buteyko Method, myofunctional therapy, and the simple, practical recommendations at the end of this chapter can play a powerful role in supporting recovery. Practicing nasal breathing during the day, building better breathing habits, and gently improving tongue posture can help your child maintain nasal breathing through the night and keep their airway more open during sleep.

Even if medical treatment is needed, breathing re-education can help reduce symptoms, improve sleep quality, and support your child's overall progress both now and in the years ahead.

Obstructive Sleep Apnea

Sleep apnea in children is a serious condition where the airway becomes partially or completely blocked during sleep, causing repeated pauses in breathing. First described in 1976 by Guilleminault et al.,[25] pediatric OSA falls on the severe end of the sleep-disordered breathing spectrum.

The interruptions in breathing, known as "apneas," can happen dozens of times a night, breaking up a child's sleep and affecting their health, behavior, mood, and development. A parent might notice their child breathing audibly, then suddenly pausing for two or more breaths. As breathing resumes, the child may shift position in the bed, followed by a gasp or a snort as their body tries to "catch up," something parents might hear as a loud breath or shifting in the bed.

At first glance, it might not seem like anything serious. It's easy to assume this is just how your child sleeps, especially if they've always snored a little or moved around a lot in bed. But that doesn't mean it's normal. Even brief pauses can disrupt deep, restorative sleep, and over time, this can have a significant impact on their overall wellbeing.

What Happens During Sleep Apnea?

- **Obstructive apnea.** A complete collapse of the airway, including the throat, causes the child to stop breathing—even though the chest and tummy are still moving as the body tries to breathe. This means airflow is fully blocked for at least two breaths.
- **Hypopnea.** A partial collapse of the airway that results in a decrease in airflow to the lungs of 50% or more, accompanied by either a drop in blood oxygen saturation of at least 3% or an EEG-detected arousal during sleep.
- **Other signs.** Loud snoring, drops in oxygen levels (oxyhemoglobin desaturation), carbon dioxide buildup (hypercapnia), and frequent nighttime awakenings.[26]

Unlike adults, who often experience daytime sleepiness, children with sleep apnea may show signs of behavioral disturbances, from subtle impairments in learning, attention, and behavior to prominent neurobehavioral deficits that may mimic ADHD or learning disabilities.[27]

When it comes to the impact of sleep apnea on a child's sleep quality, research has shown some clear and concerning patterns. In a study by Durdik and colleagues, researchers examined how OSA affects sleep in children aged three to eight years old.[28] They found that children with OSA spent significantly less time in deep, restorative sleep (stage NREM 3) and more time in light sleep (stage NREM 1). They also took longer to fall asleep and had poorer sleep efficiency overall, meaning their sleep was more fragmented and less effective.

In simple terms, even though they may have been in bed for the required number of hours, their bodies weren't getting the full benefits of sleep. Deep sleep is where the body grows, repairs, and resets. It supports growth, learning, memory, and emotional regulation. When that part of sleep is reduced, children may appear tired during the day, find it harder to concentrate, become more irritable, or struggle to manage their emotions.

Dr. Peter Durdik, the lead researcher, pointed out that it's this loss of deep sleep, the part of sleep when the brain and body do their most important recovery work, that may explain why so many children with sleep apnea struggle during the day.

How Common Is Sleep Apnea in Children and Teens?

Sleep apnea affects 1 to 5% of children,[29] though the actual number may be higher due to underdiagnosis. The likelihood of developing OSA changes with age and certain risk factors:

- **Ages three to six.** OSA is most common in younger children, as this is when the tonsils and adenoids reach their largest size, often leading to airway obstruction during sleep.[30]
- **Teenagers.** As kids grow, factors like obesity, changes in facial and jaw structure, and hormonal shifts can increase the risk of OSA.

Despite how common it is, OSA in children and teens is frequently overlooked. Symptoms like snoring, restless sleep, or behavioral challenges can be mistaken for normal childhood sleep issues or even misdiagnosed as ADHD. Other symptoms include nocturnal enuresis (bedwetting), sleep terrors, sleepwalking, confusional arousals (where a person wakes up in a confused or disoriented state), depression, insomnia, and even psychiatric problems.[31]

What Causes Sleep Apnea in Children?

As with other forms of sleep-related breathing disorders, the causes of OSA often trace back to factors that compromise the airway or disrupt the natural mechanics of breathing.

The underlying factors involved in OSA can be divided into:[32]

- **Anatomical factors.** Anatomical factors that effectively narrow the airway can contribute to sleep-disordered breathing in children. These include structural issues such as a small or recessed lower jaw (mandible), excess fat deposits around the throat (pharyngeal fat pads), tongue tie, and enlarged lymphoid tissues in the upper airway, particularly the adenoids and tonsils. These physical features can narrow the airway, making it harder for your child to breathe easily and quietly through the night.

    If a child regularly breathes through their mouth while growing, it can shape the way their face and jaws develop and not in a good way. Over time, this can narrow the airway and make breathing during sleep more difficult.[33]

- **Non-anatomical factors.** Factors such as inflammation in the upper airway (e.g., due to asthma) and neurological disruptions that affect the muscles responsible for keeping the airway open also narrow the airway passage and compromise breathing stability during sleep, increasing the likelihood of airway obstruction.

Looking at these factors, it's clear that the causes of sleep apnea in children are varied. Just like in adults, it's important to recognize the individual contributing factors rather than relying on a single treatment approach.

The History and Role of Adenotonsillectomy in Pediatric Sleep Apnea

Since enlarged adenoids and tonsils are the most common cause of upper airway obstruction, the gold standard treatment for pediatric sleep apnea has traditionally been adenotonsillectomy—surgical removal of the adenoids and tonsils. This procedure dates back to the 1800s, and considering modern anesthetics were not yet available, one can only imagine how painful and traumatic it must have been for children at that time.

Adenotonsillectomy has a long history, and its use increased significantly from the 1970s onward, following Dr. Christian Guilleminault's description of pediatric obstructive sleep apnea.

The adenoids are tissue located at the back of the nose where it meets the throat, while the tonsils are positioned in the throat. If either of these structures becomes enlarged, which often occurs together, it can reduce airway size, making breathing more difficult. As resistance to airflow increases, the airway becomes more prone to collapse, further restricting breathing during sleep.

Rethinking Adenotonsillectomy: The Need for a More Comprehensive Approach

At first glance, removing the adenoids and tonsils seems like the obvious solution. However, as research evolves, it is becoming increasingly clear that this approach may not be as effective as once believed. Studies show that these lymphatic tissues play an important role in immune system function, and their removal may lead to potential health consequences later in life. Furthermore, unless nasal breathing is restored after surgery, the long-term success of the procedure may be limited, reinforcing the importance of addressing both the anatomical and functional aspects of breathing in treatment strategies.

In a 2010 paper by Dr. Bhattacharjee et al. published in the *American Journal of Respiratory and Critical Care Medicine*, the authors state:

"The overall efficacy of adenotonsillectomy (AT) in the treatment of obstructive sleep apnea syndrome (OSAS) in children is unknown."[34]

What makes this particularly striking is that it was written as recently as 2010, despite adenotonsillectomy being performed for nearly 40 years as the standard treatment for pediatric sleep apnea. This raises an important question: Were doctors simply in the dark? Had the procedure been widely accepted without sufficient research into its long-term effectiveness?

The study reports that while adenotonsillectomy can be beneficial, it does not always fully resolve OSA in children. Researchers analyzed 578 children, approximately 50% of whom were obese. The results showed that adenotonsillectomy led to a significant reduction in the apnea-hypopnea index (AHI).

However, only 157 children (27.2%) achieved complete resolution of OSA, defined as an AHI of less than 1 event per hour post-surgery.

While 73% of children still had sleep apnea post-surgery, their condition improved, with AHI dropping from 18 to 4 events per hour. However, 4 events per hour in children is on the borderline of moderate sleep apnea, meaning many still experienced breathing disruptions during sleep.

If enlarged adenoids and tonsils were the sole cause of sleep apnea in children, then their removal should have completely resolved the condition. Yet this was not the case. Other factors such as obesity, asthma, poor craniofacial development, poor muscle tone, and dysfunctional breathing patterns likely contribute to persistent sleep apnea, even after adenotonsillectomy.

This challenges the long-held assumption that removing the adenoids and tonsils alone is a sufficient treatment. Instead, it highlights the need for a more comprehensive assessment to determine the most appropriate interventions, which may include jaw and airway development by airway-focused dentists, myofunctional therapy, Buteyko training to help asthma, oral breathing and dysfunctional breathing, and weight management—all of which are essential for achieving long-term success in treating pediatric sleep apnea.

The Overlooked Role of Adenoids and Tonsils in Long-Term Health

There is a common belief that removing the adenoids and tonsils has little impact on long-term health. However, little is known about the lasting consequences of these procedures beyond perioperative risks. This lack of awareness is significant, as these lymphatic organs play a crucial role in both the development and function of the immune system.

According to the authors of a study analyzing 1.2 million people born in Denmark between 1979 and 1999, this ignorance is particularly concerning.[35] Their research highlights the important immunological functions of the adenoids and tonsils, raising questions about the long-term health implications of their removal.

The study analyzed 17,460 children who had their adenoids removed, 11,830 who had their tonsils removed, and 31,377 who had both their tonsils and adenoids removed.

The researchers found that adenoidectomy and tonsillectomy were associated with a twofold to threefold increase in diseases of the upper respiratory tract, including chronic sinusitis, rhinitis, bronchitis, and pneumonia, and even an increased risk of chronic obstructive pulmonary disease (COPD) later in life. Given that the adenoids and tonsils play a crucial role in immune defense, their removal may compromise the body's ability to filter and respond to airborne pathogens, making individuals more vulnerable to recurring infections and long-term respiratory issues. These are not small side effects. For many children, it could mean a lifetime of dealing with more colds, congestion, and respiratory challenges that could have been reduced or avoided.

Based on their findings, the authors state:

> "This suggests that any immediate benefits of these surgeries may not extend into adulthood."

These findings challenge the long-standing belief that removing the adenoids and tonsils has minimal long-term health consequences. Instead, they highlight the importance of carefully weighing the risks and benefits before proceeding with surgery, particularly given the essential role these tissues play in immune defense during early development.

The Key to Lasting Results: Restoring Nasal Breathing After Surgery

It is worth emphasizing that for any child experiencing sleep problems, the number one priority is to address the child's poor sleep quality. The effects of sleep disturbances in children can be devastating, impacting not only their quality of life but also long-term brain development. Sleep problems in childhood do not simply resolve with age—they can carry into adulthood, affecting cognitive function and emotional regulation.

There are cases where removal of the adenoids and tonsils is necessary for a child to develop properly, both physically and mentally.

But here's where many children fall through the cracks. If adenotonsillectomy is performed, it is essential that the child undergoes nasal breathing training—such as the techniques provided in this book—after surgery. Without this step, the benefits of the procedure may be short-lived, and sleep-disordered breathing can return in as little as three years.

A study following 88 children who underwent adenotonsillectomy examined them at 6 months, 12 months, 24 months, and 36 months post-surgery. Researchers observed that the apnea-hypopnea index was 3.47 events per hour 6 months after surgery but worsened to 6.48 events per hour after 36 months.[36] This data demonstrates a decline in sleep quality within just 3 years, with the primary cited reason being continued mouth breathing post-surgery.

To quote the late Dr. Christian Guilleminault, a pioneer in sleep medicine:

"Treatment of pediatric obstructive sleep apnea (OSA) and sleep-disordered breathing (SDB) means restoration of continuous nasal breathing during wakefulness and sleep."[37]

It is interesting that Dr. Guilleminault didn't just emphasize nasal breathing during sleep. He specifically included the restoration of nasal breathing during the day as well. This distinction is crucial because breathing habits during wakefulness directly influence breathing patterns during sleep. For many parents, the idea of "training your child to breathe through their nose" might sound unusual but this is often the missing step after surgery.

A key part of this retraining process is myofunctional therapy, which focuses on strengthening the tongue and orofacial muscles, improving tongue posture, and promoting correct swallowing patterns. By guiding proper tongue placement on the roof of the mouth and reinforcing nasal breathing, myofunctional therapy plays an essential role in stabilizing the airway, reducing the risk of relapse, and supporting long-term breathing and sleep health.

FROM SLEEP APNEA AND ALLERGIES TO RESTFUL NIGHTS AND A NEW BEST FRIEND: HENRY'S JOURNEY

Henry, a bright and energetic 13-year-old from Northern Ireland, didn't always have the easy, active life he enjoys today. From infancy, he struggled with a range of health issues—digestive problems, allergies, asthma, and severe sleep apnea. The toll of poor sleep affected not only Henry but his entire family.

But through a combination of Buteyko breathing exercises, MyoTape mouth taping, and a tonsillectomy, Henry's life changed dramatically. His mother, determined to find a solution, introduced breathing exercises in a fun and engaging way, helping him retrain his body to breathe through his nose—a small change that made a world of difference.

The Early Struggles: Allergies, Asthma, and Sleep Apnea

Henry's journey began when he was just a baby.

"At three months old, he developed digestive issues and was diagnosed with cow's milk protein allergy. Later, tests showed he was also allergic to dogs and house dust mites. By age two, he was diagnosed with asthma, and on top of it all, he was a baby who simply did not sleep. And if a baby isn't sleeping, no one in the house is sleeping."

As Henry grew, his sleep problems worsened. He snored heavily and woke up frequently throughout the night. Eventually, his doctor diagnosed him with sleep apnea.

The Turning Point: Breath Training and Mouth Taping

With few treatment options available, Henry's mother took matters into her own hands. Having already seen benefits from mouth taping in her own sleep, she decided to try it with Henry.

"I was hesitant at first, but knowing how much it had helped me, I felt confident it would be safe and beneficial for him, too."

She also introduced Buteyko breathing exercises, adapting them into fun activities Henry could enjoy.

"We turned it into a game—like 'Teddy on the Tummy,' where he'd practice gentle nasal breathing while keeping his stuffed animal still on his belly. He loved it, and over time, his sleep improved."

At age four, Henry underwent a tonsillectomy, which helped significantly. But the real magic happened when they combined surgery with consistent breathing exercises and nighttime mouth taping using MyoTape.

The Life-Changing Results

By age five, everything had changed.

"His asthma improved, his sleep transformed, and he was finally getting the deep, restorative rest he had missed for years. Our ENT consultant had told me, 'By the time your child is five, all these problems will probably be gone.' I was skeptical—but they were right!"

Today, Henry is a thriving teenager—healthy, athletic, and excelling in sports and academics. And in a heartwarming twist, his old dog allergy disappeared!

"A few years ago, we tested it out with a trial period, and to our amazement, he had no reaction! Now, we have a family dog, and he's Henry's best friend."

Henry's mother credits breathing re-education, MyoTape, and the power of nasal breathing for their life-changing results.

"I'm so grateful to Patrick McKeown and the Buteyko breathing technique. It transformed my sleep and health and did the same for my son. Having these tools at your disposal can make all the difference. They worked for us—and I know they can work for anyone."

ASSESSING SLEEP PATTERNS IN CHILDREN: WHAT DO PARENTS NEED TO LOOK FOR?

So, how might you know if a child has sleep-disordered breathing?

Common symptoms during *sleep*:[38,39]

- Snoring (often loud and habitual)
- Periodic gasping, choking, or pauses in breathing (apneas)
- Restless sleep with frequent tossing and turning
- Mouth breathing and audible breathing

- Bedwetting or waking up to use the bathroom
- Nightmares or night sweats
- Sleeping in unusual positions to improve airway patency

Common *daytime* symptoms of sleep-disordered breathing include:

- Excessive daytime sleepiness or fatigue (though this is uncommon in young children)
- Difficulty waking up in the morning
- Behavioral issues such as hyperactivity, irritability, or aggression
- Trouble focusing and poor academic performance
- Frequent headaches, particularly in the morning
- Dry mouth or sore throat upon waking

If you suspect a child has a sleep disorder, consult a pediatrician or sleep specialist for diagnosis or referral for further investigation. Your physician may use some of the following diagnostic tools to form a comprehensive picture of the child's sleep health:

- **Parent and child history.** Detailed accounts of sleep habits, bedtime routines, and any symptoms.
- **Medical evaluation.** To rule out any underlying conditions.
- **Sleep diaries.** Parents or caregivers are typically asked to record bedtimes, wake-up times, night awakenings, naps, and any bedtime behaviors or difficulties over one or two weeks. These diaries provide valuable insights into a child's sleep habits and help clinicians identify issues like insomnia, irregular sleep schedules, or behavioral factors affecting sleep.
- **Completion of assessment tools.** The *Children's Sleep Habits Questionnaire* is one of the most commonly used assessment tools for pediatric sleep.[40] It assesses the type and frequency of common sleep issues experienced by children, including bedtime resistance, sleep onset delay, sleep duration, sleep anxiety, night wakings, parasomnias, sleep-disordered breathing, and daytime sleepiness.

- **Referral for a sleep study.** A sleep study is a non-invasive test conducted overnight in a sleep lab to monitor sleep patterns and identify sleep disorders like OSA. The child is connected to sensors that measure brain activity, breathing, heart rate, oxygen levels, and muscle movements. Parents are often allowed to stay with younger children to ease anxiety. The goal is to gather detailed data to guide treatment for sleep-related issues.

Early recognition and treatment of sleep disorders are critical. Australian doctor and researcher Colin Sullivan, who invented the CPAP device to treat obstructive sleep apnea, highlighted the importance of early intervention in children with sleep-disordered breathing:

> "I've spent a lot of my career looking at pediatric sleep apnea, sleep disorder breathing, and I do think that trying to intervene early, identifying kids who have the risk factors, gives us a chance of preventing it."[41]

Promoting Functional Nasal Breathing

Encouraging nasal breathing and addressing early signs of sleep-disordered breathing in children is key to supporting children in reaching their full developmental potential, and improving their sleep quality and overall health for life.

What Does the Research Say?

A randomized controlled trial by Mendonca et al. explored how the Buteyko Method can help children with asthma and mouth breathing.[42] The results were promising, showing that simple breathing exercises can make a big difference in breathing efficiency, asthma control, and overall well-being. The children who practiced the Buteyko Method experienced fewer asthma symptoms and relied less on medication. Many who were habitual mouth breathers learned to breathe through their nose. Breathing through the nose helped improve sleep quality, reduce snoring, and lower airway resistance. This study suggests that retraining how kids breathe—focusing on nasal breathing and reduced over-breathing—can significantly improve respiratory health and overall quality of life.

How Can Pediatric Dentists and Healthcare Providers Help Children Breathe Better?

Pediatric dentists, orthodontists, and other health professionals can play a crucial role in diagnosing and managing sleep-related breathing disorders. The American Dental Association encourages dentists to screen for sleep-related breathing disorders as part of a comprehensive medical and dental history, recognizing symptoms such as daytime sleepiness, choking, snoring, or apneas witnessed by parents/caregivers, identifying anatomical factors like suboptimal craniofacial growth and development, and evaluating risk factors.[43] By identifying these signs early, dentists can help interrupt the progression of childhood sleep-disordered breathing into more complicated OSA in adulthood by breaking the vicious cycle between craniofacial deformation and respiratory function aggravation, thereby improving the quality of life in childhood.[44]

> "Ever since taking Patrick's course for dental professionals in 2019, my sleep quality has improved significantly. I wake up feeling more rested and refreshed and spring out of bed between 5:30am and 6:30am without an alarm. This program has changed my life, my business and my clients who see me for this work."

If a risk for sleep-related breathing disorders is determined, dentists should refer to the appropriate physician for diagnosis and treatment. This is key, as early intervention can significantly improve outcomes for children. Dentists and health professionals can also educate families about the impact of breathing habits on sleep, behavior, and overall development.

CHAPTER 13

CONCLUSION

THE BREATH OF BETTER SLEEP—FOR EVERY AGE

Sleep is one of the most fundamental functions of life; yet for many, it remains a nightly struggle. What often goes unnoticed is the profound connection between how we breathe and how well we sleep. Whether you're the parent of a restless child, a teenager feeling overwhelmed by school and social life, or an adult juggling work, family, and a never-ending to-do list, your breathing influences not just your sleep but your overall well-being.

The goal of this book has been to bring awareness to this connection—how you breathe, whether through your nose or mouth, in your upper chest or diaphragm, fast and hard or slow and light. The Buteyko Method, a physician-developed breathing technique with nearly 70 years of clinical application, has helped millions of people worldwide, from young children with restless sleep to high-performing athletes seeking better recovery. What makes the Buteyko Method unique is its emphasis on nasal breathing at all times—during rest, physical activity, and most importantly, during sleep. But there's more to it than just breathing through the nose. Another key part of the method is learning to breathe light and slow, so you're not taking in more air than your body actually needs. Of all the breathing approaches to support better sleep, the Buteyko Method makes a great deal of sense. Breathing through an open mouth, or breathing too fast and hard, increases resistance in the airways and triggers a stress response in both the body and mind, neither of which support restful, restorative sleep. The Buteyko Method takes the opposite approach: it helps the breath soften, and the nervous system shift into a calmer, more balanced state, the kind of state that naturally supports deeper, more peaceful sleep.

Nasal breathing is no longer a niche idea; it's becoming mainstream. Thanks to research-backed discussions and books like *Breath* by James Nestor, more people are waking up to the reality that how we breathe profoundly shapes our health. For years, I knew that breathing techniques, when applied with scientific understanding, had life-changing potential. I sometimes wondered when this knowledge would be widely embraced. Now, I no longer have doubts. Breathing re-education, including the Buteyko Method for health and the Oxygen Advantage® for mental and physical performance, is here to stay.

A SIMPLE, LIFELONG PRACTICE

Breathing should be simple, and the best part is that these techniques can be applied at any age. Children can develop healthy breathing habits early, preventing common sleep-disordered breathing issues like snoring, mouth breathing, and even behavioral challenges linked to poor sleep. Teenagers, often facing increased stress and screen time, can benefit from conscious breathing to improve focus, energy, and sleep quality. And for adults, whether struggling with fatigue or insomnia or simply looking for better recovery, small changes in breathing can create a profound impact.

It doesn't take hours of practice or drastic lifestyle changes—just small, mindful shifts in how you breathe. A simple way to start is by wearing MyoTape at night to ensure nasal breathing, promoting correct tongue posture and reducing sleep disruptions. It's a practical solution that can support children, teenagers, and adults alike.

And during the day? Look for the little windows. Instead of mindlessly scrolling through your phone, take a moment to check in with your breath. When walking, try breathing through your nose and keeping it light and slow. These little moments add up, reinforcing good breathing habits without requiring extra effort. Poor sleep already costs you time—in the form of fatigue, brain fog, and low energy. But when you take even a small step to improve your breathing, you start gaining that time back in clearer thinking, better focus, and deeper rest.

A BREATH-BASED REVOLUTION

We can no longer ignore the far-reaching benefits of breathing retraining—for sleep, for respiratory health, for mental well-being. The science is clear, and the solution is accessible to everyone. Children, teenagers, and adults alike can all benefit from something as simple as breathing the way we were designed to—through the nose, lightly, slowly, and deeply.

That's it. Just start. Try something small from this book and notice the difference. If we all do this, awareness will continue to grow, and more people will have access to a science-based, practical approach to breathing that improves health at every stage of life.

I encourage you to put these techniques into practice. Any attention you give to your breath will reward you. It might even change your life.

Breathe well. Sleep well.

Patrick McKeown
Galway, Ireland

APPENDICES

APPENDICES

APPENDIX A

RESOURCES FOR BETTER SLEEP AND BREATHING

Free Guided Audio Sessions

A series of guided audios is available to help with falling asleep more easily, getting back to sleep if you wake during the night, or achieving deep rest to support better energy during the day. There are versions created for both children and adults. The audios are written and spoken by Patrick McKeown and Tiger Bye, and have already been used by tens of thousands of people to improve breathing patterns, ease into deep rest, and make falling asleep easier. They're free to use, can be downloaded to your phone, and played in flight mode. Just scan the QR code to access them.

Breathing Tools and Educational Resources

MyoTape: Encouraging Nasal Breathing

Developed by Patrick McKeown, MyoTape promotes nasal breathing during sleep. Unlike traditional mouth tapes, it gently surrounds the mouth, bringing the lips together with light elastic tension without covering them, allowing for comfortable nasal breathing throughout the night. This practice can lead to improved sleep quality, reduced snoring, and enhanced overall health.

To purchase MyoTape, visit ***www.myotape.com***. Use the discount code *Myo10* at checkout to receive a 10% discount on your order.

ButeykoClinic App: Guided Breathing Exercises

The ButeykoClinic app, available on both iTunes and Android platforms, offers a comprehensive suite of resources to improve your breathing patterns. The app features guided audio exercises for adults and instructional videos demonstrating various breathing techniques. Additionally, it includes a dedicated children's section where Patrick McKeown teaches his daughter, Lauren, how to unblock her nose, transition to nasal breathing, and improve her breathing habits. This resource is very helpful for individuals and families aiming to incorporate effective breathing practices into their daily routines.

Buteyko Clinic Sleep Courses and Consultations

For those seeking structured guidance to address sleep-related concerns, ButeykoClinic.com offers specialized sleep courses designed by Patrick McKeown:

- **Recorded sleep workshop.** Access a recorded workshop by Patrick McKeown that guides you through all the exercises detailed in this book. Ideal for learning at your own pace and revisiting the material as needed.
- **Live sleep workshop.** Participate in a live Zoom session where Patrick McKeown personally leads attendees through the exercises and addresses individual questions, offering real-time feedback and personalized instruction.

Additionally, one-to-one consultations in the Buteyko Method are available with Ciaran McKeown, Patrick's brother, who has been teaching the method since the early 2000s. Ciaran is a formally trained mental health counselor and breathwork instructor who specializes in assisting individuals with conditions linked to dysfunctional breathing, such as asthma, anxiety, sleep apnea, and chronic fatigue syndrome.

For more information and to enroll, visit ***https://buteykoclinic.com***.

APPENDIX B

ORGANIZATIONS DEDICATED TO AIRWAY, SLEEP, AND BREATHING

Academy of Orofacial Myofunctional Therapy

The Academy of Orofacial Myofunctional Therapy (AOMT) is a leading postgraduate training academy dedicated to educating allied health professionals in the treatment of orofacial myofunctional disorders. Founded by Joy Moeller, BS, RDH, a dental hygienist and myofunctional therapist with over 39 years of experience, and Marc Richard Moeller, who serves as the Managing Director, the AOMT offers comprehensive courses designed for professionals such as speech-language pathologists, dental providers, occupational therapists, and physical therapists. These programs focus on the evaluation, diagnosis, and treatment of orofacial myofunctional disorders, emphasizing a multidisciplinary approach to patient care.

Samantha Weaver, MS, CCC-SLP, a practicing myofunctional therapist since 2009, is also a director at AOMT. She has been instrumental in developing the academy's curriculum, which incorporates the latest evidence-based research on breathing remediation, sleep disorders, TMJ disorders, posture, fascia release, and frenulum inspection and surgery. AOMT's instructors are located across the United States and internationally, providing accessible training opportunities worldwide. To contact AOMT, you can visit their website at *https://aomtinfo.org/*.

American Sleep and Breathing Academy

The American Sleep and Breathing Academy (ASBA) is dedicated to strengthening the field of sleep health by promoting a multi-disciplinary approach to sleep medicine. Recognizing that effective sleep care requires input from multiple specialties, ASBA fosters collaboration between dentists, physicians, myofunctional therapists, respiratory specialists, and other healthcare professionals. Rather than limiting sleep care to a single profession, ASBA encourages team-based treatment strategies to improve patient outcomes.

ASBA also serves as a hub for professional networking and education, expanding involvement to any healthcare professional or administrator working in sleep health. Through conferences, training programs, and certifications, ASBA helps practitioners stay at the cutting edge of sleep disorder treatments, airway health, and integrative approaches to sleep medicine. By bringing together experts from diverse backgrounds, the academy is advancing a more comprehensive, research-driven approach to diagnosing and managing sleep disorders.

One of the academy's strongest proponents of breathing re-education for sleep disorders was Alan Hickey, a fellow Irishman who lived in the United States. Alan was a passionate advocate for the role of functional breathing in sleep health, recognizing that dysfunctional breathing patterns contribute to a wide range of sleep-related issues, including snoring, sleep apnea, and daytime fatigue. He worked tirelessly to raise awareness about the connection between airway health, breathing patterns, and restorative sleep, encouraging both professionals and individuals to rethink their approach to sleep medicine.

Sadly, Alan passed away in January 2025, but his dedication to breathing science and sleep health continues to inspire those who knew him and those who benefited from his work. His advocacy within ASBA and the broader sleep health community played a significant role in expanding the conversation around the importance of breathing in sleep medicine.

To learn more about ASBA, explore training opportunities, or connect with like-minded professionals, visit *www.asba.net.*

American Academy of Physiological Medicine & Dentistry

The American Academy of Physiological Medicine & Dentistry (AAPMD) is a leading organization dedicated to promoting interdisciplinary collaboration and education for optimal airway growth, development, and function. Established in 2012, AAPMD brings together professionals from various healthcare fields— including dentistry, medicine, myofunctional therapy, breathing re-education, physical therapy, and more—to address airway-related issues through a comprehensive, team-based approach.

Recognizing that airway health significantly influences sleep quality and overall well-being, AAPMD emphasizes the importance of a collaborative model in both awareness and treatment of airway dysfunction. By fostering cross-disciplinary partnerships, the organization ensures that patients receive holistic, evidence-based care aimed at improving breathing, sleep, and long-term health outcomes.

AAPMD is committed to providing its members with the latest tools and knowledge to recognize the critical role of optimal airway physiology and sleep in health, development, performance, and function. Through innovative educational programs, public awareness initiatives, and a multidisciplinary referral network, AAPMD strives to advance the standards of care in airway health.

For a discussion on the importance of multidisciplinary approaches to sleep and health, particularly within the context of the AAPMD, refer to the conversation between Dr. Steve Carstensen, DDS, and Patrick McKeown in Appendix C of this book.

For more information about AAPMD's mission, membership opportunities, and educational resources, visit their website at *www.aapmd.org* or contact them via email at *info@aapmd.org*.

The Vivos Institute

The Vivos Institute, established in 2016 by Vivos Therapeutics, Inc., is a premier private research and training institution located in Denver, Colorado. Its mission is to advance sleep therapeutics by providing advanced postgraduate education to dentists, dental teams, and other healthcare professionals. The Institute offers a range of accredited courses focusing on sleep, Buteyko breathing and airway management, aiming to enhance clinical skills and patient care. Attendees include dental and chiropractic professionals seeking to expand their expertise and earn continuing education credits.

For more information or to contact The Vivos Institute, you can visit their website at *https://thevivosinstitute.com/* or reach out via email at *ce@thevivosinstitute.com*. Their state-of-the-art campus is located at 7001 Tower Road, Suite B, Denver, CO 80249. You can also call them at 720-399-9322.

Buteyko Clinic International

The Buteyko Clinic International is a globally recognized training and education center specializing in breathing re-education for health, sleep, and performance. Founded in 2002 by Patrick McKeown, a leading expert in breathwork and author, the clinic is dedicated to teaching the Buteyko Method, a science-backed approach to improving breathing patterns for better respiratory function, nervous system regulation, and overall well-being.

The Buteyko Clinic offers dedicated professional training, particularly for airway-focused dentists, myofunctional therapists, and other healthcare professionals looking to integrate breathing re-education into their practice. In addition to courses for sleep and respiratory health, the clinic has recently launched a new program called "Psychophysiological Breath Training," designed for professionals working in mental health. This course focuses on using breathing techniques to help manage stress, anxiety, trauma, and emotional regulation, providing therapists and clinicians with practical tools to support their clients.

For those looking for individual guidance, Buteyko Clinic International has a network of certified instructors worldwide who specialize in applying breathing techniques for asthma, sleep-disordered breathing, and mental health concerns. Whether you need help improving your breathing for better sleep, reducing breathlessness, or managing stress and anxiety, you can find an instructor to guide you through the process.

Beyond education, the Buteyko Clinic has also developed a range of breathing support products, including MyoTape, to encourage safe nasal breathing during sleep, the Buteyko Belt to promote diaphragmatic breathing, and the SportsMask for respiratory muscle training.

To learn more about Buteyko Clinic International, explore professional training programs, or find an instructor near you, visit *www.buteykoclinic.com* or contact the clinic directly at *info@ buteykoclinic.com*.

APPENDIX C

NO PROFESSION CAN GO IT ALONE

I had a conversation with Dr. Steve Carstensen, a dentist with decades of experience in airway health and sleep dentistry, and he shared something that resonated with me:

> "Even after graduating from dental school, from my very first days in practice, it was obvious that I needed more education if I truly wanted to help my patients. For years, I took classes that expanded on what we learned in dental school—teeth, materials, gum disease, jaw joint comfort. But something kept nagging at me: none of those classes ever addressed how my patients developed these dental issues in the first place.
>
> The American Academy of Physiologic Medicine & Dentistry (AAPMD), attracted me to a meeting one year by offering talks by non-dentists talking about why people developed disease in the first place. I had experience with my own American Dental Association leadership wondering why I wanted to put on a program that included physicians, asking, 'Why would a dentist want to listen to a doctor?' It seemed obvious to me that healthcare professionals should learn from each other.
>
> Increasingly, it's become understood that homeostasis depends on proper breathing and good nutrition to provide the basis for health. Classes for dentists at most conferences stick

to the basics. Searching for who could teach me about nutrition, breathing, and professional collaboration has opened whole new avenues for addressing the health concerns of the person in my clinic.

Sleep is another physiologic process never mentioned in dental school, but it turns out nearly half the population doesn't breathe well during sleep. Disruptions to physiology during this critical 'rest' period form the basis of many chronic illnesses, so getting this sleep-breathing problem under control is vital if we want to address community health. As a physiology geek, digging into the implications of poor sleep breathing became fascinating, and it turns out dentistry has an entry point: keeping the airway open during sleep is routinely done by using custom-fitted oral devices. Only dentists can make these specialized appliances, so that means dentistry must take that role. But we are now affecting whole-person physiology, from understanding the diagnosis to the implications of non-treatment to the health benefits of proper management. Therefore, it's imperative for dentists to collaborate with physicians, speech pathologists, physical therapists, nutritionists, communication specialists, functional medicine experts, and other dedicated professionals within the AAPMD.

Embracing an overlap of health responsibilities does not come easy for any highly trained professional. Silos, turf, fear of the unknown, and other limitations provide the opportunity for AAPMD to bring many of us together to share the goal of meeting people where they are and addressing concerns from basic physiology all the way to our specially trained procedures. People need to breathe, a natural process that can be coached to improve, and they need dental care that only a narrowly trained professional can provide. When we all share in the knowledge of what is available in our collaborative provider network, we can direct the people trusting us to help them to the right person at the right time in an improvement journey.

Sleep cannot be avoided. Good sleep, however, is missing from many people's lives. Improving sleep begins with identifying why it's not good, and addressing the found problems from root to branch. If all any health provider knows is the skillset they were trained in, they may not be able to see what else is possible, or necessary. Getting together with like-minded professionals allows everyone to learn more, see more, and point the way to a more precise solution for the people who trust them."

Dr. Carstensen's website is *https://tmjsleepsolutionsnw.com*.

The American Academy of Physiological Medicine & Dentistry's website is *https://aapmd.org/*.

REFERENCES

Available at *https://buteykoclinic.com/pages/*
thebreathingcureforbettersleep

Accessed via the QR code

ACKNOWLEDGMENTS

This book is the result of the collective efforts of many talented individuals, and I feel truly fortunate to collaborate with such a dedicated team.

A grateful thanks to my publisher, Humanix Books, and particularly to Keith Pfeffer, for believing in this project and supporting not only this title but also two of my earlier books.

Particular thanks are due to Catherine Bane for her diligent contributions as coauthor, researcher, and editor. Thanks to Bex Burgess, whose illustrations add an extra dimension to this book. Thanks also to Patricia Wallenburg for expertly formatting the text.

During the research phase of this book, we reached out to you, our global network, inviting you to complete an online survey or share your experiences through an interview with our research team. Thank you to the incredible 800+ members of the Buteyko Clinic, Oxygen Advantage®, and MyoTape communities who generously shared their sleep stories and real-life insights. A particular thank you to Alina, Simon, Davina, Sean, Lisa, Marinka, and Liam, who participated in interviews and shared their experiences in-depth. Their insightful stories, featured throughout this book, show just how simple and even life-changing these practices can be.

Thanks also to Dr. Steve Carstensen for the insightful interview, included in Appendix C.

I would like to acknowledge the significant contributions of Joy Moeller, Marc Moeller, and Samantha Weaver from the Academy of Orofacial Myofunctional Therapy (AOMT). Their unwavering dedication has been instrumental in advancing the fields of myofunctional therapy and the Buteyko Method, bringing these practices into greater public awareness.

I also extend my appreciation to the exceptional team at Oxygen Advantage® and Buteyko Clinic International. Special thanks to Jon Murray, Audrey Keogh, Eoin Tonge, Tijana Krstović, Ruth Gibney, Orla Kyne, Ronan Maher, Ciaran Lohan, Martin Levanti, Sean Hayes, Catherine Bane, and Alessandro Romagnoli—your unwavering support and commitment are invaluable.

A special thank you to my friend Tom Herron. An expert psychotherapist and Master Oxygen Advantage® Instructor, Tom is always on hand to offer sage guidance and encouragement.

To Tiger Bye, breath educator and yoga instructor, thank you for providing audio recordings to add to our library of relaxing audio resources.

A sincere thank you to the 10,000+ Buteyko Clinic and Oxygen Advantage® Instructors who have joined us on this journey and continue to spread the message of better breathing.

Thanks to the thousands of clients I have worked with over the past 23 years, who have placed their trust in me to help them improve their breathing and sleep. Your stories and successes are the driving force behind this work.

As always, my deepest gratitude goes to my wife, Sinead, and my daughter, Lauren.

Catherine would like to thank her husband Tristan for picking up on everything else while she worked on the book. Thanks also to her boys, Torin and Arlo, and her friends for their support and encouragement every step of the way.

Finally, enormous thanks to you, the reader, for supporting this work—I hope it will bring you many restful nights of sleep.

ABOUT THE AUTHORS

PATRICK McKEOWN is Director of Education and Training at Buteyko Clinic International, an organization dedicated to breathing re-education for health and the professional training of instructors worldwide. The clinic specializes in teaching the Buteyko Method, a science-based approach to functional breathing that supports the management of a wide range of conditions, including asthma, anxiety, panic attacks, snoring, and sleep apnea.

He is also Director of Education and Training at Oxygen Advantage®, a performance-based breathing program that enhances mental and physical resilience, energy, focus, and athletic performance. His clients include world-class athletes, elite military personnel, and internationally renowned musicians, all seeking to unlock their full potential through breathing training.

To date, more than 13,000 health, wellness, and fitness professionals have trained in breathing re-education through the combined instructor programs of Buteyko Clinic International and Oxygen Advantage. In the world of breathing, these programs are recognized as market leaders in e-learning, with millions of people worldwide reading Patrick's books and participating in online trainings.

Patrick is the author of 11 books, including *The Breathing Cure: Develop New Habits for a Healthier, Happier, and Longer Life*, *The Breathing Cure for Yoga: Apply Science Behind Ancient Wisdom for Health and Well-Being*, and *Mouth Breather—Shut Your Mouth: The Self-Help Book for Breathers*. He has also written three Amazon category bestsellers, *Close Your Mouth*, *Asthma-Free Naturally*, and *Anxiety Free: Stop Worrying*, and *Quiet Your Mind*. His international bestseller, *The Oxygen Advantage* is widely regarded as a leading resource on breathing for athletic performance and is now available in 16 languages.

Patrick's work has been featured on CNN, BBC, TEDx, *The New York Times, USA Today, The Times, Men's Health, Women's Health, Dr. Oz Magazine,* Mercola, and Mind Body Green.

He is also the inventor of several breathing tools, including MyoTape to support nasal breathing during sleep, the SportsMask to strengthen respiratory muscles and simulate altitude training, the Buteyko Belt to improve diaphragm awareness, and a nasal dilator to make nasal breathing easier during exercise.

When asked what he has learned most from over 20 years of teaching breathing, Patrick says simply:

"It got me out of my head. Doing so is the greatest gift available to everyone. Life becomes that bit softer—and you're more likely to reach your full potential."

www.oxygenadvantage.com
www.buteykoclinic.com

CATHERINE BANE, PH.D. has spent over 20 years working in public health and research. She holds a Ph.D. from Queen's University, Belfast, and is a member of the British Psychological Society and the Division of Health Psychology. A lifelong good sleeper—aside from the early years of motherhood—she was floored by the unexpected sleep challenges that surfaced in her early forties. This personal experience, combined with her professional expertise, deepened her interest in sleep and its impact on well-being.

Once her forties arrived, the things Catherine had once juggled effortlessly felt overwhelming. Waking at 2 a.m. and lying awake for hours became her new reality. No matter what she tried—sleep hygiene, meditation, yoga, breathing exercises, supplements—nothing worked. Fatigue became a daily occurrence and crept into every aspect of her life, making even simple things feel insurmountable. She knew something had to change.

That change came unexpectedly when Catherine stumbled upon Patrick McKeown's work while listening to a podcast. Intrigued by the Buteyko Breathing Method, she decided to give it a try. Unlike other techniques she had explored, this one felt different—it was science-backed, practical, and, most importantly, effective.

She began with *Breathe Light by Relaxation*, a guided audio practice on the Buteyko app. For the first time, practicing breathing exercises didn't feel like another task on her endless to-do list. Instead, they became a welcome means to calm her busy mind and enhance her sleep.

Eager to deepen her understanding, Catherine pursued further training, completing the Oxygen Advantage® Advanced Instructor Training with Patrick McKeown and psychotherapist Tom Herron in 2022. She felt the benefits of these exercises ripple throughout her life. Now, on the odd occasion when she does wake up at night, she has the tools to ease back into restful sleep effortlessly.

Collaborating with Patrick McKeown, Catherine has contributed to several publications, including *The Breathing Cure for Yoga* (McKeown & Tzanis, 2025), *Mouth Breather—Shut Your Mouth: The Self-Help Book for Breathers* (McKeown & Dunne, 2024), and *The Buteyko Method Psychophysiological Breath Training Manual* (McKeown, Romagnoli, Bye, Herron & Bane).

Catherine also remains actively involved in health research. She holds an Evidence Synthesis Ireland Evidence Review Fellowship funded by the HSC R&D Division of the Public Health Agency and is collaborating with Warwick University on an evidence review of health screening.

Through both personal experience and professional expertise, Catherine is dedicated to helping others reclaim their sleep, health, and well-being.

https://buteykoclinic.com/pages/instructor-profile/
catherine-bane